Exercise Psychology

Joe D. Willis, PhD
Georgia State University

Linda Frye Campbell, PhD
University of Georgia

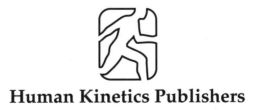

Human Kinetics Publishers

Library of Congress Cataloging-in-Publication Data

Willis, Joe Don, 1936-
   Exercise psychology / Joe D. Willis, Linda Frye Campbell.
     p. cm.
   Includes bibliographical references (p.) and indexes.
   ISBN 0-87322-366-7
   1. Exercise--Psychological aspects. 2. Physical fitness-
-Psychological aspects. I. Campbell, Linda Frye, 1947-
II. Title.
GV481.2.W55   1992
613.7'1--dc20
                                         92-15246
                                            CIP

ISBN: 0-87322-366-7

Acquisitions Editor: Rick Frey, PhD
Developmental Editor: Christine Drews
Assistant Editors: Kari Nelson, Moyra Knight,
  Laura Bofinger, and Dawn Roselund
Copyeditor: Anne Dueweke
Proofreader: Karin Leszczynski
Indexer: Theresa J. Schaefer
Production Director: Ernie Noa
Typesetters: Yvonne Winsor and Kathy Fuoss
Text Design: Keith Blomberg
Text Layout: Yvonne Winsor
Cover Design: Jack Davis
Cover Photo: Wilmer Zehr
Illustrations: Gretchen Walters
Interior Photos: Photos on pages 19, 79, 173, and 199 courtesy
  of Bluefield Regional Medical Center, Bluefield, WV.
Printer: Braun-Brumfield

Printed in the United States of America   10 9 8 7 6 5 4 3

Human Kinetics
P.O. Box 5076, Champaign, IL 61825-5076
1-800-747-4457

Canada: Human Kinetics, Box 24040, Windsor, ON N8Y 4Y9
1-800-465-7301 (in Canada only)

Europe: Human Kinetics, P.O. Box IW14, Leeds LS16 6TR, England
(44) 532 781708

Australia: Human Kinetics, 2 Ingrid Street, Clapham 5062, South Australia
(08) 371 3755

New Zealand: Human Kinetics, P.O. Box 105-231, Auckland 1
(09) 309 2259

In loving memory of
Betty
And, for their unwavering support,
encouragement, and caring,
we also dedicate this book to
Alan and *Nell*

Contents

Part II

Applying Psychological Principles   **93**

Preface

With the tremendous growth of interest in exercise and fitness over the past 3 decades, exercise science has developed into a viable academic discipline to prepare people for careers in fitness management, health promotion, and wellness-related programs. Parallel with the growth of exercise science, health psychology and behavioral medicine have become increasingly important in helping to solve problems in medicine and other health-related fields. It was probably inevitable that exercise psychology, a new hybrid discipline that combines exercise science and psychology, would emerge to address the behavioral and psychological implications of exercise participation. Exercise psychology, as we interpret it in this text, is the study of psychological processes and behaviors related to exercise participation.

Exercise psychology is rapidly becoming an important dimension of exercise science. Although researchers have sporadically investigated various psychological dimensions of exercise participation for several decades, only in the last few years has there been sufficient breadth and depth of research to make a synthesis such as this possible. It should be pointed out, however, that exercise psychology is still in a very early stage of development and will undoubtedly continue to evolve if researchers and practitioners maintain their high levels of interest. The body of knowledge as we have identified it in this work is likely to grow and change considerably over the next several years.

The expansion of the literature on exercise psychology has come from several disparate sources. The disciplines of exercise science, health education, sport psychology, health psychology, behavioral and psychosomatic medicine, clinical and counseling psychology, and nursing have all made significant contributions to the growing body of knowledge. At the moment, exercise psychology is genuinely interdisciplinary with quality research coming from many areas and an extensive exchange of ideas and information across disciplines. Also significant is the lack of dominance by a single group or professional entity.

The impetus for this book grew out of the experience one of the authors has gained from 10 years of teaching exercise psychology courses for undergraduate and graduate students in exercise science. At first, the course depended most heavily on the sport psychology literature for its subject matter. However, over the years there has been a distinct change in the course content as other disciplines have become interested in exercise as a way to improve certain aspects of human functioning. One of the difficulties in developing and teaching an exercise psychology course has been the absence of a suitable text. Although several excellent anthologies have covered selected aspects of exercise psychology quite well, none of these collections has provided the breadth of coverage we consider essential to prepare the exercise practitioner. This text attempts to remedy this deficiency.

Because this is the first attempt to synthesize the exercise psychology literature into textbook form, some important topics may have been omitted. Because there is not a highly circumscribed body of knowledge that is widely recognized as essential to the discipline, the contents reflect our judgments of what should be included. However, we do not presume to define the boundaries of the growing discipline of exercise psychology.

The major purposes of the text are to provide prospective fitness and exercise professionals with essential theoretical information and to offer suggestions of practical value in leadership roles in exercise, wellness, health promotion, corporate fitness, cardiac rehabilitation, commercial fitness, and other related areas. The text is intended for upper-level undergraduate and beginning-level graduate courses, as well as for practitioners who seek additional knowledge to help them function more effectively.

The book is organized into two parts consisting of five chapters each. Part I addresses research-based and theoretical topics. However, we have attempted to infuse suggestions for practical application throughout this section. Part II has an applied focus and discusses the skills and techniques for effective exercise leadership. However, because we wanted this text to be more substantive than a "cook book" of practical suggestions, we have included sufficient theory for the reader to understand the topics under discussion. Hence both theory and applications are provided throughout the text.

Acknowledgments

We are grateful to the people who gave of their time, expertise, and encouragement in the development and completion of this project. The faculty and students in the Department of Health, Physical Education, Recreation, and Dance at Georgia State University and the Department of Counseling and Human Development Services at the University of Georgia have been instrumental in technical and editorial support in the content development of the book. They have also motivated us with their interest and enthusiasm for the project.

We wish to thank several people who worked on various phases of the book along with us. Shahla Khan, Bobby Gonzales, and Alan Stewart gave generously of their time in performing library searches, proofreading, and providing research support. Jane Hobson and her colleagues of the inter-library loan staff (Georgia State University) gave invaluable assistance in acquiring materials, and Anna Bowen (University of Georgia) worked diligently on the manuscript preparation of select chapters. Our developmental editor at Human Kinetics, Chris Drews, has shared with us both her exceptional technical expertise and her professional support, encouragement, and empathy. She has greatly enhanced the quality of our product and the quality of our experience in writing it.

Finally, we thank the many other colleagues and practitioners who have given of their expertise to help us achieve our goal of providing a text that addresses both the theoretical and applied aspects of exercise psychology.

Part I

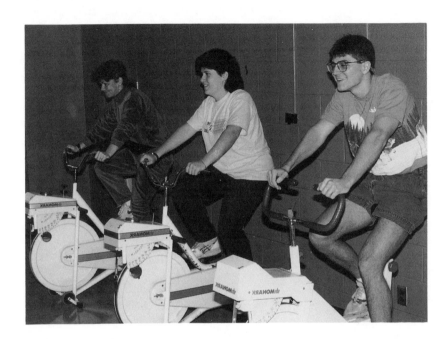

Theoretical Foundations of Exercise Psychology

To be effective, the exercise professional needs to know how exercise affects the body generally, and how it is likely to affect a particular client. In this text, we make the case that the exercise professional needs substantive knowledge and skills in the psychological domain as well. Unless the practitioner can attract clients to exercise programs, maintain their participation over time, meet their individual exercise needs, and assure them of an enjoyable, beneficial experience, the practitioner will not be successful. No matter how knowledgeable in exercise physiology or how proficient in applying technical skills learned in an exercise science preparation program, the practitioner must know how exercise is likely to affect a person psychologically, both immediately and over the long-term. The successful practitioner will plan, organize, and conduct the program on sound principles that address psychological as well as physiological outcomes.

Part I provides an overview of the research literature in several important areas. Chapter 1 explores the reasons why people exercise. After identifying major motivational themes and their implications for the practitioner, we summarize the reasons most often given for not exercising. The difficulties of maintaining exercise behaviors are examined in chapter 2. Exercise adherence is one of the most important, and certainly the most persistent, problems facing the exercise practitioner. Chapter 2 outlines the factors considered important in maintaining exercise behaviors and gives several suggestions for promoting adherence.

In chapter 3 we review the acute and chronic psychological effects of exercise. In the burgeoning literature on the relationship between exercise and mental health, we are particularly interested in the effects of exercise on mood, depression, anxiety, and stress. Chapter 4 discusses the relationships between exercise participation and aspects of personality and self-concept. This chapter also looks at aspects of personality, such as Type A behavior, locus of control, hardiness, and personality disorders, and how they are affected by exercise.

The final chapter in Part I considers the value of theory in understanding and predicting exercise behavior. Chapter 5 presents theoretical models that have been specifically developed to explain exercise, as well as other generic theories. The health belief model, the theory of reasoned action, and self-efficacy theory are especially applicable to exercise programming.

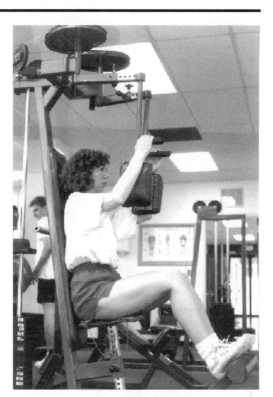

Chapter 1
Why People Exercise: Motives for Fitness

In the past 20 to 30 years, the world has witnessed a phenomenal growth in interest and involvement in physical activity. More particularly, forms of exercise that promote physical fitness and favorably affect one's health and overall functioning have become central to the lives of many people. In this book, we explore the psychological effects of exercise and how psychological factors influence exercise behaviors.

Because we will be using the concepts of *physical activity*, *exercise*, and *physical fitness* throughout this work, perhaps it would be appropriate to

clarify each of these terms. Although the terms *physical activity* and *exercise* are frequently used interchangeably, we have adopted the interpretation of Caspersen, Powell, and Christenson (1985), which distinguishes between the two concepts. *Physical activity* is perceived as any bodily movement produced by skeletal muscles that results in energy expenditure. *Exercise* is defined as a subset of physical activity. It is planned, structured, and repetitive, and has a primary objective of improving or maintaining physical fitness. For example, people who work in their gardens for enjoyment without concern for other possible outcomes would be engaging in physical activity. If a gardener systematically engages in the activity for the express purpose of maintaining or improving physical fitness, it would be considered exercise.

Physical fitness refers to a person's ability to perform physical activity (Caspersen et al., 1985). A distinction is often made between *health-related* physical fitness and *skill-related* physical fitness. Health-related components of physical fitness include cardiorespiratory endurance, muscular endurance, muscular strength, body composition, and flexibility. Although not of central importance in this book, skill-related fitness includes the components of agility, balance, coordination, speed, power, and reaction time.

EXERCISE INVOLVEMENT IN NORTH AMERICA

The fitness movement in the United States began in the mid-1950s with a chain of events that brought national attention to exercise and fitness. In 1954, results of fitness tests that compared European and American school children led to a public demand for programs to improve the low levels of fitness among America's youth (Kraus & Hirschland, 1954). A second influential event in the initiation of the fitness movement was the heart attack of President Eisenhower followed by his highly visible exercise rehabilitation program. Shortly thereafter, a White House conference on youth fitness was convened, which culminated in the establishment of the President's Council on Youth Fitness. The continuing emphasis on physical fitness during the Kennedy administration maintained national interest (Kennedy, 1960). Other events, such as the first Surgeon General's report on smoking released in the 1960s, encouraged more active and healthy lifestyles, and led to the increased fitness participation of people of all ages, which continued well into the 1970s and 1980s.

In a review of trends in adult physical activity, Stephens (1987) concluded that there was strong evidence of an increase in leisure time physical activity during the past 2 decades. He characterized this growth as a "genuine phenomenon." In commenting on Stephens's work, Blair, Mulder, and Kohl (1987) agreed with the conclusion, and Shephard (1988b) used data from Canadian sources to extend this conclusion to Canada.

Some experts question these figures on fitness and exercise, particularly with respect to the degree of participation that can be demonstrated. An analysis of eight national surveys (Stephens, Jacobs, & White, 1985) conducted in the United States and Canada between 1972 and 1983 showed that only about 20% of North America's population exercised enough to achieve cardiovascular benefit. An additional 40% were active to a lesser degree but may still have received some health benefits, and at least 40% were entirely sedentary. Analyses of this sort are fraught with methodological difficulties, such as different definitions of key terms like *physically active* and highly variable results. This point is well illustrated in Table 1.1 in which the figures representing "level of activity" range from 15% all the way up to 78%.

Recent analyses of surveys in the United States (Stephens, 1987) and Canada (Shephard, 1988b) have indicated that the rapid growth in exercise and fitness activities observed in the 1970s and 1980s may be leveling off, or even slightly declining. A summary of Stephens's findings is shown in Table 1.2. These observations are strong reminders that the exercise professional still has much work ahead in educating the public about the health benefits of exercise. Major segments of the population, such as the aging, the poor, and blue-collar workers, have yet to be reached. The deplorable physical condition of children and young people is also of considerable concern. However, one should not be discouraged about the future status of exercise programs. As we shall demonstrate, the benefits of exercise are many, and as more people become aware of these benefits, the need for trained leaders will continue to grow.

THE NATURE OF MOTIVES AND MOTIVATION

The mysteries of human behavior have preoccupied scholars for centuries. We try constantly to understand the behavior of others as well as our own behavior. One place to begin the search for understanding is with the word itself. The term *motivation* has evolved from the Latin root of the verb *movere*, which means *to move*. Certainly motivation implies movement or activation. Terms such as *aroused, incited, energized, activated*, and *intense* are used to describe a highly motivated state. Motivated states related to activities that require less effort and produce less dramatic outcomes are harder to detect. Nonetheless, the behaviors of

Table 1.1 Proportion of Population Physically Active During Leisure Time, Grouped by Rigor of Definition, United States and Canada, 1972–83

Survey	Definition of active (key terms in quotes)	Percent active
	Most rigorous definitions	
CDC-State BRF Survey	3 or more kcal per kg per day of expenditure on single major activity	21
Perrier-1[a]	1,500 kcal per week or 3 or more kcal per kg per day on sports and conditioning for an average size person	15
Miller Lite	Athletic index score = 12 or above, where 1 point given for weekly participation, 4 points for "daily or almost daily" participation in 29 listed activities	19
	Less rigorous definitions	
PCPFS-1	"Now participate" in 1 or more of 16 listed sports	51
PCPFS-2	"Now doing" 1 or more of 6 listed exercises	55
NHIS-1	Participation in 1 or more of 6 listed exercises "on a regular basis"	49
NSPHPC	"Often" participate in 1 or more of 7 listed activities	78
Perrier-2	Participated "on a regular basis any time during the past year" in 1 or more of 37 listed activities	53[b]
Canada Fitness Survey-1	Participated in sport or conditioning for 3 or more hours per week during 9 or more months per year	56
	Least rigorous definitions	
NHIS-2	Any participation in 1 or more of 14 listed sports in last 12 months	42
F&AS-1	Any participation in 1 or more of 8 listed sports in last 12 months	50
F&AS-2	Any participation in 1 or more of 8 listed conditioning activities in last month	59
Canada Fitness Survey-2	Any participation in 1 or more of 90 listed sports in last 12 months	68
Canada Fitness Survey-3	Any participation in 1 or more of 14 listed exercise activities in last month	58

Note. BRF = Behavioral Risk Factor; F&AS = Fitness and Amateur Sport; NHIS = National Health Interview Survey; NSPHPC = National Survey of Personal Health Practices and Consequences; PCPFS = President's Council on Physical Fitness and Sports.

[a]Numbers after studies indicate different definitions of "active" used.

[b]This percent excludes unknowns which are treated as "low active" in report.

From "A Descriptive Epidemiology of Leisure-Time Activity" by T. Stevens, 1985, *Public Health Reports*, **100**(2), p. 149. Reprinted by permission.

people who are "motivated" to engage in exercise and other forms of physical activity are, for the most part, observable and likely to be distinguished by significant effort.

There is currently little agreement among scholars as to the nature of motivation, the factors involved in motivated behavior, or the relationships among these factors. In a review article, Kleinginna and Kleinginna (1981b) cited 102 definitions of *motivation* and *motives*. Even the consensual definition attempted in the review article seemed unable to capture the essence of motivation. The authors used *motivation* to refer to "those energizing/arousing mechanisms with relatively direct access to the final common motor pathways, which have the potential to facilitate and direct some motor circuits while inhibiting others" (p. 272). Similarly, there is little

agreement on how best to obtain data on motivational phenomena, or on how to use that data to bring about desired behavioral changes.

Despite the diverse ideas on the nature of motivation and the varied approaches to the study of that topic, motivation remains a very relevant subject for the exercise practitioner and the exercise scientist. Understanding why some people choose to exercise while others do not, or why a large percentage of those who begin to exercise drop out within a short time, would be of great practical value. This knowledge would enable exercise professionals to conduct more effective programs, both in terms of human outcomes and economic costs. Some progress has been made in answering the complex questions related to motivation for exercise and fitness, but much work is yet to be done.

Table 1.2 Summary of Findings

Known

Adult leisure-time activity has increased in the United States in the last two decades.

Women have increased their activity levels more than men.

Older Americans (age 50 and over) have increased their activity levels more than younger adults.

The increased participation is not confined to low- or moderate-intensity activities.

There currently exist no satisfactory time series on adult activity at the national level.

Overall quality of measurement of physical activity is improving.

Suspected

The rate of increase was most pronounced in the 1970s, and has slowed recently.

Participation in some activities has begun to decline.

This trend toward greater activity is not confined to the 1970s and early 1980s, but dates to at least the early 1960s.

There has been a greater increase in vigorous activities (e.g., jogging) and active sports than in moderate- or low-intensity activities (e.g., walking).

Time series data on leisure activity will improve.

Unknown

Whether the education gap is closing.

What the rate of increase has been.

Whether current levels of participation can be sustained or increased further.

From "Secular Trends in Adult Physical Activity: Exercise Boom or Bust" by T. Stevens, June 1987, *Research Quarterly for Exercise and Sport*, **58**(2), p. 103. Reprinted by permission.

Although the exact meaning of *motivation* remains elusive, it generally refers to *causative* factors, or factors that initiate behaviors, direct actions, and influence when a specific behavior is discontinued. Put more succinctly, motivation is concerned with arousal, direction, and persistence of behavior (Franken, 1982). Of primary interest are the influences that incite action and determine the direction, intensity, and persistence of the action. Past learning and immediate influences also combine with other factors to determine the initiation, intensity, and persistence of behavior on any particular occasion (Atkinson, 1978).

We shall deal with each of these aspects of motivation in a different chapter. The present chapter will consider the initiation of exercise behaviors by reviewing motives for exercise and fitness participation. Chapter 2 will deal with long-term involvement in exercise behaviors (persistence) by exploring exercise adherence, and chapter 6 will discuss the intensity of exercise behaviors in relation to motivational techniques.

It is important for the exercise professional to understand why people choose to exercise or become involved in fitness activities. Knowing a person's motives enables the practitioner to better plan the individual's program. Also, knowing the range of motives represented in a group of exercise clients enables the exercise professional to offer sufficient variety to maintain interest. Understanding people's motives also helps practitioners plan strategies to help clients maintain exercise behaviors. Because motives change over time, programs must be flexible to encourage continued involvement.

REVIEW OF RESEARCH ON EXERCISE AND FITNESS MOTIVES

The work of Gerald Kenyon (1968a) was among the earlier and more influential scholarly efforts to classify the reasons why people engage in physical activity. Kenyon developed a theoretical model that hypothesized six subdomains to explain the value of physical activity. The subdomains are summarized in Figure 1.1. A brief description of each follows:

■ *Physical activity as a social experience.* It is believed that involvement in some forms of physical activity can meet some of the social needs of certain participants. Some physical activities provide a medium for meeting new people or perpetuating existing relationships.

■ *Physical activity for health and fitness.* This subdomain relates to involvement in physical activity primarily for the development or enhancement of physical fitness.

■ *Physical activity as the pursuit of vertigo.* Kenyon modified the more traditional definition of the term *vertigo* to mean activities involving risk, danger, or a thrill derived from speed or acceleration. Activities in this category include skiing, mountain climbing, and sky diving.

■ *Physical activity as an aesthetic experience.* This subdomain pertains to physical activities that appeal to participants because of their characteristics of beauty, grace, symmetry, or other artistic qualities. Ballet, synchronized swimming, gymnastics, and aerobic dance are representative of physical activity as an aesthetic experience.

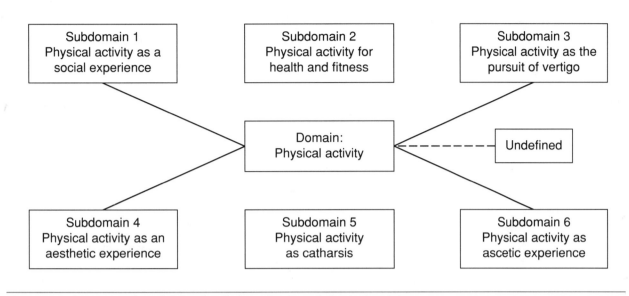

Figure 1.1 Structure of model for the characterization of physical activity.

From "Conceptual Model for Characterizing Physical Activity" by G.S. Kenyon. This article is reprinted with permission from the *Research Quarterly for Exercise and Sport, 39* (1), 1968, pp. 96-100. *Research Quarterly* is a publicaton of the American Alliance for Health, Physical Education, Recreation and Dance, 1900 Association Drive, Reston, VA 22091.

■ *Physical activity as catharsis.* This subdomain refers to participation in physical activity to release tension and pent-up emotions.

■ *Physical activity as an ascetic experience.* The willingness or desire to endure long, strenuous, and often painful training in pursuit of a particular goal characterizes physical activity as an ascetic experience. Training for a marathon, running up Pikes Peak, or preparing for a decathlon are examples.

After completing his model for characterizing physical activity, Kenyon (1968b) developed an instrument to measure attitudes based on the model. This instrument, or modifications of it, has been used in many of the studies on participation motives. One of the earlier studies using Kenyon's instrument for measuring attitudes employed 699 male college students (Dotson & Stanley, 1972). These students chose pursuit of vertigo, catharsis, and social interaction as the strongest perceived values of physical activity. Ascetic, fitness, and aesthetic outcomes were the lowest ranked values in the study. More recently, Adamson and Wade (1986) used a modified version of the instrument to study participation motives of Australian health science students. They found that the most important motives were to become fit, to maintain a healthy lifestyle, to have fun, and to meet people.

Although the Kenyon instrument has been used extensively in the study of exercise motives, the results have not been particularly enlightening. The disappointing results are due in large part to the ill-conceived or inappropriate use of the instrument. As Godin and Shephard (1986) point out, instruments such as the Kenyon inventory are designed to test cultural changes in attitudes toward physical activity rather than individual attitude changes. Nevertheless, Kenyon's conceptualization is helpful in understanding basic motives for participation. We shall be referring to this model throughout the text.

A variety of other approaches have been used to study motives for exercise. Brunner (1969) used the Adjective Check List and a questionnaire to study the differences between men who exercised regularly and inactive men. The men in the study were of comparable age and had similar occupations. Brunner found that the physically active group identified the primary benefits of exercise as physical fitness, feeling better physically and mentally, fun and enjoyment, and weight control. The inactive group ranked relaxation, feeling better, fun and enjoyment, and being outdoors as the main benefits of exercise.

An extensive survey of 1,708 Finnish executives found that improved health, physical fitness, improved working capacity, and weight control were the primary motives among those who were willing to participate in an exercise program (Teraslinna, Partanen, Koskela, & Oja, 1969). As a participant observer in various informal exercise groups, Roth (1974) identified several recurrent motivational themes. He found that although physical pleasure and pain are sensory outcomes of exercise, most subjects said they adopted strategies to distract themselves from the pain and learned to emphasize feelings of increased well-being after exercise. Other motivational themes Roth identified were the desire for health, social approval, and self-approval.

Sex Differences in Exercise Motives

In a study of a group of male and female college students, health and fitness, competition, and social experience were rated as the most important reasons for participating in physical activities (Mathes & Battista, 1985). Females in the study ranked health and fitness, social experience, and competition in that order, while males chose competition first, followed by health and fitness, and social experience. A comparison between athletes and nonathletes showed that athletes assigned significantly higher values to the competition motive. However, there were no differences between the groups in scores assigned to social experience. Both athletes and nonathletes identified health and fitness as being of highest importance. The athletes' next highest priority was competition followed by social experience, while nonathletes rated social experience higher than competition.

When looking at sex differences in motives and in other factors which affect one's participation in sport and exercise in physical therapy students, Adamson and Wade (1986) found only 1 of 15 items that differed between men and women. Women perceived their teachers to be more encouraging of participation. With respect to participation motives, however, there were no sex differences. In contrast, in a 1985 study of two British exercise classes—one for men and one for women—Biddle and Bailey (1985) found significant sex differences in motives. Women favored aesthetic and cathartic activities, while men placed higher value on health and fitness, and competition. It was suggested that different emphases in the classes could account for the differences in the motives. The class for men was described as competitive, goal-oriented exercise typified by self-monitored circuit training, while the class for women contained noncompetitive dance-related activities.

In a group of 411 male and female runners, Harris (1981a) found that the major reasons for running were to feel better physically and psychologically, followed by weight control and relaxation. Women were more likely than men to report that they ran to become more fit, control weight, look better, or because they had friends or relatives who ran. A related study of female runners (Harris, 1981b) revealed that most saw themselves as stronger, happier, more relaxed, and more energetic as a result of running. Of particular interest was the finding that running made the women feel more attractive and feminine. These results sharply contrasted with the view of running as a masculine activity. Another finding of interest was the report that 95% of female runners received social support for their running from family members and friends, and fewer than 20% reported any opposition. The reported effects of exercise cessation were mostly negative, such as reduced energy, feelings of guilt, depression, feeling fatter, and increased tension.

Sex differences in exercise motives will be discussed in more detail later in conjunction with the work of Johnsgard (1985a, 1985b). However, it seems safe to say that there are few important differences between men and women with regard to motives for exercise and fitness. Motives related to health and fitness seem to predominate among both men and women. There are slight differences in secondary motives, which tend to be related to the type of activity experienced.

Motives of Runners

We have focused on the motives of runners because running is one of the more popular participant sports in North America. It is also often the activity of choice for the development of aerobic fitness in organized as well as in self-directed fitness programs. Moreover, runners are well organized and cohesive, with many well-established running clubs and a growing body of literature. Most importantly, runners have been the focus of more research, especially motivational and other psychological research, than other mass participation sports.

Of the motivational research done with runners, that of Johnsgard probably has the best potential for application. Data obtained from a study of older runners led to the development of a questionnaire designed to measure motives of runners in the general population (Johnsgard, 1985a). The 10 motives included in the instrument, called the Runner Motivation Test (RMT), were

■ afterglow—the elevated mood and feeling of relaxation after running;

■ fitness—cardiovascular and general physical fitness;

■ centering—space to be alone and to experience self;

■ challenge—to challenge or improve self;

■ competition—to measure self against others;

■ fame and fortune—to make money or win fame;

■ feels good—how one feels during a run;

■ identity—the definition of self as a runner;

■ slim—to control weight; and

■ social—to make new friends or maintain old friendships.

The RMT along with an invitation to participate in the study was published in a leading running magazine (Johnsgard, 1983). In all, 574 men and 149 women responded. For both sexes, the main motive for running was to challenge oneself. It was clear that to run regularly, or to run farther or faster than before was more important than running farther or faster than someone else. As shown in Table 1.3, running for fitness was more important for men, who ranked it second, than for women, who rated it fifth.

Table 1.3   Mean Running Motives for Men and Women

Motive	Men	Women	F
Challenge	7.59	7.33	2.74
Fitness	6.99	6.03	19.50**
Afterglow	6.21	7.26	20.01**
Centering	6.13	6.10	.06
Competition	5.61	4.27	32.75**
Feels good	5.60	5.63	.00
Identity	5.48	5.90	3.56
Slim	5.35	6.55	18.88**
Social	3.58	3.96	3.02
Fame and fortune	2.46	1.97	5.42*

*$p < .05$. **$p < .001$.

From "The Motivation of the Long Distance Runner" by K. Johnsgard, 1985, *Journal of Sports Medicine and Physical Fitness*, **25**, pp. 135-139. Reprinted by permission.

"Centering," or the need to be alone when training, was ranked fourth in importance by both sexes. Women scored "afterglow" and "slim" significantly higher than men. Competition with others was rated fifth by men and eighth by women. Apparently, fraternization was not an important motive of experienced runners; both men and women cited social reasons for participation as ninth in importance. Rated last by both sexes was "fame and fortune." Johnsgard concluded that although there were some sex differences in motives, both sexes shared a common core of central motives. Stated simply, people run for physical fitness and to feel good physically and emotionally.

In a subsequent study, Johnsgard (1985b) revised the Runner Motivation Test to apply to any sort of endurance training, and renamed the instrument the Test of Endurance Athlete Motives (TEAM). The major modification involved dropping "fame and fortune" because of its lack of relevance and adding a new motive called "addictions." "Addictions" was included as a motive because some runners reported that they began running to stop or control unhealthy habits such as smoking, drinking, and drug use.

Targeting members of the Fifty-Plus Runners Association, Johnsgard attempted to differentiate current motives for running from those which prompted experienced runners to start running in the first place. As shown in Table 1.4, the results suggested that initially important motives seemed to retain their importance. However, some original motives did change in their degree of importance as running experience increased. Fitness and weight control, which were central beginning motives, diminished in importance with running experience. It was speculated that this might occur because experienced runners come to take fitness and weight control for granted as other rewards of running become apparent.

Both sexes were found to have parallel increases in "afterglow" and "identity," which was interpreted as positive changes in mood, self-control, and self-concept. Only a small percentage of men and women reported that they began running to stop or control unhealthy, nonfood addictions, and "addictions" was shown to be even less important as a current motive of experienced runners. Comparing the results with the earlier study, Johnsgard suggested that older runners of both sexes value competition less than younger runners, and that weight control is less important to older women than to younger women. It was concluded that among older dedicated runners, the reasons for beginning to run are closely related to motives for continuing. However, there are parallel shifts in the strengths of some motives for both sexes as running becomes more established as part of their lifestyle.

Using an open-ended survey that enabled comparison between early reasons for jogging with current reasons, Vitulli (1987) found that health and fitness remained the top priority. In support

Table 1.4   Mean Retrospective and Current Running Motives

	Men			Women		
Motive	Began	Now	t	Began	Now	t
Fitness	7.99	7.42	3.59***	7.19	6.39	2.38*
Challenge	6.08	5.46	4.08***	5.48	5.74	.27
Slim	5.42	4.89	2.71**	6.06	4.52	3.97***
Feels good	4.81	5.11	1.83	5.19	5.13	.14
Afterglow	4.56	5.32	4.22***	5.06	6.26	2.41*
Identity	4.37	4.79	2.17*	3.68	4.74	2.67*
Centering	4.33	4.57	1.20	4.77	5.74	2.03*
Competition	3.11	3.57	2.59**	2.06	2.84	1.91
Social	2.64	2.95	1.90	3.06	2.74	.94
Addictions	1.58	.65	4.58***	1.81	.71	2.80**

*p < .05. **p < .01. ***p < .001.

From "The Motivation of the Long Distance Runner II" by K. Johnsgard, 1985, *Journal of Sports Medicine and Physical Fitness*, **25**, p. 141. Reprinted by permission.

of Johnsgard's results, Vitulli found that relatively high status was given to self-esteem, personal identity, and improved state of mind as motives for continued participation in jogging. In a study of commitment to running, Carmack and Martens (1979) asked 250 men and 65 women about their reasons for beginning to run and reasons for presently running. Getting in shape or maintaining fitness again topped the list of motives for both. Enjoyment was ranked second as a motive for beginning and continuing to run. Weight control, which was listed third as a motive for beginning to run, dropped to fourth as a motive for presently running. Although competition was not on the list of motives for beginning to run, it moved to the third most important motive for experienced runners.

A more recent study reported three motives to be particularly important in running: challenge, health and fitness, and personal well-being (Clough, Shepherd, & Maughan, 1989). It was suggested that similarities between the motives for running and motives for other leisure activities emphasized the need to examine running within the wider context of leisure.

RECURRING MOTIVES FOR EXERCISE

From the previous review, it seems that there are four or five primary motives for exercising. Most reasons could be included under the general topics of increased health and fitness, improved appearance, fun and enjoyment, social experience, and psychological benefits. Each of these major themes will be discussed individually although it should be kept in mind that there is a great deal of interaction among them. For example, weight control affects health and fitness as well as appearance, and probably affects how a person feels. It should also be remembered that most people exercise for more than one reason, and that these reasons tend to change over time.

Health and Fitness

It is increasingly clear that the population is generally aware of the health benefits of exercise. Most people now believe that they should exercise, even though they may not have a definite idea of what they should be doing. The medical profession, despite tentative early support of exercise, now wholeheartedly endorses exercise as a means to promote the general health and well-being of the populace. As people learn more about the health benefits of regular physical activity, many are motivated to begin exercising. Unfortunately, large population segments, particularly blue-collar workers, low-income groups, and the elderly, have not joined the fitness movement in any significant way. This will be a major challenge for fitness and health professionals in coming years. At present, regular exercise is associated with people of higher income, education, and occupational status (Stephens et al., 1985).

Haskell (1984) stated that of all claims regarding health benefits of exercise, those with the most substantial scientific basis include the maintenance of optimal body weight or body composition, the prevention of coronary heart disease, and the normalization of lipid and carbohydrate metabolism. Although lacking in persuasive data, other likely benefits of exercise are the prevention of high blood pressure or hypertension, the maintenance of bone density, and the prevention of lower-back syndrome. Several other conditions show improvement with exercise, although there is no evidence that exercise prevents these disorders. These conditions include chronic obstructive lung disease, kidney failure, and arthritis.

Results from animal, experimental, observational, and clinical research led Haskell (1984) to conclude that physical activity can help delay the onset or reduce the severity of several major chronic degenerative diseases. He also stated that the type, intensity, and amount of exercise needed to achieve these potential health benefits were well within the capabilities of most healthy adults. Indeed, as we shall see in chapter 10, exercise may forestall the physiological decline associated with aging.

For many people, health and fitness is a primary motive for exercise, especially for those beginning an exercise program. Research to date suggests that the general public is not only aware of the health benefits of exercise, but is also beginning to do something about it.

Exercise as a Means to Improve Appearance

Exercise is one of the more frequently relied upon means of enhancing appearance. Weight loss and improved muscle tone are typically what people have in mind when they speak of "shaping up." Although physical appearance concerns both women and men, it is somewhat more important to women.

Improved body image is another way of describing the desired changes brought about through training. Body image, or the perceptions and evaluations of one's body, is also an important factor in self-concept and personality. Secord and Jourard (1953) found that body satisfaction was closely related to self-satisfaction in a group of female students. A follow-up study (Jourard and Secord, 1955) revealed a shared ideal of female body dimensions. As shown in Table 1.5, the study found that the subjects' ideal dimensions were smaller than their actual body measurements, with the exception of bust size.

Secord and Jourard (1953) speculated that the restrictiveness of the ideal dimensions could cause anxiety and insecurity for some women. If a woman's status and security are dependent on her attractiveness and she does not feel attractive, there is an attendant loss of self-esteem. The authors described the concept of a perceived ideal as a "tyrannical should," that is, one *should* be 5 ft 5 in. tall, weigh 122 lb, and measure 34.83 in. in the bust. Self-hate, guilt, and insecurity are often the result if one fails to achieve the ideal. According to the authors, such a strong imperative probably accounts for widespread efforts among women to sculpture their bodies toward the ideal through surgery, corsetry, dieting, exercise, and camouflage.

More recently, Garner, Garfinkel, Schwartz, and Thompson (1980) associated female body shape with social status. While special emphasis is placed on the appearance of women, the relation of male physical attractiveness to role status, money, and power is not as strong. For women, pressure to be thin, which is a characteristic of higher social class, is cited as a strong motive to lose weight and appear young, beautiful, and sexy. Concepts of female beauty vary from culture to culture, and sometimes change over time. In recent years, the North American concept of female beauty has shifted from the voluptuous, curved, soft physique to a more angular, lean, "tubular" appearance.

An article titled "New Ideal of Beauty" in *Time* magazine (1982) declared the new standard of beauty to combine thinness and muscularity. Weight training and other vigorous forms of exercise were cited as ways to attain this ideal. Indeed, many female celebrities have become exercise role models. Not only have they adopted exercise as important aspects of their lives, but some have even become successful fitness gurus, developing and marketing videotapes and books. Jane Fonda was probably the first and undoubtedly the most successful of the celebrity fitness entrepreneurs. Others seeking to capitalize on their popularity to promote fitness products include Raquel Welch, Victoria Principal, Debbie Reynolds, Olivia Newton-John, and even Angela Lansbury. Unfortunately, many of these celebrity packages contain inaccurate and potentially harmful information.

The perceived need to be thin has been increasingly linked to anorexia nervosa and other eating disorders. The current obsession with weight and the resulting eating disorders are rooted in societal pressures on women (Silverstein, Peterson, & Perdue, 1986). A study of high school girls (Garner et al., 1980) showed that 70% were unhappy with

Table 1.5   Mean Difference Between Measured (and Estimated) Size and Ideal Size of Five Body Aspects

Body aspect	Size[a]	Ideal size	Mean difference (measured)	Mean difference (estimated)	CR	p
Height	65.69	65.33	.16	.20	.30	> .10
(inches)	65.52		.01			
Weight	125.42	122.48	2.94	1.49	1.98	.05
(pounds)	126.97		4.49	1.35	3.32	< .01
Bust	34.14	34.83	.69	.20	3.45	< .001
(inches)	34.28		.55	.19	2.89	< .01
Waist	25.45	24.27	1.18	.18	6.36	< .001
(inches)	25.57		1.30	.18	7.22	< .001
Hips	37.43	35.06	2.37	.29	8.17	< .001
(inches)	36.84		1.78	.23	7.74	< .001

[a]The first entry is the measured size, the second, the estimated size.

From "Body-Cathexis and the Ideal Female Figure" by S. Jourard and P. Secord, 1955, *Journal of Abnormal and Social Psychology*, **50**, pp. 243-246.

their weight and wanted to be thinner. The researchers called this phenomenon a "sociocultural epidemic" in which fashion's ideal may affect vulnerable adolescents who believe that thinness will lead to beauty and success.

The necessity for women to be thin is communicated through a constant barrage of messages carried by magazines, movies, and television. These messages expose women to a standard of bodily attractiveness that is slimmer than at any time since the 1930s (Silverstein et al., 1986). Popular mass market books that promote unusual diet or exercise plans have also been implicated in the increase in eating disorders. One such book has been called a form of direct training in anorexic behaviors and attitudes (Wooley & Wooley, 1982).

That messages to be slim are aimed at women much more than at men was demonstrated forcefully by a content analysis of 48 women's and 48 men's magazines (Silverstein et al., 1986). The researchers found 96 articles and advertisements about the body in the women's magazines and only 12 in the men's. Even more amazing was the discrepancy between the number of advertisements and articles related to food in the different magazines. There were a total of 1,407 such articles in the women's magazines and only 25 in the men's. These disproportionate numbers clearly show how much more important slimness is for women than for men.

Despite these findings, however, men as well as women seem to be increasingly concerned with appearance and body weight. Two related studies of readers of *Psychology Today* conducted 13 years

apart (Berscheid, Walster, & Bohrnstedt, 1973; Cash, Winstead, & Janda, 1986) revealed dramatic growth in dissatisfaction in appearance. In the earlier survey, 35% of men and 48% of women expressed dissatisfaction with body weight. The later survey found that the dissatisfaction had grown to 41% and 55%, respectively. Unhappiness with overall appearance increased from 15% to 34% for men and from 34% to 38% for women.

A survey of 33,000 readers of *Glamour* magazine ("Feeling fat," 1984) corroborated the results of the previously mentioned study. Seventy-five percent of respondents said they were too fat, although only 25% were overweight according to conservative height-weight tables. Even 66% of underweight women reported that they were too fat and dieted often. Only 6% reported feeling very happy about their bodies and 15% said their bodies were "just right." Among the numerous weight-loss techniques reported, exercise was the method most universally used.

With such importance attached to physical appearance, it is understandable that it would be a major motivating factor to exercise. Although this may be encouraging to the exercise professional in terms of numbers of participants, there is a down side to society's preoccupation with appearance. Many people who would like to be physically active probably fail to participate because of their embarrassment over how they look in a leotard, running shorts, or a bathing suit. The exercise professional must work to overcome oversensitivity to appearance by emphasizing other benefits of exercise programs. They must counsel clients to take a more rational view of the importance of appearance and to deal better with their limitations.

Exercise for Enjoyment

Many people begin exercise programs to improve their health or to lose weight, but few people continue these programs unless they find a form of exercise that they enjoy. Rather than answering the "stern call of cardiovascular duty" (Massie & Shephard, 1971), most people engage in physical activity over a long period because they have found something that gives them a sense of fun or happiness. Joe Henderson, an author of popular running books, contends that fitness is a stage that runners pass through on the way to becoming runners, and that most would continue to run even if they found out that running wasn't good for them (Perry, 1987). According to Henderson, they would continue to run for other reasons, such as fun and personal satisfaction.

Several studies of adult participation in regular exercise have pointed out the importance of childhood involvement (Krotee & La Point, 1979; Snyder & Spreitzer, 1979; Yoesting & Burkhead, 1973). The play of young children, especially spontaneous play, is motivated solely by pleasure and personal satisfaction. As children move into organized play such as youth sports, other motives become operative, although having fun remains a major objective (Passer, 1982). In reviewing the studies of participation motives of young athletes, Gould and Horn (1984) concluded that most had several motives for participation. Those motives that were consistently rated highest were improving skills, having fun, being with friends or making new friends, experiencing thrills or excitement, attaining success, and developing fitness. As one might expect, many individual differences in motives as well as some group differences were found. Young female athletes placed more emphasis on having fun and making friends. In a summary of 12 studies of participation motives of young athletes, Carron (1984) found that having fun was listed first in six of the studies and second in another.

Perhaps as people mature their priorities change and they come to believe that having fun is no longer appropriate for "grownups." As they acquire the work ethic through education and socialization the need for play and spontaneity may be programmed out and replaced by the need to be productive, acquisitive, and successful. When carried over to exercise programs, these values fail to maintain their interest over time.

Wankel (1985) suggested that instead of the usual focus on the health outcomes of a fitness program, the emphasis might better be placed on the enjoyment or quality of the experience. He also maintained that health and enjoyment need not be contradictory objectives. A person may reap the health benefits of exercise while experiencing the pleasurable aspects of activity. For most people, however, the symbiotic relationship of exercise, health benefits, and enjoyment is achieved only after extended involvement. Typically, the first stages of an exercise program are not perceived as enjoyable, but rather as something to be endured because it is "good for you." Wankel pointed out that this perception directly parallels the high dropout rate during the first weeks of a program.

If exercise practitioners want to maximize continued participation, enjoyment must be a major focus of exercise programs from the outset. To make a fitness program enjoyable it is necessary to understand the distinction between *intrinsically motivated* activities and *extrinsically motivated* activities.

Intrinsic motivation refers to benefits and satisfactions inherent in the activity, while *extrinsic motivation* concerns reasons not directly involved with the activity (Deci, 1975). People who exercise for the enjoyment of the sensations that accompany the activity are participating for intrinsic reasons. People who exercise to lose weight, improve health, or feel better are participating for extrinsic reasons. Earning a T-shirt, pleasing a boss, or being with friends are also extrinsic motives.

Although some of these are good reasons to exercise, they are not important enough to most people to sustain their participation for long. Too often, the exercise professional emphasizes extrinsic values of physical activity to the exclusion of other outcomes. They champion the physiological benefits of exercise because they know that their clients' health will improve if they exercise appropriately. This approach, which Bain (1985) calls the rational-scientific approach, assumes that one merely has to explain the health benefits of exercise to motivate people. The high dropout rate from most exercise programs suggests that this is not a good strategy. Perhaps a better approach would be to stress extrinsic values to attract people, but then to switch to a more intrinsic focus.

The work of Csikszentmihalyi (1975) is particularly important to understanding the enjoyment of physical activity. In his theoretical model of enjoyment, Csikszentmihalyi developed the concept of flow, which is based on the tenet that self-rewarding involvement is the key to human development. The flow model defines *enjoyment* as a balance between the challenges of an activity and the skills of the participant. Two other concepts important to the model are *anxiety* and *boredom*. *Anxiety* is viewed as an imbalance between challenges and skills, that is, when one's skills are inadequate for the challenge at hand. *Bordeom* occurs when one's skills are greater than the challenges of an activity. When challenges and skills are equal and greater than zero, the experience is considered optimal and is called a flow experience (Chalip, Csikszentmihalyi, Kleiber, & Larson, 1984).

Rudnicki and Wankel (1988) have successfully related the flow concept to fitness programming. In a recent study, they found self-challenge to be a primary predictor of long-term exercise involvement. They suggested that fitness programs include challenging and interesting experiences within the participants' capabilities. When one achieves the level of competence necessary for a flow experience, enjoyment and satisfaction are likely to result. To maintain interest over time, it is necessary to increase the level of difficulty of the activity as one becomes more competent. The study also found that nonhealth factors (such as enjoyment) and "programmatic" factors (such as convenience, regularity of an organized program, and leader encouragement) were important in the re-enrollment of clients.

It is often difficult for the practitioner to promote the fun and enjoyment of certain fitness activities. Most people who are beginning fitness programs find calisthenics and jogging boring. Rather than insisting that clients perform these activities, the practitioner should find more enjoyable activities that yield similar physiological outcomes. The popularity of aerobic dance can probably be attributed to the elements of rhythm and music, which make the experience more interesting for many people. The challenge for the exercise professional is to match the client to program activities that yield maximum satisfaction while providing enough exercise to achieve a training effect.

Exercise as a Social Experience

For many people, the social aspects of exercise are an important reason for their participation. Social reasons for physical activity range from meeting new people (exercise facilities have been called the singles clubs of the eighties) to fighting loneliness and social isolation. The relaxed atmosphere of a fitness class makes social interaction easier for some people. Sharing the group exercise experience often leads to camaraderie and friendship among regular participants. Opportunities for socializing occur before, during, and after participation. Indeed, the socializing associated with some activities has become institutionalized. Expressions such as "19th hole" and "apres-ski" indicate the enjoyment of the congenial companionship of like-minded participants (Stiles, 1967).

Regular exercise participants often observe how much more enjoyable the experience is when others share it. Heinzelmann and Bagley (1970) found that almost 90% of their 195 program participants preferred to exercise with someone else or with a group rather than work out alone. They also found that when people exercise together, they enjoy the experience more, derive social support, feel a sense of personal commitment to continue, and welcome the opportunity to compare their progress and level of fitness with other participants.

The companionship that often comes of shared participation may lead to long-term friendships and mutual esteem. Snyder and Spreitzer (1979) found that for golf partners who play at a regular time for many years, social attachment becomes the primary factor in their continued participation. In such groups, the absence of a member is keenly felt and the permanent loss of a group member has a lasting effect on those remaining.

Social experience as an important motive for participation is evident at all ages. *Affiliation*, or the desire to be part of a team, to be with friends, or to make new friends, is a leading motive for participation in youth sports (Gould & Horn, 1984; Passer, 1982). College students, both athletes and nonathletes, have indicated that social interaction is an important part of their attraction to sport. Students value the opportunities to interact and form relationships (Mathes & Battista, 1985). Older adults also identify social motives as important (Heitmann, 1986). Although the pattern of participation motives for boys and girls is quite similar (Passer, 1982), adult women typically rate the social experience slightly higher than men do (Biddle & Bailey, 1985; Mathes & Battista, 1985).

Practitioners should always promote the social dimension in their fitness programs. Ways to foster a social atmosphere include using the names of the participants, employing "mixer" activities in the early phases, using small group and partner activities, establishing buddy systems, celebrating birthdays and other special occasions, and scheduling social events such as weekend outings. By creating a "family" atmosphere, the exercise professional increases the likelihood that participants will continue in the exercise program.

Exercise for Psychological Benefits

Although the psychological benefits of exercise are widely recognized among participants, the many ways in which the benefits are described make them difficult to characterize. The psychological benefits that people cite range from "feeling good" to claims of a "cathartic effect" or a "runner's high." Somewhere in between lie the beliefs that exercise reduces tension and anxiety, elevates mood, improves one's coping ability, increases self-worth, and promotes feelings of happiness. Despite this diversity, it is obvious that people generally believe regular exercise brings about beneficial psychological changes.

Age and sex are factors that seem to influence the importance assigned to the psychological outcomes of exercise. Older adults tend to place greater importance on psychological benefits (Heitmann, 1986), while children give this outcome among the lowest of values (Passer, 1982). Women seem to appreciate the potential psychological benefits more than men do (Biddle & Bailey, 1985; Johnsgard, 1985b; Sidney & Shephard, 1976).

People must experience exercise before they can appreciate how it can positively alter their moods and self-concepts (Johnsgard, 1985b). People's identities may be enhanced as they realize that they can control and change their lives, and identity may be further enhanced as they become fit and trim. Johnsgard points out that although exercise can be inconvenient and physically uncomfortable, people persist because they have learned that it usually makes them feel better emotionally.

However nebulous the concept of psychological benefits, studies show that people believe exercise makes them feel better. In Brunner's (1969) study, "to feel better physically and mentally" was rated second in importance of the 23 benefits listed by regular exercise participants. Harris (1981a) found that 87% of her subjects recognized some psychological benefits of running, and many felt depressed or guilty if they did not run.

In recent years, considerable attention has been given to the concept of *exercise addiction*, or *exercise dependence* as some prefer to call it (Pargman, 1980). According to Pargman (1980), those who are "hooked" exhibit a strong degree of reliance on exercise to provide the pleasurable feelings or sensations they are seeking. These findings closely parallel Glasser's (1976) ideas about *positive addiction*. The type of exercise most often associated with exercise dependence is running. Another interesting aspect of positive addiction is that people frequently report withdrawal symptoms after missing one or more workouts (Morgan, 1979). Indeed some runners persist in training despite illness and even serious injury. Although the scientific understanding of exercise addiction is incomplete, we will review the existing studies on this topic, as well as other aspects of the psychological effects of exercise in chapters 3 and 4.

Because of the personal nature of the exercise experience, the practitioner has limited control over the psychological benefits experienced by participants. One strategy might be to discuss the "feeling good" phenomenon with clients to promote expectations of feeling better after exercise. Pointing out the use of exercise as effective stress management would also help enhance the expectation that exercise reduces tension. Exercise professionals should also apprise clients of problems related to exercise dependence. The physical, social, and psychological implications of exercise dependence, its symptoms, methods of avoiding the problem, and approaches to rehabilitation should all be covered.

REASONS FOR NOT EXERCISING

Despite information about the benefits of exercise, personal appeals, and social pressures, some people still fail to exercise. Understanding the reasons why may help the exercise professional plan strategies to counter or negate them. The most frequently cited reasons for inactivity include lack of time, fatigue, inadequate facilities, lack of knowledge about fitness, and lack of "willpower" (Fitness Ontario, 1981; Goodrick, Hartung, Warren, & Hoepfel, 1984). The exercise leader must take seriously each of these barriers to exercise participation and deal with them creatively. Following are suggestions for addressing some common reasons for not exercising.

Lack of Time

Lack of time is by far the most frequently cited reason for not exercising. Business or career responsibilities, family obligations, or just "too busy" in general are the usual justifications for inactivity. However, having no time for exercise is often more of a perception than a reality. Few people are scheduled so tightly that they cannot work in some exercise breaks. If governors, senators, and even the president of the United States can find time to exercise, others should be able to work it into their daily routines as well.

Time management training may help some clients find time for exercise. Workshops may be offered as part of a comprehensive lifestyle program, or simplified techniques for managing time may be discussed as part of the counseling process. Unless the client believes that exercise can be "worked in," the practitioner is practically guaranteed that the person will drop out of the program.

However, lack of time is not the real issue for most people. Choosing not to exercise is more a matter of priority. People find time to watch TV, read the newspaper, go to the movies, stop off at the bar, and engage in a host of other pastimes. People do what they enjoy, and the fitness professional should not ignore this fact. To attract and hold the attention of a typical client, the practitioner must offer a program that provides enjoyment and personal satisfaction.

Fatigue

Being too tired is the second most common excuse for not exercising. However, feeling tired is usually a matter of mental rather than physical fatigue. The demands of everyday life tend to be more psychological than physical, exacting an emotional toll that makes people want to collapse in front of the TV at day's end.

The fitness practitioner must make people aware of the great restorative benefits of exercise. A brisk walk, a couple sets of tennis, or a bicycle ride would do more to relieve feelings of fatigue than several hours of television viewing. Again, the emphasis should be on enjoyable activities. A person who has had a day full of "hassles" does not want to be faced with another "chore" at the end of the day. An activity that is anticipated with pleasure is much more likely to encourage regular participation.

Lack of Facilities

People often claim that they cannot exercise because they have no access to facilities. They may believe that exercise facilities are nonexistent, inconvenient, or inappropriate. However, few communities are totally void of public facilities for fitness and sports activities. Parks, recreation centers, tennis courts, and swimming pools are almost always available. Similarly, nonprofit organizations such as the YMCA provide facilities and programs in many cities, and, increasingly, churches are providing recreation facilities and programs. The for-profit fitness and health club industry is flourishing throughout North America. The claim therefore that facilities are not available is rarely valid.

People may often say that facilities are not available when they really mean that they are not convenient. The perception of convenience is very important. In their study of 1,708 Finnish manager-executives, Teraslinna, Partanen, Koskela, and Oja (1969) found that those who lived closest to an exercise facility were more willing to participate in an exercise program. Another aspect of convenience has to do with other services offered by the fitness center. A person with young children will be more likely to come if baby-sitting services are available.

Concern about inappropriate facilities has to do with the amount of space, the features of the facility, attractiveness, and ambiance. Facility characteristics generally matter a great deal and may be the difference in whether people come to a facility or not. Knowing this, the exercise professional should provide a clean, spacious, and tastefully decorated facility, and a wide array of exercise equipment.

Of course, access to elaborate facilities is not really necessary to enjoy the benefits of exercise. One can walk, bike, jog, or do any number of activities in and around the home. However, few people have enough motivation to stay with an exercise program on their own, especially in the beginning stages. For this reason, good facilities and professional instruction play an important role in establishing the exercise habit. Nevertheless, unsupervised programs can be successful (Gettman, Pollock, & Ward, 1983) and should always remain an option. Either way, periodic follow-up of some sort is desirable. With continuing access to an exercise professional or a "home base" facility, the independent exerciser can be periodically evaluated, pick up information, or simply receive encouragement. For example, the Canada Life Assurance Company provides counseling services to approximately 300 employees who do not participate in the company's group fitness program (Cox, 1984). If a person's circumstances dictate that they exercise alone, it is comforting to know that resources are accessible if needed.

Lack of Knowledge About Fitness

Many people simply do not know what form of exercise they should choose or how much to do.

How to check their level of fitness or improve areas of weakness can be equally mystifying. Fitness as an area of study has often been either ignored or inadequately presented in formal education. To fill this information void, people may turn to friends, purchase books on fitness, or rely on their intuition. If organized programs are convenient and accessible, some will seek these out.

Unfortunately, there also exists an immense amount of misinformation concerning all aspects of exercise. With celebrity and other self-styled "experts" dispensing fitness advice, it is hard for the uninformed to know what is correct. People will often accept as credible, information from someone who looks as though they know what they are doing. The exercise professional should be prepared to deal with these misconceptions in a straightforward, factual manner. Clients must be made to understand that bulging biceps or a trim physique do not necessarily qualify a person to give fitness advice.

Of course, all organized exercise and fitness programs seek to educate clients in a number of ways. An educational component is typically part of each class period in group programs. Special programs such as clinics and workshops can provide more in-depth information. Guest speakers have successfully promoted interest in special topics. Free printed materials, a lending library, and even audio and video resources can also help satisfy the demand for accurate information about exercise and fitness.

Exercise professionals should also make a greater effort to share fitness information and counter the effects of the untrained "experts." Practitioners could write exercise and fitness articles for the popular press instead of leaving these topics to feature writers. Appearing on television talk shows is another means of disseminating accurate information. In some cities, fitness experts who appear regularly on local television do a very good job of educating people about exercise. Outreach programs such as "fit fairs," exercise demonstrations in shopping malls, free exercise workshops, and clinics for church and civic groups are other ways to communicate knowledge about fitness and exercise.

Lack of Willpower

Willpower is traditionally considered a personality trait or psychic force that enables a person to control his or her actions (Thoresen & Mahoney, 1974). It is often assumed that people can effect major behavioral changes by simply "putting their minds to it," implying a repository of inner strength that allows them to transcend problems (Williams & Long, 1975). Many also believe that willpower is something you are born with. Of course, this does not bode well for individuals who would like to change but believe they lack this characteristic.

Unfortunately, attributing failure to lack of willpower falls short of identifying the factors that led to failure. Moreover, a person who incorporates the perception of "lack of willpower" into their self-concept severely hampers future efforts to change. The exercise professional must often deal with clients who have tried many times and failed, and who have subsequently come to believe that failure is inevitable due to their lack of willpower. Because low self-esteem associated with perceived lack of willpower decreases enthusiasm for future efforts, the practitioner must coax and cajole to get such a person to try one more time. If there is to be any measure of success, the practitioner will have to re-educate the client with respect to willpower.

Rather than focusing on willpower, the practitioner should promote the concept of self-control, which assumes that the ability to change behavior is based on knowledge and control of current situational factors (Thoresen & Mahoney, 1974). To exercise self-control, a person must understand what factors influence his or her behavior and learn how to alter these factors to bring about the desired changes. This approach gives the client a much clearer idea of what must be done to effect change. Then when temporary setbacks arise, the person does not attribute them to a lack of willpower.

SUMMARY

An exercise practitioner must understand why people exercise to help those with low motivation. This chapter has provided an overview of the motives for participation in exercise and fitness activities. For adults, regardless of age or sex, the most common motive for exercise is improved health and fitness. Improved appearance is also a strong motivating factor, especially for women of all ages. Other motives for participation are enjoyment, social experience, and psychological benefits. The practitioner should keep in mind that people usually exercise for more than one reason and that time and situational influences tend to change motives. Also, the importance of client enjoyment and intrinsic satisfactions should not be underestimated.

The most common reasons for not exercising include lack of time, fatigue, inadequate facilities, lack of knowledge about fitness, and lack of willpower. Suggestions for overcoming barriers to participation include assistance in developing time management skills, educating clients about the benefits of exercise, providing alternatives to traditional group programs, and providing individual counseling to help clients solve their problems.

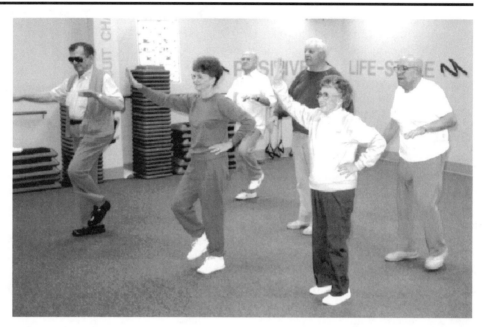

Chapter 2

Factors in Continued Exercise Behaviors: Exercise Adherence

The high rate of attrition in exercise programs is perhaps the greatest concern of the fitness professional. This problem affects virtually all programs. Even clients with access to the finest fitness facilities with the best evaluation, instruction, and member services are subject to the dropout phenomenon.

Millions of people begin to exercise each year, but for most the commitment fades as quickly as the typical New Year's resolution. Even people who have experienced myocardial infarction are prone to drop out of cardiac rehabilitation programs despite the extremely high health risks of not exercising. What accounts for this major discrepancy between wanting to exercise and the inability to stay with an exercise regimen? Although the fledgling discipline of exercise psychology cannot supply a

definitive answer at this point, some of the factors that influence exercise adherence are beginning to become clear. Before discussing these factors, however, an overview of the nature and scope of the attrition problem would be helpful.

THE DROPOUT PHENOMENON

Most exercise professionals find attracting people to a program to be much easier than keeping them there. Typically, about half of those who begin an exercise program drop out within the first 6 months (Wankel, 1987). The dropout rate is similar even for cardiac patients who have entered exercise rehabilitation programs (Oldridge, 1984a). Attrition rates, however, vary considerably from program to program. After reviewing 10 studies of

19

primary prevention exercise programs, Oldridge (1982) found dropout rates that ranged from 13% to 75%. His data on compliance in 18 secondary prevention programs showed dropout rates ranging from 3% to 87%. In reviewing this literature, Franklin (1988) found a mean dropout rate of 46% for healthy adults and 44% for cardiac patients. Although the studies varied considerably as to what constituted a "dropout," the message was clear: Exercise practitioners must find better ways to maintain their clients' interest.

Not only are dropouts frequent, they occur early on. The rate of attrition is typically greater in the first 2 to 4 months and then levels off to about 50% after 6 months. Consequently, one of the major challenges facing the exercise practitioner is to get people over the "hump" of the first few weeks, thereby increasing their chances of continuing compliance.

Representative data on compliance rates for one group of healthy adults are given in Figure 2.1. The rate of attrition for cardiac rehabilitation patients resembles that for healthy adults. Figure 2.2 chronicles the compliance rates of four groups of patients over a 4-year period. Two of the groups participated in the extensive Ontario Exercise Heart Collaborative Study (OEHCS), which followed 731 subjects. The other two groups were composed of 112 cardiac patients in a Swedish hospital program (Oldridge, 1982).

Clarification of Terms

There has been little consistency in the definitions of key terms in studies of exercise continuity. To avoid confusion, we would like to clarify some important terms before continuing this discussion.

Adherence

Common usage of the term *adherence* implies "sticking to" or faithfully conforming to a standard of behavior in order to meet some goal. *Adherence to exercise* has most often been defined for research purposes as a percentage of attendance. For example, a person who has attended 10 out of 20 sessions would have an adherence rate of 50%. However, some researchers have approached the concept of adherence in more black-and-white terms. Either a person achieves a pre-set standard of attendance, say 70% of all classes, or he or she is considered a dropout. We prefer to rate adherence on a continuum that ranges from complete nonadherence to total adherence. If we were to use attendance as the measure of adherence,

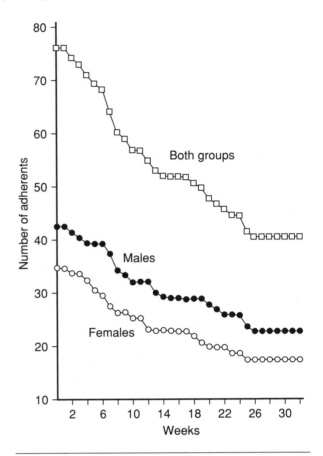

Figure 2.1 Adherence curves for male (n = 42) and female (n = 34) participants across the 32-week exercise programs.

From "Adherence Patterns of Healthy Men and Women Enrolled in an Exercise Program" by A. Ward and W.P. Morgan, 1984, *Journal of Cardiopulmonary Rehabilitation*, 4, p. 145. Reprinted by permission.

we might define low adherence as less than 40% attendance and high adherence as attendance over 80%. Such an approach was used by Gale, Eckhoff, Mogel, and Rodnick (1984). They classified subjects who attended less than 10% of exercise sessions as early dropouts, 10% to 49% were considered to be nonadherers, and subjects attending 50% or more were considered adherers.

Although attendance is often used as a measure in adherence studies, Wankel (1984) correctly pointed out that attendance is a "dirty" measure of adherence because it assumes that all types of nonattendance are equivalent. Typically, no leeway is given for unavoidable and discretionary absences. Wankel suggested a system that incorporates the concept of *excused absences* to more accurately reflect motivation or commitment to exercise.

Martin and Dubbert (1982) introduced the concept of *ideal adherence*, which is expressed as a

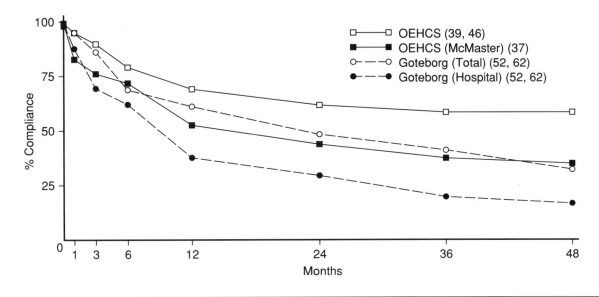

Figure 2.2 Compliance rates in two long-term (4-year) clinical trials of exercise and rehabilitation following myocardial infarction. Reference numbers are in parentheses.

From "Compliance and Exercise in Primary and Secondary Prevention of Coronary Heart Disease: A Review" by N.B. Oldridge, 1982, *Preventive Medicine*, **11**, p. 62. Reprinted by permission.

percentage of overall adherence. Success at achieving *ideal adherence* would be determined by comparing the *observed adherence* of an individual with a pre-set criterion. This approach has been operationalized by comparing the person's frequency of aerobic exercise sessions in a given week with the ideal standard of 3 per week. A definition of *ideal adherence* could also include a provision for duration and intensity of exercise as well as frequency (i.e., the percentage of sessions in which 60% to 65% of maximum heart rate is achieved for at least 15 to 30 minutes). As Martin and Dubbert (1985) pointed out, attendance does not necessarily constitute adequate exercise adherence unless people exercise appropriately when they do attend. By the same token, program "dropouts" may actually be complying with the exercise prescription on their own at home. Not all program dropouts abandon exercise entirely. Both of these examples point out some of the weaknesses of using program attendance to measure adherence. Nevertheless, if one believes that habitual exercise helps sustain meaningful exercise involvement over time, then attendance can be considered a useful measure of adherence.

Compliance

In the scientific literature on exercise, the terms *adherence* and *compliance* are often used interchangeably, although there are some exceptions.

For example, Oldridge (1979a) defined *compliance* as the degree to which subjects adhere to a protocol or treatment. He later defined *compliance* as "the continued participation in the exercise program at some minimal frequency with an attendance rate of "x" number of sessions out of "y" maximum number of sessions" (Oldridge, 1982, p. 56). More recently, Oldridge (1988b) differentiated between the terms by using *compliance* to describe behaviors related to following "immediate or short-term health and medical advice and direct prescription to relieve symptomatology" (p. 286), and using *adherence* in reference to long-term behavioral changes associated with ameliorating or preventing symptomatology. Another interesting distinction was made by Hindi-Alexander and Throm (1987). They interpreted *compliance* as a "sense of coercive obedience to orders" and *adherence* as "negotiated agreement." Although in some instances there may be good reason to differentiate between adherence and compliance, we shall use the terms interchangeably throughout this text.

Dropout

Typically, the term *dropout* applies to clients who have been active for a time and then have quit. Sometimes a distinction is made regarding the time of involvement, for example "subjects who participated for 2 months or less and then dropped out" (Shephard & Cox, 1980, p. 70), or subjects who miss "more then 2 consecutive weeks of sessions for reasons other than sickness, travel, or injury" (Ward & Morgan, 1984, p. 149). Some definitions of *dropout* are quite specific, such as "not attending a single supervised session for eight weeks for reasons other than myocardial infarction or death" (Oldridge, 1979a, p. 373), while others are more general, such as one who "stopped attending the program prior to the completion of the one year prescribed treatment regimen" (Blumenthal, Williams, Wallace, Williams, & Needles, 1982, p. 521). We will define program dropouts as individuals who have been active for some specified time and then, for one reason or another, have ceased to participate.

Reasons for Dropping Out

In studies of healthy adults, the primary reason given for dropping out of a program is lack of time. In a representative study, participants said that the program took too much time away from work and family (Gettman et al., 1983). Illness in the family, lack of interest in the program, and travel to the exercise center, which was considered too time consuming and expensive, were other reasons cited for dropping out. Table 2.1 summarizes the reasons given for dropping out of a corporate exercise program (Song, Shephard, & Cox, 1983).

Table 2.1   Reasons for Dropping out of an Employee Fitness Program

Reason	Men	Women
Loss of interest	7	9
Lack of time	16	20
Joined another health club	0	4
Joined community fitness program	0	2
Exercising on my own	3	5
Other	4	9
Total	30	49

From "Absenteeism, Employee Turnover and Sustained Exercise Participation" by T.K. Song, R.L. Shephard, and M. Cox, 1983, *Journal of Sports Medicine and Physical Fitness*, **22**, p. 394. Reprinted by permission.

Cardiac rehabilitation patients have identified similar reasons for dropping out. Figure 2.3 depicts some of these. The "psychosocial" category in the figure includes lack of interest and family problems. "Unavoidable" reasons refer to work conflicts, change of job, or change of residence

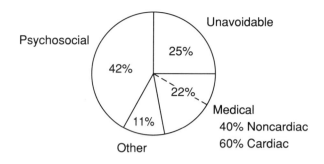

Figure 2.3   Reasons for dropout.

From "Compliance of Post Myocardial Infarction Patients to Exercise Programs" by N.B. Oldridge, 1979, *Medicine and Science in Sports*, **11**(4), pp. 373-375. Copyright © 1979 by the American College of Sports Medicine. Reprinted by permission.

(Oldridge, 1979a). A later summary of reasons for dropping out of a rehabilitation program also included program inconvenience and transportation difficulties as significant problems (Oldridge, 1982).

Of particular importance to this discussion are the initial objectives of people who subsequently drop out. Danielson and Wanzel (1977) established that most dropouts have two to four objectives in mind when they begin an exercise program, which indicates that they entered the program for some expected results. It is significant that people who did not attain their objectives dropped out at a much faster rate than those who did meet their goals. By 6 months, over 92% of non-goal attainers had dropped out, while over 60% of goal attainers remained in the program. This evidence dramatically demonstrates the importance of personalized, attainable goals in reducing dropout rates.

INDIVIDUAL FACTORS IN EXERCISE ADHERENCE

Few topics in exercise science have received the level of attention that has been focused on exercise adherence in recent years. Certainly we know more now than we did 10 years ago. We will begin a review of the extensive literature on exercise adherence with a look at factors relating to the individual.

Exercise History

Opinions differ as to the relation of childhood exercise experiences to exercise adherence as an adult (Dishman, 1985). One of the first studies to consider the influence of past involvement found that physically active men were more likely to have been high school athletes than sedentary men. The active men were also more likely to have participated in physical activity programs while in college (Harris, 1970). The study also found that 70% of the active men had received parental encouragement for physical activity, while only 40% of the inactive men had been encouraged by their parents. Snyder and Spreitzer's research (1979) supported the finding that parental encouragement influences future activity. A different study of 376 college professors also found a relation between prior experiences in high school and college recreational and varsity sports and more extensive exercise involvement later in life (Krotee & La Point, 1979). In the same vein, Yoesting and Burkhead (1973) found a direct relationship between the activity level of an individual as a child and the activity level of that individual as an adult.

Two findings from a survey conducted by the President's Council on Physical Fitness and Sports also support the importance of prior exercise experience (Clarke, 1973). One conclusion was that those who participated in school sports were more likely to be currently exercising than those who did not. The second finding was that people who had physical education classes were more likely to be currently exercising than those who did not have such classes.

Because early involvement is so important to a lifelong commitment, parents should be made aware of the importance of early exposure and encourage their children in all types of physical activity. Schools must also assume a greater role in helping children establish exercise habits and in promoting the benefits of an active lifestyle. To increase the probability of children becoming active adults they must be exposed to fun exercise experiences throughout their childhood and youth. Exercise and health professionals should promote these principles in every way possible.

Recent Exercise Behaviors

Another aspect of the question of the influence of prior experience on present exercise behavior relates to the recency of the experience. In a study that followed up on 250 subjects who had completed a comprehensive physical fitness evaluation and received an exercise prescription, it was found that the best predictor of current level of activity was one's exercise level just before the evaluation. Those who were most active before the evaluation continued to be the most active, and those the least active continued that pattern (Kruse & Calden, 1986). Other studies have reiterated the importance of recent experience and habit on present and future exercise behaviors (Godin & Shephard, 1986; Valois, Shephard, & Godin, 1986).

Active Versus Inactive Leisure Time

Research shows that people who are inactive in their leisure time are more apt to drop out of exercise programs than those who are active during leisure time. This pattern applies to postmyocardial infarction patients as well as to healthy adults (Andrew et al., 1981; Oldridge, 1982; Oldridge, Wicks, Hanley, Sutton, & Jones, 1978; Snyder, Franklin, Foss, & Rubenfire, 1982; Teraslinna, Partanen, Koskela, & Oja, 1969).

Current Level of Fitness

Although it might be assumed that a person's level of fitness upon entering an exercise program would influence their tendency to remain in the program, current research suggests that beginning fitness level has little to do with exercise adherence. One study that did find differences between regular participants and dropouts was that of Young and Ismail (1977). They reported significantly higher performance levels on a submaximal exercise test for continuing participants. Most studies, however, find no initial fitness differences between adherers and dropouts (Blumenthal et al., 1982; Epstein, Koeske, & Wing, 1984; Massie & Shephard, 1971; Ward & Morgan, 1984; Wilfley & Kunce, 1986). In fact, a few studies have found program adherers to be initially less fit than dropouts (Dishman, 1981; Gale et al., 1984).

If future exercise behaviors are highly dependent on present and past behaviors, the sedentary person who has little exercise background probably would have more difficulty establishing an exercise habit. The decision to adopt an active lifestyle would require more commitment for the chronically inactive than for the individual with an established exercise habit (Godin, Valois, Shephard, & Desharnais, 1987). Because a chronically inactive person would also be more likely to drop out, such a person would warrant special attention from the exercise professional. On the other hand, clients with a good physical activity background and a good record of recent involvement would start and sustain an exercise program more easily.

Smokers and Nonsmokers

Nearly every study we reviewed found a link between smoking and dropping out (Gale et al., 1984; Knapp, Gutman, Squires, & Pollock, 1983; Massie & Shephard, 1971; Oldridge, 1984b; Oldridge & Jones, 1983). Smokers are much more likely to drop out in the first few weeks of a program than are nonsmokers (Oldridge et al., 1978) and have also been found to be 2.46 times more likely to be program dropouts than nonsmokers (Oldridge et al., 1983). The one study that failed to show a relationship between smoking and nonadherence to exercise involved post-coronary males (Shephard, Corey, & Kavanagh, 1981). However, this study did find that smoking habits had a marked effect on prognosis, with recurrence of infarction being least likely in those who cut back or stopped smoking entirely.

Demographic Factors

Being able to rely on population profiles as indicators of program adherence would help exercise professionals identify clients "at risk" and design special programs for them. In this section, we will review current information on the importance of demographic factors in program adherence.

Age

Involvement in physical activity generally declines as people age. This contention is supported by various surveys done in the United States and Canada (Clarke, 1973; Fitness Ontario, 1983; Miller Brewing Company, 1983) as well as by a review of data on the exercise habits of North Americans (Stephens et al., 1985). However, does the tendency to decrease activity with age necessarily mean that older adults are more likely to drop out of exercise programs than younger ones? The literature on this is equivocal at the moment. Some studies of healthy adults find age to be a factor in compliance while others do not. Ward and Morgan (1984) found that program adherents were older than dropouts, and Gale and colleagues (1984) reported similar results. In contrast, Kruse and Calden (1986) found significant differences favoring younger participants.

Other studies have found no relationship between age and program maintenance. Research on 124 firefighters did not find age to be a factor in program compliance at a 3-month post-check, although at the 6-month follow-up the noncompliers were significantly younger than the compliers

(Reid & Morgan, 1979). An extensive community survey found that age had no bearing on program maintenance, nor did it affect maintained or decreased activity levels (Sallis et al., 1986).

Results of studies of patients in cardiac rehabilitation programs are also contradictory. Two studied identified age as a factor in dropping out (Baun, Bernacki, Riggins, & Landgren, 1983; Knapp, Gutman, Squires, & Pollock, 1983), while others failed to find differences in compliance based on age (Blumenthal et al., 1982; Stern & Cleary, 1981; Tirrell & Hart, 1980).

Based on this information, exercise professionals should avoid preconceived notions of their clients' adherence based on age.

Gender

While research shows marginal gender differences in exercise involvement with men being slightly more active than women (Brooks, 1988; Stephens et al., 1985), whether gender is important in exercise adherence is not entirely clear. A 1-year community study of 1,411 adults found no differences between men and women in global activity change or in rate of dropout from regular activity (Sallis et al., 1986). Ward and Morgan (1984) reported nearly identical adherence patterns for men and women. Kruse and Calden (1986) also found that gender was not a factor in predicting current exercise compliance. Consequently, the exercise practitioner should probably not be concerned with gender differences as a factor in program compliance.

Marital Status

Do single people exercise more and adhere to programs better than married people? Recent North American surveys typically show that single people are more active than married people (Wankel, 1987). However, this data can be misleading. Because marital status is affected by age, education, and income, it can be only negligibly associated with physical activity (Brooks, 1988). Two other exercise adherence studies that considered marital status reported contradictory results. One study showed no difference in adherence based on marital status (Oldridge & Jones, 1983), while the other study found that more dropouts were single (Gale et al., 1984). Because marital status is associated with so many other factors, it is probably not a good indicator of adherence.

Socioeconomic Factors

Personal factors such as educational background, occupation, and income would seem to be reasonable variables to study when looking for predictors of exercise and program adherence. Overall, however, socioeconomic characteristics have not been researched to a desirable degree with respect to adherence.

Education

Although there is considerable evidence that involvement in physical activity is influenced by level of education (Brooks, 1988; Fitness Ontario, 1983; Miller Brewing Company, 1983), few studies have addressed the role of education in exercise adherence. In a study of 120 male cardiac rehabilitation patients, Oldridge and Jones (1983) found that 51% of those with less than a high school education dropped out, while only 36% of those with at least a high school education were dropouts. In contrast, a study of healthy adults found that education was not a predictor of adherence (Gale et al., 1984). It appears, therefore, that the role of education in program compliance requires further study before it can be of value to the practitioner. However, when education is combined with other factors, its predictive value may increase considerably.

Income and Occupation

Participation in various forms of exercise and sport seems to be influenced by income and occupation (Brooks, 1988; Clarke, 1973; Fitness Ontario, 1983; Miller Brewing Company, 1983). A review of North American participation surveys (Stephens et al., 1985) found three indicators of socioeconomic status—income, education, and occupation—to be positively associated with exercise. In other words, people of higher income, education, and occupational status are more likely to be physically active. Income and occupation factors have also been considered in several exercise adherence studies that yielded mixed results (Friedman & Hellerstein, 1973; Gale et al., 1984; Massie & Shephard, 1971; Stern & Cleary, 1981). By far the most consistent finding in studies relating income and occupation to exercise compliance was that blue-collar workers are more likely to drop out of exercise programs than white-collar workers (Gale et al., 1984; Oldridge, 1979b; Oldridge, 1984b; Oldridge et al., 1983; Oldridge & Jones, 1983). This finding seems to apply to both healthy adults and cardiac rehabilitation patients. In an attempt to explain the blue-collar dropout phenomenon, Allison and Coburn (1985) pointed out that many blue-collar workers believe they get enough exercise through their work, and therefore need not exercise in their leisure time. Other possible explanations they gave

were the workers' lack of awareness of the benefits of exercise and their lower inclination to engage in preventive health behaviors in general. The latter reason may be due to a lower sense of personal control.

Nevertheless, high dropout rates among blue-collar workers are not an entirely foregone conclusion as illustrated by an extensive study of over 7,000 blue-collar employees at three sites (Cox, 1984). Using an approach that stressed counseling and tailoring programs to individual needs, researchers allowed employees to choose from program components that included recreational and competitive activities, fitness classes, individual and home programs, and educational interventions. After 2 years, the dropout rate ranged from just 17% to 30%. In some instances, participation rates were as high as 75% of the total work force, moreover, those involved in the program participated an average of twice a week. It appears, therefore, that blue-collar workers can be meaningfully involved through counseling and program planning based on individual needs and interests. Table 2.2 summarizes data from a study that addresses several of these factors (Oldridge & Jones, 1983).

Physical Factors

Physical characteristics would be another logical focus in research on factors that predict exercise adherence. Some of the more objective and reliable measures of individual differences currently available are of physical characteristics. However, studies using physical characteristics as indicators of exercise adherence have not been very successful. The single exception is angina, which consistently has been found to adversely affect exercise compliance among myocardial infarction patients (Bruce, Frederick, Bruce, & Fisher, 1976; Oldridge, 1984b; Oldridge et al., 1983; Shephard et al., 1981). The higher dropout rate of patients with angina is not surprising, because the symptoms most often occur during exercise (Oldridge et al., 1983).

Among the physical factors initially thought to affect exercise adherence were body weight and a high percentage of body fat (Dishman & Gettman, 1980; Dishman, Ickes, & Morgan, 1980; Massie & Shephard, 1971; Young & Ismail, 1977). However, other researchers have not been able to verify that these factors predict adherence (Baun et al., 1983; Shephard & Cox, 1980; Ward & Morgan, 1984). It appears that more study is needed. Furthermore, as Ward and Morgan (1984) have suggested, different adherence models for men and women may be required.

Table 2.2   Differences Between Compliers and Dropouts: Sociodemographic Characteristics at Entry

Characteristic	Total (N = 120)	Dropout (N = 62)	Complier (N = 58)	X^2
Education				
< High school	34%	51%	49%	
≥ High school	49%	36%	64%	$p \geq .15$
Missing	17%			
Marital status				
Married	68%	42%	58%	
Unmarried	15%	44%	56%	$p \geq .80$
Missing	17%			
Occupational status				
Employed	62%	42%	58%	
Unemployed	21%	46%	54%	$p \geq .80$
Missing	17%			
Occupation				
White collar	58%	41%	59%	
Blue collar	42%	63%	37%	$p \leq .01$
Smoking				
Yes	27%	77%	23%	
Never or quit	73%	43%	57%	$p \leq .005$
Leisure				
Active	38%	36%	64%	
Inactive	61%	62%	38%	$p \leq .01$

Note. Missing data are due to dropout before the questionnaires were completed.

From "Improving Patient Compliance in Cardiac Exercise Rehabilitation: Effects of Written Agreement and Self-Monitoring" by N.B. Oldridge and N.L. Jones, 1983, *Journal of Cardiopulmonary Rehabilitation, 3,* p. 259. Reprinted by permission.

Several additional physical factors have been investigated, with either conflicting or inconclusive results. Among these factors are height (Bruce et al., 1976; Dishman, 1981; Shephard & Cox, 1980; Ward & Morgan, 1984), blood pressure (Blumenthal et al., 1982; Oldridge & Jones, 1983; Ward & Morgan, 1984) and cholesterol and triglycerides (Blumenthal et al., 1982; Stern & Cleary, 1981).

There has been limited success in distinguishing between adherers and dropouts using the left ventricular ejection fraction (LVEF) as assessed through radionuclide angiography. But the impracticality of this measure negates its utility for practitioners (Blumenthal et al., 1982; Knapp et al., 1983). With the possible exception of angina, individual physical factors apparently provide little information of practical value in predicting adherence.

PSYCHOLOGICAL FACTORS IN EXERCISE ADHERENCE

There have been numerous attempts to identify key psychological factors that would help explain the complex issue of exercise adherence. Unfortunately this considerable research has not yet yielded consistent results that could be of practical value to exercise professionals. Despite these discouraging research outcomes, however, it would be instructive to review the psychological factors that have been studied so far.

Personality

Several aspects of personality have been investigated with respect to exercise adherence. Young and Ismail (1977) used the Cattell 16PF, a personality test consisting of 16 personality factors, to compare regular exercisers, exercise dropouts, and exercise converts. Regular exercisers were found to have greater self-confidence and emotional stability than either the converts or the dropouts. The study also found that exercise converts were initially much more philosophically conservative and traditional than regular exercisers, but that over a 4-year period they became more liberal and analytical, consistent with the personalities of regular exercisers.

Several studies have used aspects of the Minnesota Multiphasic Personality Inventory (MMPI) to gain insight into the adherence question. An extensive study of patients with prior myocardial infarctions found that those who dropped out of a low-level exercise program were more anxious and depressed than those who remained in the program (Stern & Cleary, 1981). Blumenthal and colleagues (1982) also used the MMPI in another study of recovering myocardial patients. The patients who dropped out of the exercise program scored significantly higher in the areas of social introversion and anxiety and significantly lower in the area of ego strength. Moreover, the dropouts' higher scores on hypochondriasis and depression approached significance. It was suggested that the people in these studies who dropped out of the group exercise programs might benefit more from individual exercise programs. However, two studies of healthy adults (Massie & Shephard, 1971; Shephard & Cox, 1980) found that anxiety, as measured by the Taylor Manifest Anxiety Scale, did not affect adherence.

Several investigators have looked for possible links between the Type A and Type B personality distinction and exercise adherence. It is generally assumed that the Type A person, characterized as aggressive, ambitious, and time conscious, is more likely to drop out of an exercise program than the more relaxed Type B person. This assumption was confirmed in a study of cardiac rehabilitation patients (Oldridge et al., 1978). The study found that program dropouts had significantly more Type A characteristics than program compliers. In a study of healthy adults, Shephard and Cox (1980) also observed significantly higher Type A scores among low adherers as compared to nonparticipants, dropouts and high adherers. Interestingly, this observation applied to male but not to female low adherers. It was suggested that the Type A subjects did not intentionally drop out, but became low adherers due to real or perceived time conflicts associated with management roles. Another explanation was that Type A people are more likely to reach upper management levels and therefore have more business-related obligations that might restrict exercise class attendance.

Researchers have also given considerable attention to self-motivation in relation to exercise adherence. Dishman et al. (1980) defined *self-motivation* as a general disposition to persevere. They hypothesized that self-motivation could be reliably measured as a stable personality characteristic that relates to adherence. The subsequent

development and validation called the Self-Motivation Inventory (SMI) led to several studies (Dishman & Ickes, 1981). One study that supported the value of the SMI for predicting adherence was reported by Knapp, Gutman, Foster, and Pollock (1984). With elite male and female speedskaters as subjects, they were able to predict adherence to the training regimen by the skaters' scores on the SMI.

However, other studies involving the SMI produced results that did not support the self-motivation construct as predictive of exercise adherence. One study found that SMI not only failed to predict exercise program adherence, but the adherent group had lower SMI scores (equal to or less than 128) than the early dropout and nonadherent groups combined (Gale et al., 1984). Two studies conducted by Wankel, Yardley, and Graham (1985) also failed to find a relationship between self-motivation and participant attendance in exercise programs.

Researchers have had some success in predicting program adherence by combining SMI scores with other variables. Using self-motivation scores together with data on percent body fat and body weight in a prediction model, investigators were able to classify approximately 80% of adherers and dropouts (Dishman & Gettman, 1980; Dishman et al., 1980). The prediction model was based on a sample that was made up entirely of men.

Ward and Morgan (1984) found the regression equation developed by Dishman and colleagues to be ineffective in predicting the dropout patterns of men and women in a study of healthy adults. Although the model accurately predicted the adherence patterns of 87% of the subjects, it correctly predicted only 25% of dropouts. It was suggested that perhaps separate prediction models were needed for women and men, because these two groups may drop out for different reasons. Another interesting suggestion was that because different factors may be correlated with adherence over time, independent models based on temporal considerations may be needed.

Results of studies on other personality traits as predictors of exercise adherence tend to be conflicting or inconclusive. The internal-external control of reinforcement construct (Rotter, 1966) has received some research attention, but none of the studies has effectively discriminated between program adherers and dropouts (Dishman & Gettman, 1980; Dishman et al., 1980; McCready & Long, 1985; O'Connell & Price, 1982). The same comment can be made with respect to self-concept (Wilfley & Kunce, 1986).

The effect of mood on adherence patterns has been of interest to some researchers. Ward and Morgan (1984) found that female dropouts and adherers had different levels of anger, with dropouts scoring higher on the factor of anger at the conclusion of a 32-week exercise program. Male adherers, however, were significantly lower in tension and depression, higher in vigor, and had more desirable global mood scores. In contrast, an 8-week investigation of an exercise program for healthy adults failed to produce any differences in mood states between subjects completing the program and dropouts (Wilfley & Kunce, 1986).

Attitude

The utility of attitude in discriminating among levels of exercise adherence has not been particularly successful. Ajzen and Fishbein (1980) defined *attitude* as a person's general feeling of favorableness or unfavorableness toward a concept. For our purposes, attitude refers to how one generally feels toward exercise and fitness-related activities. Most researchers interested in the role of attitude in adherence have used Kenyon's Attitude Toward Physical Activity Scales (Kenyon, 1968a, 1968b). Massie and Shephard (1971) found no differences between dropouts and continuing participants on any of the six attitude scales. Similar results were recorded by Dishman and colleagues (Dishman & Gettman, 1980; Dishman et al., 1980). McCready and Long (1985), using a revised version of the Kenyon instrument, found an association between percentage of attendance and the attitude variables of catharsis (release) and social continuation (being with friends). One interesting finding was that subjects who had a less positive initial attitude for social continuation and a more positive attitude for catharsis, had better attendance records.

Some researchers have recently demonstrated that attitudes defined more specifically in terms of action, target, context, and time can effectively predict exercise behaviors (Godin & Shephard, 1986; Godin et al., 1987). These researchers used an adapted version of Fishbein and Ajzen's theory of reasoned action (Ajzen & Fishbein, 1980), to show that attitudes can help predict and explain exercise behaviors. Moreover, they successfully opened up one of the more promising avenues of research on exercise adherence. The theory of reasoned action will be discussed in more detail in a later section.

Health Knowledge and Beliefs

An important component of most fitness programs is instruction on the various health benefits of exercise. If people believe that regular exercise will improve their health, it is presumed that they would be more likely to exercise than people who believe that exercise has no bearing on health.

Reid and Morgan (1979) were able to increase compliance in an experimental group of firefighters by providing them with a 1-hour program that included verbal and written information, and a film about why and how to exercise. A control group received a one-page sheet that gave some exercise suggestions. At 3 months, the compliance rate for the experimental group was 55% and only 29% for the control group. This effect, however, proved to be temporary. The experimental group eventually lost 40% of its previous compliers, thereby reverting to approximately the same level as the control group. In an extension of this study, Lindsay-Reid and Osborn (1980) produced some unexpected results with respect to the relationship between health beliefs and exercise behavior. Perception of susceptibility to heart disease and other illnesses was negatively associated with exercise adherence. Tirrell and Hart (1980) obtained similar results in a study of patients recovering from coronary bypass surgery. Patients who perceived themselves as most susceptible to heart disease were the least compliant, and those who worried less about health or who believed they had little control over their health were more compliant. In reaction to these unexpected results, researchers wondered about the patients' interpretations of the questions relating to health beliefs. It was also suggested that the rigidity of the compliance measure influenced the level of compliance. There were also barriers to participation, such as weather and illness, that affected compliance.

A study of healthy adults enrolled in an employee fitness program revealed a somewhat different pattern (Morgan, Shephard, Finucane, Schimmelfing, & Jazmaji, 1984). For men, program initiation was linked to their beliefs about the health benefits of exercise and to confidence in their ability to control health outcomes. Program adherence, on the other hand, was related to their perceived ability to attend and to realize program expectations. In contrast, women were motivated to enroll in the program by perceived poor health. This finding was consistent with another study in which perceived vulnerability to a health threat enhanced the intentions of college women to begin a regular exercise program (Wurtele & Maddux, 1987). Table 2.3 compares beliefs about exercise for sedentary and active subjects.

Until more definitive conclusions are established to the contrary, the exercise professional should continue to provide sound scientific information

Table 2.3 Average Belief Scores for Sedentary and Active Subjects

Belief	Sedentary (N = 89) x ± s.d.	Active (N = 83) x ± s.d.
Help me fill free time	0.88 ± 1.74	1.53 ± 1.28**
Help me to control my body weight	2.07 ± 1.10	2.28 ± 0.88
Be healthy	2.71 ± 0.53	2.81 ± 0.40
Be physically damaging	–2.24 ± 1.23	–2.31 ± 1.24
Relieve tension	2.06 ± 1.11	2.33 ± 0.80
Improve my physical appearance	2.10 ± 0.98	2.12 ± 0.88
Help me to feel better	2.38 ± 0.78	2.49 ± 0.63
Help me meet people	1.12 ± 1.36	1.04 ± 1.12
Be time consuming	0.96 ± 1.33	1.16 ± 1.27
Improve my mental performance	1.80 ± 1.12	2.13 ± 0.87*
Help me to be physically fit	2.55 ± 0.66	2.76 ± 0.43*

Note. All scales range from +3 to –3.

*$p < .05$. **$p < .01$.

From "The Impact of Physical Fitness Evaluation on Behavioral Intentions Towards Regular Exercise" by G. Godin, M.H. Cox, and R.J. Shephard, 1983. *Canadian Journal of Applied Sports Science*, **8**(4), p. 244. Reprinted by permission.

about exercise. However, one should not assume that because information is presented the clients will act on the information or incorporate it into their personal belief systems.

Multiple Individual Factors

To this point, we have focused on the ability of single characteristics, such as attitude or body weight, to predict exercise adherence. As you have seen, however, the process is much more complicated than that. Realizing the complexity of adherence, several researchers combined selected individual factors to improve their ability to predict adherence.

As mentioned earlier, scores on the Self-Motivation Inventory have been combined with the factors of body weight and percent body fat to create a prediction model that has had some success in predicting adherence, but has done less well in predicting potential dropouts (Dishman & Gettman, 1980; Dishman & Ickes, 1981). However, factors that help predict potential dropouts from exercise rehabilitation have been identified in the extensive Ontario Exercise-Heart Collaborative Study (Oldridge et al., 1983). A multivariate analysis determined that 58% of noncompliers were smokers. By adding the factor of blue-collar occupational status, the dropout rate increased to 69%. Also including the characteristics of inactive leisure and jobs that require little effort, the success rate for predicting dropouts increased to 95% (Oldridge, 1979b). A

subsequent study of graduates of cardiac rehabilitation found that the presence of any two of the following factors—smoking, blue-collar occupation, or inactive leisure habits—correctly identified 81% of dropouts (Oldridge & Spencer, 1985). In a study of patients recovering from myocardial infarction, Blumenthal and colleagues (1982) found that the combination of the physical factor of left ventricular ejection fraction (LVEF), which is an aspect of heart output, and the psychological factors of social introversion and ego strength predicted 90.4% of the compliers and 78.6% of the dropouts.

By presenting these few multidimensional models, we have intended to demonstrate the complexity of the adherence phenomenon, but also show that there is hope of eventually arriving at a better understanding of the phenomenon. Although the results of some of these studies are encouraging, there is much yet to be done. The search for interdependent factors needs to be expanded, and existing research replicated and extended. In addition, refinement of the current predictive models and the development of new ones is also needed. Better understanding of all the factors and processes involved in adherence is a matter of considerable urgency to the exercise professional.

SOCIAL FACTORS IN EXERCISE ADHERENCE

In the literature on exercise compliance, social factors have not received the degree of attention that individual or program factors have received. The exercise practitioner should keep in mind that people do not operate in a social vacuum. It would be naive to ignore the influence of the social milieu in which exercise program clients live and work. Most people belong to several social networks that affect them in very pronounced ways. What happens to an individual at home, at the office, or in other social settings can significantly affect that person's involvement in an exercise program.

Spousal and Family Social Support

A recurring social factor related to adherence is the degree of social support that the noninvolved spouse exhibits for the exercise behaviors of the involved spouse. *Spousal social support* is generally defined as the demonstration of a positive attitude toward an exercise program and the encouragement of the spouse's involvement in it. Spousal social support is evidenced by an expressed interest in program activities, a pronounced enthusiasm for the spouse's efforts and progress, and a willingness to accommodate the spouse's exercise involvement within the family routine. Presumably, the support of family members other than the spouse is important also, although there is less information about how other family members affect adherence. It is probably safe to assume, however, that the support of more family members increases a person's chances of successful adherence. Increasingly, therapy programs are tapping the power of family relationships to change behaviors (Epstein et al., 1984; Monahan, 1986).

Some of the earliest research that addressed this factor found that adherence patterns in males were influenced significantly by their wives' attitudes (Heinzelmann & Bagley, 1970). As demonstrated in Figure 2.4, 80% of the participants whose wives had positive attitudes toward the program had good adherence patterns, while only 40% of those whose wives had neutral or negative attitudes had good program adherence. The Ontario Exercise-Heart Collaborative Study (Oldridge et al., 1983) demonstrated even more dramatic effects of spousal support. The dropout rate for patients whose spouses were indifferent or negative toward the program was 3 times that of patients whose wives were supportive of the program. Several other researchers (Andrew & Parker, 1979; Godin & Shephard, 1985; Wankel, 1985) have supported these findings. To take advantage of the benefits of spousal support, exercise professionals should try to promote such support in participants' families. One way to elicit spousal support is to involve

spouses in the program. Involvement may range from an orientation session for family members to parallel exercise programs. An important objective when involving spouses is to fully educate them about all aspects of the exercise program. This helps reduce the potential for conflict between participant and spouse by promoting mutual understanding of the nature of the program (Oldridge, 1984a). In the cardiac rehabilitation program described by Oldridge, the spouse was offered a program at the same time as the patient. This program has had a very positive effect on patient compliance. Before the program for spouses was established, there was a dropout rate of 56%. The rate was cut to 10% for patients with a spouse in the support program (Erling & Oldridge, 1985).

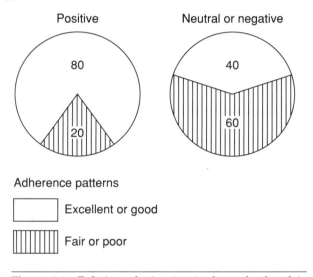

Figure 2.4 Relation of wives' attitudes to husbands' adherence in a physical activity program.

From "Social and Psychological Factors That Influence the Effectiveness of Exercise Programs" by F. Heinzelmann. In *Exercise Testing and Exercise Training in Coronary Heart Disease* (p. 280) by J. Naughton (Ed.), 1973, New York: Academic Press. Copyright 1973 by Academic Press. Reprinted by permission.

Peer Social Support

Although not extensively documented at present, peer influences on exercise behaviors are probably significant for many people. Friends, neighbors, and colleagues can all influence how people spend their discretionary time. "Significant others" probably influence people's behaviors in ways in which they are not even aware. Moreover, as participants in ongoing social systems people tend to conform to behavioral norms. Indeed, the theory of reasoned action (Ajzen & Fishbein, 1980) includes normative beliefs as one of the components to predict behavior. Although there are stages in life when peers play a more important role (for example, in adolescence), most people are always conscious to some degree about what others may think. One of the more consistent findings related to peer support is the strong preference of most people for group exercise programs as opposed to working out alone. This underscores the degree to which we depend on others for support and encouragement to continue.

Wankel's (1985) study of adult university employees yielded some interesting insights into the role peers play in exercise adherence. Continuing program participants cited significantly higher amounts of encouragement from nonwork friends and from their work supervisor. In fact, the encouragement of the work supervisor was the second most important factor distinguishing between continuing participants and dropouts among the 23 variables studied. The encouragement received from work friends was slightly, but not significantly, higher for continuing participants than for dropouts, although scores for both groups were relatively high.

Social support, whether it is family, peer, or work-related, is clearly an important factor in exercise persistence. Developing innovative means to increase all forms of social support should be a priority of exercise professionals.

Work Demands

As we discussed in chapter 1, the most prevalent reason for failing to exercise or dropping out of exercise programs is lack of time. Obviously, work places significant demands on people's time. Table 2.4 shows that 56% of absences in one program were work related. Work is important to most people not only as the source of livelihood, but as an important element of identity. The exercise professional should make every effort to accommodate clients by tailoring programs to their specific work needs. Extensive travel, physically demanding work, frequent meetings, long hours, and demanding supervisors are all work characteristics that can interfere with participation in an exercise program. Exercise professionals can use insights gained into people's work situations in the entry interview to develop exercise prescriptions with individualized strategies for accommodating work schedules.

Andrew and colleagues (1981) found that recovering myocardial infarction patients were more likely to drop out if they thought exercise sessions

Table 2.4   Reasons for Absences From the Training Sessions

Reason	%
Work	31
Work trip	25
Illness	22
Vacation	12
Injury or soreness due to exercise	5
Tiredness or undefined unwillingness	1
Other	4
Total	100

From "Feasibility of an 18 Month's Physical Training Program for Middle-Aged Men and Its Effects on Physical Fitness" by P. Oja et al., 1974, *American Journal of Public Health*, **64**, p. 461. Reprinted by permission.

interfered with their work. Interestingly, they were also somewhat more likely to drop out if they felt that work was interfering with the exercise program. Conflict with work schedule was a major reason given for dropping out of another large cardiac rehabilitation program (Bruce et al., 1976). In apparent contradiction, this study also found that 67% of those remaining in the exercise program were working while only 38% of dropouts were employed. Time interference with work and family life is also a major barrier to participation in programs involving healthy adults (Gettman et al., 1983).

In corporate fitness programs, uncooperative managers can effectively dampen the enthusiasm for program participation (Adams & Landgreen, 1988). It is not surprising that the enthusiastic endorsement of a supervisor can have a very positive influence on program compliance (Reid & Morgan, 1979). It is, however, the scheduling problem that clients perceive as the single largest barrier to program participation (Desharnais, Bouillon, & Godin, 1987).

PROGRAM FACTORS AFFECTING ADHERENCE

Individual and social factors affect the clients' initial and early participation in exercise programs, however, program characteristics assume greater significance in compliance the longer a person stays in the program. Several aspects related to how a program is organized and conducted have been shown to affect adherence. In this section, we shall discuss program components that are most important to continuing participation. The setting characteristics that will be discussed first assume a facility-based, supervised group program. Unsupervised, nonfacility-based programs will be addressed later.

Convenience

There are two interrelated aspects of convenience that are crucial to program adherence: time convenience and location convenience. Structured exercise programs for normal, busy people must be offered at times when people are available, and at an easily accessible location. A study of business executives found that of the 11 variables included, the distance from one's residence to the exercise facility was the single most important factor in determining willingness to participate in a preventive exercise program (Teraslinna et al., 1969). Convenience has been cited as a crucial factor in corporate (Cox, 1984) as well as community programs (Goodrick, Hartung, Warren, & Hoepfel, 1984). In a study of healthy volunteers, Wankel (1985) found that dropouts and participants differed in their perceptions of time and location convenience. Differences were more pronounced for time inconvenience than for inconvenience of location. Times when classes are offered is not the only aspect of time convenience that should be considered. Length of class period and perceptions of a tight schedule are also important aspects. A person who races against the clock to squeeze in an exercise class and then dashes off to make a business appointment will probably conclude that it is not worth the hassle. Indeed, one study noted that the inconvenience of trying to fit in an exercise class during the lunch hour affected the decisions of several corporate employees to drop out (Song et al., 1983).

Dropping out of an exercise rehabilitation program is also related to convenience of location (Andrew & Parker, 1979; Prosser et al., 1985). Apparently, the difficulty of arriving on time can distinguish between program compliers and dropouts. One study (Andrew et al., 1981) showed that those who had difficulty being punctual were more than twice as likely to drop out than those who had no trouble arriving on time. Dropouts were also more likely to cite inconvenience of location and parking difficulties as major obstacles than were program adherers.

The Exercise Facility

In addition to scheduling and location, physical characteristics of the facility affect the attendance of many people. Factors such as ambiance, floor space, ventilation and lighting, and the types and amount of exercise equipment are important considerations. Many features, such as a swimming pool, racquetball courts, tennis courts, clean locker facilities, and an appropriately floored aerobics area with good acoustics, as well as amenities, such as a snack bar, lounge, child-care facilities, whirlpools, and saunas, all combine to create an impression that affects how a person feels about going there. Of course, the ideal facility just described is not possible in many corporate, community, or agency situations. A successful program can be staged with much less. Indeed the facility is probably less important than other program components, such as program leadership. Still, to maximize participation and long-term involvement, the program administrator should strive to create a pleasant environment with as many amenities and facility features as situationally feasible. Somewhat in disagreement with this point of view, Shephard (1988a) states that "once a certain minimum investment has been made in space and equipment, any further increase in the size or luxury of the facility has little influence upon program adherence" (p. 309). Since both of these positions are based upon opinion rather than specific data it would appear that the role of facilities could benefit from scientific inquiry.

Research concerning the importance of facilities in exercise attrition is practically nonexistent. In one of the few existing studies, ex-participants of an employee fitness program cited physical features of the facility as contributing to their decision to drop out (Song et al., 1983). Reasons such as lack of air, crowded changing areas, and the unavailability of bicycle ergometers were noted.

Program Social Support

Earlier we discussed the importance of family and peer support in continuing exercise behaviors. We shall now address the importance of the social support received from fellow participants and the class leader. Although social reasons are typically not high on the list of priorities for those beginning exercise programs, it has been consistently demonstrated that the group tends to assume considerably more importance as social relationships are formed and group camaraderie is established. Wankel (1985) found "friendship within the program" to be one of the better predictors of program adherence. This phenomenon has been consistently observed in groups of healthy adults (Bain, 1985; Heinzelmann & Bagley, 1970; Martin et al.,

1984; Massie & Shephard, 1971) as well as in cardiac rehabilitation patients (Prosser et al., 1985).

Some beginning exercisers are in need of strong social support from the outset. A major research report (Fitness Ontario, 1981) observed that people tend to join an organized group with someone else, perhaps a friend or acquaintance, and are more likely to begin an exercise program if someone else in their family or circle of friends is already active. This observation was corroborated by Danielson and Wanzel (1977) who found that women in particular were more likely to attend with a companion than were men. A study that reported an unusually high adherence rate (94%) cited group composition and group dynamics as having a particularly important influence (Gillett, 1988). Moreover, carpooling emerged as a factor that facilitated program attendance. There is also, however, the occasional exception of the individual who never really participates in the dynamics of the group and remains independent and aloof.

Program content can be an important factor in group social support. Activities like aerobic dance that are characterized by a narrow external focus and a large percentage of "time on task" do not permit much time for social interaction. However, the typical exercise class that consists of a warm-up period, 30 to 40 minutes of aerobic activity, a cool-down period possibly with some group discussion, and several minutes in the shower and locker room affords many opportunities for social contact. This social process becomes important to many participants and is a major factor in exercise continuance.

Carron, Widmeyer, and Brawley (1988) addressed the need for developing the exercise group into a cohesive social unit. Other studies (Wankel, 1984; Wankel et al., 1985) employed a structured social support program that consisted of the following elements: leader, class, exercise partner, and home support. With the exception of home support, participants found the support program very effective. Program instructors also found the social support program to help promote a positive class atmosphere and enhance attendance.

Group Versus Individual Programs

Whether there are any differences in adherence between supervised group programs and unsupervised individual programs is an important question. Most exercise practitioners are probably biased toward group programs. We have already seen the importance of group dynamics to continuing participation. As one study found (Heinzelmann & Bagley, 1970), almost 90% of those surveyed preferred to exercise with a group or with another person rather than exercising alone. The reported advantages of the group program were more enjoyment, social support, an increased sense of personal commitment to continue, and a welcomed opportunity to compare one's progress and level of fitness with that of others. Group programs are also more cost effective in terms of instruction, monitoring, and evaluation. Individual programs, however, provide maximum flexibility with respect to time and convenience.

One of the few studies to address this issue directly compared a YMCA group program to an individual program based upon Kenneth Cooper's (1970) aerobics point system, which assigns a point value to aerobic exercise based upon duration and intensity (Massie & Shephard, 1971). The dropout rate for the individual program was 52.6% compared to only 18.2% in the YMCA group. Subjects in the individual program reported more discomfort and injury. Other impediments cited in the individual program were loneliness, boredom, ridicule, and the dangers of winter darkness and ice. Studies of recovering cardiac patients have recommended group programs (Prosser et al., 1985; Tirrell & Hart, 1980). Mutual support, individual satisfaction, avoidance of boredom, greater opportunities for educating patients about the exercise prescription, and overcoming barriers were the advantages of group programs.

Although some individual programs report high rates of attrition (Jarvie & Thompson, 1985), some researchers have observed considerably different results. An investigation that compared supervised group programs of circuit training and jogging with unsupervised individual programs, revealed no appreciable differences in attendance between the two group programs and the individual program (Durbeck, Heinzelmann, Schacter, & Haskell, 1972). Subjects in all three groups attended about half the number of exercise sessions recommended. They cited work-related problems as the primary reason for absences. Another study of 47 police officers revealed a dropout rate of 35% for those in an unsupervised program while officers participating in a group program dropped out at a rate of 45% (Gettman et al., 1983). Both groups had received 4 weeks of supervised training during which the basic program principles were explained. Subsequently, the supervised program was held at a central exercise facility while the unsupervised group trained independently at a location of their choice, typically neighborhood streets or school tracks. The unsupervised group would return to the central facility every 2 weeks for a supervised session and progress check.

Because time and commitment conflicts prohibit many people from participating in group programs and because some people prefer to exercise alone, there is a definite need to accommodate both individual and group approaches in exercise and fitness programs. Suggestions for a successful unsupervised program include: (a) teach clients how to start a program, (b) provide supervision early in the program, (c) have clients report progress periodically, and (d) encourage a home-based program for clients' convenience (Gettman et al., 1983).

Table 2.5   Best Liked Program Features

Features	Percent of participants
Organization and leadership	32
Exercising in general	31
Recreation—games	29
Social aspects—camaraderie	26
Health and fitness benefits	14
Regularity of exercise	12
Medical evaluations	9
Feeling of accomplishment	6

From "Response to Physical Activity and Their Effects on Health Behavior" by F. Heinzelmann and R.W. Bagley, 1970, *Public Health Reports*, **85**(10), p. 906. Reprinted by permission.

Program Leadership

Effective leadership is a key variable in exercise adherence. Indeed, some consider it to be the single most important ingredient. A good leader can compensate to some extent for other program deficiencies, such as lack of space or equipment, with creative programming. By the same token, weak leadership may result in program atrophy or even demise regardless of how elaborate the facility. Moreover, no other factor has quite the potential for eliciting change in a client as a competent and enthusiastic exercise leader. As Presbie and Brown (1977, p. 67) have said, a leader is a "walking, talking, independent variable." In other words, a knowledgeable leader can have a deliberate effect on the behaviors (the dependent variable) of a client. The exercise leader must serve as an educator, counselor, cheerleader, and sometimes stern-visaged taskmaster to facilitate the changes the clients want to make. In later

chapters we will present some of the skills and strategies needed for effective exercise leadership. For now, however, we shall concern ourselves with the rather sparse data on the effect of leadership on adherence. Although several researchers have addressed the importance of leadership on adherence, it has generally received little attention (Cox, 1984; Franklin, 1988; Oldridge, 1977, 1984a).

In one of the first studies to address the importance of program leadership, Heinzelmann and Bagley (1970) found that program organization and leadership was the most important factor identified by participants (see Table 2.5). Reid and Morgan (1979) demonstrated that a 1-hour educational program presented by an exercise professional is more conducive to adherence than written information. Some research has focused on the impact of specific leadership techniques on program adherence. Martin and colleagues (1984) found that individual feedback and praise during exercise, flexible goal-setting, and training in distraction-based cognitive strategies enhanced adherence. A recent study cited other beneficial leader characteristics, including concern for participant safety and psychological comfort, expertise in answering questions about exercise, and personal qualities with which participants could identify (Gillett, 1988).

Wankel and colleagues have demonstrated the efficacy of several leadership interventions. Specifically, they demonstrated a decision-balance technique (Wankel & Thompson, 1977), perceived activity choice (Thompson & Wankel, 1980), and structured social support (Wankel, 1984; Wankel et al., 1985). Briefly, the decision-balance technique involves having the client complete a grid that assesses their perceptions of gains and losses associated with exercise participation. A participant observation study (Bain, 1985) recommended that exercise leaders place greater emphasis on the subjective-affective dimension as opposed to the traditional technical-rational approach.

Perhaps empathetic leadership is even more crucial for those working with the chronically ill. In an extensive study of post-coronary patients, those who perceived a lack of individual attention were almost twice as likely to drop out than patients who perceived a high level of attention from exercise leaders (Andrew et al., 1981). There is little question but that more research should be done on exercise leadership, particularly on intervention techniques that apply to healthy people as well as to those suffering some impairment.

Program Intensity

One salient aspect of exercise, especially for the inexperienced, is discomfort and pain. Often, people who are just beginning an exercise program try to do too much and end up with sore muscles, injuries to soft tissues, or orthopedic problems. This type of pain or injury is often the only excuse they need to abandon the program. Overdoing it is not only painful, it is also unnecessary. It is well established that only a minimal level of intensity, usually expressed as a percentage of maximal heart rate, is required to produce a training effect. However, would a lower level of intensity also enhance program adherence? Dishman (1982) observed that there was little evidence to indicate the appropriate exercise "dosage" for optimal adherence. However, he did suggest that the ideal physiological prescription might not be optimal with respect to adherence. For most people, exercise that is perceived as too intense will likely result in discomfort and cessation of exercise.

Martin and Dubbert (1982) considered overall exercise intensity to be an important predictor of adherence. Higher intensity exercise tends to be associated with lower adherence. Epstein and colleagues (1984) corroborated this observation in their studies of obese children. A low-intensity exercise program resulted in significantly better adherence than a high-intensity program. Similarly, in a community sample, adult dropout rates from vigorous activity were 50%, but only 25% to 35% for moderate activities (Sallis et al., 1986).

Based on his experience at the Aerobics Institute, Pollock (1978) stated that adults do not seem to enjoy or even tolerate high-intensity programs. He reported that the dropout rate for a high-intensity interval training program was twice that for a lower intensity continuous jogging program. It was observed that by lowering the intensity level and extending the duration of the workout, a person could achieve approximately the same results as they could from a high-intensity workout (Pollock, 1978). This approach has important implications for compliance.

In contrast to the findings, the Ontario Exercise Heart Collaborative Study observed no appreciable differences in adherence between a high-intensity exercise group, which exercised at an intensity of between 65% to 85% of estimated $\dot{V}O_2max$, and a low-intensity exercise group, which performed activities designed to keep heart rate below 50% of estimated $\dot{V}O_2max$ (Oldridge, 1984b). It was suggested that individuals will adhere to either a high- or low-intensity program providing there is sufficient motivation, variety, and enjoyment, and especially if it is in a group setting.

Enjoyment

As we discussed in chapter 1, although most people begin exercise programs for health-related reasons, factors such as fun and social experience tend to assume greater importance over time. If an exercise program is perceived as unpleasant, adherence becomes a problem (Franklin, 1986). A program that emphasizes pleasurable activity and repeated success is more likely to foster continued participation. Consistent with this point of view, Franklin has developed a "Games-As-Aerobics" approach in which flexibility and endurance activities are disguised as games, relays, stunts, and recreational activities. This approach minimizes the importance of skill and competition, and focuses on participant success and enjoyment.

Massie and Shephard (1971) observed that perhaps too much emphasis had been placed on the health benefits of exercise and recommended that more attention be given to the fun element to sustain interest. Similar conclusions have been reached by other researchers (Cox, 1984; Godin et al., 1987; Heinzelmann & Bagley, 1970; Oldridge, 1984a). After interviewing program participants and dropouts, Wankel (1985) found that factors other than the desire to be healthy were central to program continuance. Objectives such as competition, curiosity, development of recreational skills, and going out with friends—all of which are related to program enjoyment—were more important to continuing participants than to dropouts. In reviewing the literature, we found no studies that contradicted the importance of enjoyment in program adherence.

Perceived Choice

A potentially important program feature that has received limited study is the role of activity choice in program continuance. It is surprising that so few researchers have addressed this important program characteristic. Perceived choice has to do with the degree of personal control people believe they have over program content. In an important study, Thompson and Wankel (1980) found that perceived choice of activities influenced attendance at a private health club. As seen in Figure 2.5, subjects who believed that their programs were based on their own activity selections attended significantly more than those who believed that

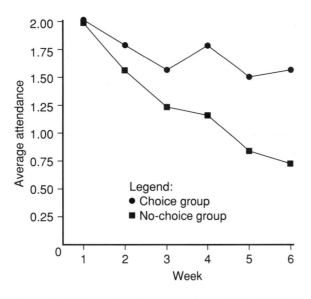

Figure 2.5 Week-by-week attendance for the choice and no-choice groups.

From "The Effects of Perceived Activity Choice Upon Frequency of Exercise Behavior" by C.E. Thompson and L.M. Wankel, 1980, *Journal of Applied Social Psychology*, **10**(5), p. 440. Reprinted by permission.

they were given a standardized program. Of considerable importance was the finding that at the end of the study the "choice" group scored significantly higher in their stated intentions for future exercise. The implications of this study are clear. The exercise practitioner must ensure that clients have a sense of choice and control over their own programs.

Relapse Prevention

In the ongoing search for ways to enhance adherence, few techniques have emerged with the potential associated with the concept of *relapse prevention*. Relapse prevention was originally developed as a behavioral maintenance program for use in addiction programs. It is a self-management program designed to maintain newly acquired behaviors (Marlatt & Gordon, 1980). The relapse prevention approach involves teaching people who are trying to change their behaviors how to anticipate and cope with relapse. The relapse prevention model contains both cognitive and behavioral components, which include behavioral skills training, cognitive interventions, and lifestyle change procedures (Marlatt & Gordon, 1985). Typically, relapse prevention programs include the identification of high-risk situations, the development of appropriate coping strategies, and anticipation of and

planning for a possible relapse. Particular attention is given to the *abstinence violation effect*, which is the tendency to let a single slip precipitate a total abandonment of the program.

However, because relapse prevention is a relatively recent development, few studies have been done on the effectiveness of relapse prevention in exercise maintenance. In one of the first studies of the effects of relapse prevention on exercise adherence, the relapse prevention intervention did not affect adherence. But this may have been due to procedural problems with the control group (Martin et al., 1984). Another study of college women in a 5-week jogging program produced mixed but encouraging results (King & Frederiksen, 1984). Two additional studies have demonstrated the potential effectiveness of relapse prevention by showing differences in class attendance that were attributed to training in relapse prevention techniques (Belisle, Roskies, & Levesque, 1987). Both studies demonstrated small but significant differences in groups who had received the relapse prevention intervention within the context of the regular program. The authors observed that although relapse prevention is not a panacea for poor exercise adherence, it is very cost effective and, when used in combination with other factors, such as social support and group cohesiveness, it has good potential for maximizing exercise adherence at minimum cost.

Though modest, the early success of relapse prevention should encourage researchers and practitioners to develop materials and techniques for the application of relapse prevention to exercise programs. As relapse prevention methodology is refined these procedures should have even greater success in promoting continuing exercise behaviors.

Cognitive Dissociation

Does what a person thinks about during exercise affect adherence? Several studies have focused on this question and have used the concepts of association and dissociation—concepts that have been used in exercise contexts for some time. Morgan (1978) described *dissociation* as a "kind of self-hypnosis" that intentionally reduces the sensory feedback received from the body during exercise. In other words, a person thinks about anything except what is occurring within the body. *Association*, on the other hand, is a process of constant monitoring of body signals relating to respiration, temperature, and other body sensations. For elite distance runners, association is apparently the strategy of choice. Although dissociation can reduce one's feelings of discomfort, Morgan cautioned that injures are more likely to occur in the dissociative state because of the lack of attentiveness to body signals of distress or to potentially dangerous external stimuli.

Martin and colleagues (1984) found that an exercise group instructed in dissociation techniques had a significantly higher rate of class attendance (76.6%) than a group instructed in cognitive association strategies (58.7%). An even greater differential was noted in the groups at a 3-month follow-up: The attendance rates were 87.5% and 37.5%, respectively. Pennebaker and Lightner (1980) conducted two experiments, both of which provided support for the position that focusing attention away from the body can reduce perceptions of fatigue. In the first study, subjects walked on a treadmill while listening to either the sounds of their own breathing or street sounds. Results indicated that paying attention to distracting sounds produced lower perceptions of fatigue and its accompanying symptoms. The second study, which compared jogging on a 200 m lap course to jogging over a cross-country course, found that times were significantly lower when students ran on the cross-country course. Although there were no perceived differences in fatigue, running the cross-country course produced significantly lower scores for boredom and frustration than running on the lap course. It was concluded that environments that decrease the amount of internally focused attention are more conducive to continuing exercise behaviors.

SUGGESTIONS FOR PROMOTING EXERCISE ADHERENCE

The literature on exercise adherence has produced a number of practical ideas for promoting continuing exercise behaviors. We shall now summarize the most relevant.

■ Programs should be scheduled as conveniently as possible for the clientele. Classes before and after work, and during the noon hour best accommodate working people, while homemakers with school-age children will probably prefer classes during school hours. Managers can help program participation by permitting flexible work hours for those who cannot otherwise be accommodated.

■ The location of the facility is a factor over which the practitioner has little control. However, the closer the facility is to work or home the better. Unsupervised program packages might compensate somewhat for those who are inconvenienced by facility location. By offering evaluation, instruction, and consulting to those who elect an unsupervised program, contact can still be maintained to monitor the individual's programs and to offer support and encouragement.

■ Facility design is another area over which the exercise practitioner has limited control. However, the practitioner should try to advocate the most comprehensive facility feasible. More space and more facility features permit a greater range of program options, thereby meeting diverse needs and interests. Services such as child care make it possible for more people to participate.

■ The ambiance of the facility is also important. Cleanliness, tasteful decor, well-kept buildings and exercise equipment, and a quality sound system all affect the clients' perceptions of the program and help determine whether they will continue to attend.

■ Because social support is important to exercise persistence, practitioners should make a concerted effort to promote support among family, staff, and other program members. Structured social support programs such as the one developed by Wankel (1984) show promise. Other approaches might include inviting family members to an orientation session in which they would be taught support techniques, or even offering classes for family members. In addition, all exercise leaders should be well trained and highly competent in social support skills. Exercise leaders should also pay attention to the group dynamics and try to develop group cohesion and morale. Staff development workshops could provide exercise leaders with the necessary training. In-class discussion of the importance of social support and how to provide it to others could also enhance the supportive behaviors of group members.

■ The program should contain enough variety to meet the diverse motives, skills, and interests of the clientele. The client should be able to choose activities in consultation with the exercise professional to fulfill the exercise prescription. Periodic evaluations should be scheduled to advise clients of progress in meeting their objectives and to help motivate continued participation.

■ Exercise programs should include an accurate system for recording aspects of client participation, such as attendance, aerobics points, physiological data, and related information. This type of data would provide valuable information about client involvement and progress, and would help identify program dropouts early. When participants record their behavior, it helps monitor progress toward exercise goals and provides a continuing source of client motivation.

■ Emphasis in program activities should be placed on enjoying the exercise experience. The class should be a fun experience. A long-term program goal should be to help clients develop a repertoire of activities from which they can derive continuing intrinsic satisfaction.

■ The level of intensity should be high enough to produce some physiological benefits, but not so high that clients will experience physical discomfort and stop exercising. Avoidance of injury should be a major concern, especially in the early stages of the program.

■ Although most clients prefer group programs, some provision should be made for individual programs. As many services as possible should be available to the individual participant. It may be necessary to provide single sex as well as mixed group classes if excessive sensitivity to the opposite sex is affecting program attendance.

■ If the program has an end point or "graduation," there should be a follow-up on clients to determine the effectiveness of the program in long-term compliance.

■ Educational programs should be part of the program. The instruction should include sound information concerning all aspects of exercise, including the "why" and "how" of exercise, injury prevention, physiological and psychological benefits, relapse prevention, cognitive dissociation, overcoming barriers to participation, time management, and other information. Educational presentations should have the objective of positively affecting attitudes and beliefs toward exercise.

■ Whenever possible, an exercise program should be coordinated with other components of a comprehensive wellness or lifestyle management program. As Epstein et al., (1984) have observed, adherence in one program area tends to generalize to other areas.

■ Lastly, exercise professionals must realize that they are important influences on client adherence. The practitioner's leadership skills, interpersonal skills, knowledge of current practice, and skillful implementation of adherence strategies may make the difference in individual success and failure and in the ultimate success or failure of the program.

SUMMARY

Exercise adherence is the single most crucial problem facing the exercise professional. We have reviewed the extent of the dropout problem and the barriers to continuance in exercise programs. A history of exercise, recent exercise involvement, and use of leisure time for physical activity are predictive of exercise adherence, while smoking is predictive of nonadherence. Demographic factors such as age, sex, and marital status are not good predictors, and only mixed success has been realized with socioeconomic factors. Although attempts to predict adherence using physical and psychological factors have been generally disappointing, program factors such as convenience, social support, and program leadership can have positive effects on program continuance. Other program factors that may promote adherence include control of exercise intensity, relapse prevention, perceived choice, cognitive dissociation, and enjoyment.

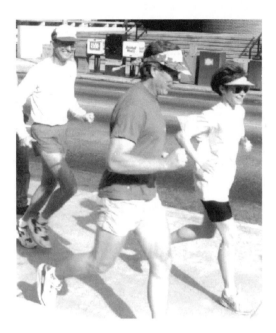

Chapter 3
Psychological Effects of Exercise

In chapter 1 we briefly discussed the notion that many people exercise regularly because it makes them "feel good." We shall now consider this phenomenon in more depth, as well as explore the broader question of the use of exercise to prevent and treat a variety of mental and emotional conditions. While it is widely believed that exercise relieves tension, improves mental functioning, and provides a sense of optimism and well-being, convincing empirical evidence to support these beliefs is not overly abundant. Nevertheless, we shall present the current knowledge regarding the effects of exercise on an array of psychological processes.

The impetus for recent interest in exercise as therapy probably comes from several sources. Dishman (1986) cited the following trends as explanations for this interest:

■ The popularity of self-help and the move toward prevention rather than treatment

■ The growing awareness of the importance of lifestyle in human longevity and quality of life

■ The growth of new fields, such as health psychology and behavioral medicine, that use exercise as a treatment and provide research results

■ The realization that traditional therapies have limitations, which has led to a search for adjunctive treatments such as exercise for some disorders

■ The staggering cost of treating mental illness in North America, which makes a low-cost, low-risk alternative treatment such as exercise attractive

Although this chapter will not provide the exercise professional with much "how to" information, it will give a current review of the scientific evidence available on the psychological effects of exercise. Unfortunately, there is an overabundance of erroneous beliefs, speculation, and misinformation related to exercise and fitness. The popular media often pick up on these mistaken notions and circulate them to the point that the public accepts them as fact. Table 3.1 summarizes some of the psychological benefits purportedly realized through exercise involvement. Which of these claims have substance and which are wishful thinking are the subject of this chapter. One role of the exercise professional is to disseminate correct information and to dispel inaccuracies. It is our intention to provide information that will enable the exercise professional to speak confidently about exercise and mental health matters.

Table 3.1 Some Proposed Psychological Benefits of Exercise in Clinical and Nonclinical Populations

Increases	Decreases
Academic performance	Absenteeism at work
Assertiveness	Alcohol abuse
Confidence	Anger
Emotional stability	Anxiety
Independence	Confusion
Intellectual functioning	Depression
Internal locus of control	Dysmenorrhea
Memory	Headaches
Mood	Hostility
Perception	Phobias
Popularity	Psychotic behavior
Positive body image	Stress response
Self-control	Tension
Sexual satisfaction	Type A behavior
Well-being	Work errors
Work efficiency	

From "The Relation of Physical Activity and Exercise to Mental Health" by C.B. Taylor, J.F. Sallis, and R. Needle, 1985, *Public Health Reports*, **100**, pp. 195-202. Reprinted by permission.

MENTAL HEALTH

Mental disorders are a major health problem. In the United States, such disorders affect an estimated 10% to 15% of the population each year. Mental health problems are a leading cause of hospitalization, accounting for approximately 30% of the total days of hospitalization of everyone hospitalized in the United States. They also account

for about 8% of total medical costs and rank third as the reason for recognition as disabled by the Social Security Administration in the United States (Taylor, Sallis, & Needle, 1985).

One in four adults at some point in life will suffer from moderate depression, anxiety, or symptoms of affective disorder. This estimate may be somewhat conservative given a survey conducted by the National Institute of Mental Health in the mid-1980s that found anxiety disorders to be the most frequently experienced mental health problem, affecting approximately 8.3% of the adult population. Alcohol and substance abuse ranked second (6.4% of adults), and depression was third, affecting approximately 6% of the adults in the study (Dishman, 1986).

Definitions and interpretations of *mental health* vary considerably. We will try to give a brief "middle of the road" definition. Mental health pioneer Karl Menninger believed that mental health involved an adjustment to the world and to other people that allows maximum effectiveness and happiness, and the ability to maintain an even temper, an alert intelligence, socially considerate behavior, and a pleasant disposition (Thackeray, Skidmore, & Farley, 1979). Layman (1960) viewed mental health as the ability to habitually meet life problems in such a way as to derive a feeling of personal satisfaction and to contribute optimally to the satisfaction and welfare of the social group. Dannenmaier (1978) presented a somewhat different perspective. He perceived mental health as a state of mind that permits the optimal exercise of one's talents and the steady movement toward the optimal satisfaction of one's needs. A simple, straightforward definition that we like interprets mental health as a "positive state of personal mental well-being in which individuals feel basically satisfied with themselves, their roles in life, and their relationships with others" (Thackeray et al., 1979, p. 8).

Following is one of the more famous characterizations of the mentally healthy person (Maslow, 1968):

- Superior perception of reality
- Acceptance of self
- Spontaneity
- Problem-centered
- Detached, desires privacy
- Autonomous, resists enculturation
- Freshness of appreciation and richness of emotional reaction

- High frequency of peak experiences
- Identification with the human species
- Good interpersonal relations
- Democratic character structure
- Creative

Mental health is not an "all or none" proposition but rather a matter of relative magnitude. Degrees of mental health and mental illness vary from person to person, and also vary from time to time in the same person. Everyone daydreams, becomes depressed, and has anxieties, and the nature and depth of these experiences varies and shifts (Thackeray et al., 1979). We shall now address whether exercise can make a difference in any of the dimensions we have identified.

Exercise and Mental Health

There are many claims about the mental health benefits of vigorous physical activity, such as improved confidence, well-being, sexual satisfaction, reduced anxiety, and positive effects on depressed moods and intellectual functioning. If substantiated, these effects would assume an important role in the primary prevention of mental illness by making people less susceptible to the factors that can cause mental disorders. Physical activity may also help improve the functioning of people with mental illness (Taylor, Bandura, Ewart, Miller, & DeBusk, 1985).

A recent survey of 1,750 physicians found that 85% prescribed exercise for depression, 60% for anxiety, and 43% for chemical dependence (Dishman, 1986). In this study, walking was the most frequently prescribed form of exercise, followed by swimming, bicycling, strength training, and running. Despite this encouraging information, many physicians prefer to use drugs to treat mental disorders, even though the side effects often pose additional problems for the patient (Dishman, 1986). For some people, exercise may reduce or preclude the need for medication while posing less risk, although the interactive effects of exercise and medication are largely unknown (Dishman 1986). Nevertheless, it is believed that physically healthy people who require psychotropic medication can exercise safely under close medical supervision (Morgan & Goldston, 1987).

Rationale for a Relationship Between Exercise and Mental Health

If exercise is to be considered seriously as a means of promoting mental health and as a treatment for mental disorders, there must be sound scientific data to back it up. Unfortunately, a cause-and-effect relationship has yet to be demonstrated. For the most part, the research has been seriously deficient in design and lacking in focus. As Folkins and Sime (1981) have pointed out, these disparate research efforts need to be organized into an integrated theoretical model. Short of this, some recurring speculations as to the processes involved have tended to emphasize either physiological or psychological perspectives (Folkins & Sime, 1981).

From a physiological standpoint, one of the better arguments for exercise as a factor affecting mental health is based on *organismic unity*. This idea maintains that people are not one-dimensional, but are physical, intellectual, and emotional beings consisting of interrelated parts. Because of this interrelatedness, the individual cannot be divided without destroying the organism. In other words, one cannot enjoy mental health if any of the other component parts of the organism are neglected (Dannenmaier, 1978).

The relationship between mind and body has interested students of human nature since the early speculations of Hippocrates, Plato, and Aristotle in the 3rd and 4th centuries, B.C. More recently, we have seen a dramatic growth in psychosomatic medicine, as well as in *holistic* health, which assumes an organismic perspective. Holistic theory maintains that no physical or mental illness may be adequately diagnosed, understood, or treated unless it is viewed as both physical and psychological (Layman, 1960).

An explanation of the mental health benefits of exercise from the psychological perspective was summarized by Folkins and Sime (1981):

- Improvement in fitness results in perceptions of control and mastery, which lead to feelings of well-being.
- Aerobic exercise provides training in biofeedback.
- Exercise is a form of meditation that can trigger an altered state of consciousness.
- Exercise provides a distraction or diversion from anxiety-producing stimuli.

We shall consider these and other possible explanations in more depth as we systematically review aspects of mental health and its relation to exercise and physical fitness. Before leaving this topic however, we should note that there is some consensus among medical and exercise scientists that physical fitness is associated with psychological well-being (Morgan & Goldston, 1987).

EMOTION

To the layman, emotion is associated with subjective feelings—feelings that are pleasant or unpleasant, mild or intense, transient or long-lasting, and that enhance or interfere with purposive behavior (Strongman, 1987). Most people identify fear, anger, shame, humiliation, joy, and sorrow as emotions. Because emotion gives the world and our place in it much of its meaning, it is intimately involved with the qualitative aspects of one's life (Strongman, 1987). According to De Rivera (1984), there are over 200 indistinguishable emotional states identified in the English language. It is not surprising that scholars have had a great deal of difficulty coming to grips with the essence of emotion due to the complexity of the topic and the various approaches from which emotion can be studied (Young, 1973). The study of emotion is also complicated by the fact that emotions are related to most other psychological processes, such as perception, memory, learning, reasoning, and action (Young, 1973).

A comprehensive review of definitions of *emotion* reveals not only a staggering number of attempts to capture the elements and essence of emotion, but also a number of prominent researchers who have either denied the existence of this phenomenon or minimized the utility of the construct (Kleinginna & Kleinginna, 1981a). Despite the lack of unanimity concerning the nature of emotion, most psychologists agree on the importance of feelings and emotions in the areas of behavior, conscious experience, individual development, and social life. Moreover, affective disturbances have been found to be important to mental health, individual adjustment, and personal happiness (Young, 1973).

Recent clinical opinion maintains that exercise has beneficial emotional effects for men and women of all ages (Morgan & Goldston, 1987). As we have seen, an exercise program that capitalizes on positive emotions such as fun, joy, self-satisfaction, confidence, pride, enthusiasm, and excitement has a decided advantage over one that focuses solely on health benefits or physiological outcomes. The high dropout rate in traditional fitness programs may be reduced by offering activities that evoke positive emotional experiences. Improvements in fitness would be an accompanying outcome of regular enjoyable activity. We have observed that people who are passionate about physical activity tend to be fit as a result of their self-generated involvement.

Exercise and Perceptions of Well-Being and Happiness

Psychological well-being, sometimes called *subjective well-being*, generally refers to satisfaction with life or degree of personal happiness. Some researchers have studied this important dimension of mental health among physically active people. It is typically assumed that physically active people see themselves more positively than those who are inactive. In a study of healthy adults, Snyder and Spreitzer (1974) found a relationship between psychological well-being, defined as perceived satisfaction with life and avowed happiness, and involvement in sports. There were also some unexpected findings, particularly with respect to sex differences. Surprisingly, the relationship between sports participation and psychological well-being was stronger among women than men. This difference may have been due to fewer culturally approved athletic opportunities for women and the tendency for women who are involved in sport to have a higher level of self-commitment than males. The researchers speculated that the positive relationship between involvement in sports and psychological well-being may be the result of the intrinsic pleasure and fun associated with games, sports, and related activities.

Whether people who exercise regularly are happier than those who do not was the subject of another study (Carter, 1977). Using a nonrandomized sample of adults, a questionnaire regarding exercise habits, and an additional question pertaining to a global measure of happiness, a low positive correlation of .27 was found between happiness and exercise involvement. The researchers offered several possible explanations for this apparent relationship between happiness and exercise, including changes in the nervous system brought on by exercise, increased self-efficacy, and more opportunities for social contact through exercise.

A survey on happiness conducted by *Psychology Today* with over 52,000 respondents found that exercise and recreation rated far below friends, home, job, and love in importance to happiness (Shaver & Freedman, 1976). Exercise and recreation, and body attractiveness were the lowest rated factors in happiness by married couples, but they were rated considerably higher by single men and women. Except for single women, health and physical condition rated surprisingly low. It is interesting to speculate on what might be different if this study were repeated with a contemporary sample. Based on the dramatic increase in interest in health, fitness, and exercise over the past 15 years, our guess is that the priority of factors related to happiness would be significantly different.

More recent research on exercise and psychological well-being has yielded some interesting results. A study that included evaluations of subjects by significant others, in addition to more traditional measures of physiological and psychological functioning, seemed to support a direct causal relationship between exercise and psychological well-being (Hayden, Allen, & Camaione, 1986). A second study that compared a group trained to increase cardiovascular efficiency with a control group trained to minimize cardiovascular conditioning revealed a marginally significant difference in subjective well-being favoring the increased cardiovascular efficiency group (Goldwater & Collins, 1985). In a community survey that used a large, representative sample to examine the effect of exercise on mental health, psychological well-being was found to be influenced by exercise, particularly in low- and middle-income groups (Hayes & Ross, 1986). In contrast to these results, Gauvin (1989) found no relationship between level of regular physical activity and subjective well-being.

If indeed exercise and physical fitness are important factors in perceptions of well-being, one would expect athletes to demonstrate a decided superiority when compared with nonathletes. Two studies have addressed this question with female athletes (Snyder & Kivlin, 1975; Rao & Overman, 1986). In the former study, the athletes were significantly more positive than nonathletes with regard to psychological well-being. This study also compared basketball players and gymnasts. The well-being scores for gymnasts were slightly higher, but the differences were not significant. The second study, which compared black female athletes with black female nonathletes, observed slight though unsignificant differences in well-being, which tended to favor the athletic group. This area would benefit greatly from additional research.

Although more and better studies are needed before the exercise practitioner can cite convincing evidence that exercise has a positive impact on one's perceptions of well-being, people who exercise tend to believe they perceive the world more positively. As far as identifying mechanisms to explain this relationship, we still do not know whether the effect is due to physiological, psychological, or social factors, or some combination of these.

MOOD

Mood is generally defined as a state of emotional or affective arousal of varying, but not permanent, duration. Moods are typically viewed as milder than emotions, which are considered more intense and of shorter duration. Moods are often thought of as *dispositions* to respond in certain emotional ways and to experience certain feelings (Wessman & Ricks, 1966). Feelings of elation or happiness that last several hours or even a few days would be an example of a mood, while anger or fear, which are more acute with a greater sense of urgency, are examples of emotions.

Exercise Induced Elation

The elevation of mood during and immediately after exercise may account for the extraordinary commitment and long-term involvement of many people. Indeed, there has been considerable discussion about two rather extreme forms of exercise-induced elation—the "runner's high" and "exercise addiction." (Because exercise addiction seems to be related to personality type, we will discuss that phenomenon in chapter 4.)

Although most people report that they feel better as a result of exercising, these reports are subjective and difficult to substantiate empirically. There is currently no methodology for measuring the "feel better" construct. As we shall see later in this chapter, however, there has been considerable research on other perceived changes in how one feels following exercise. Reductions in anxiety and tension, decreases in depression, and positive mood changes are no doubt associated with "feeling better." A thorough understanding of the phenomenon, however, awaits future research.

Runner's High

Despite the numerous articles and studies that have attempted to understand the runner's high phenomenon, it has proved to be an elusive construct. Accounts of runner's high reveal that something very positive happens occasionally to some people during runs. The feeling is not only psychologically uplifting, but frequently borders on being a mystical experience or even an altered state of consciousness. The recountings of runner's highs typically describe a very personal sense of wonder and amazement.

In many ways, the runner's high is similar to Maslow's (1968) concept of *peak experience*. Peak experiences occur in moments of most intense happiness and fulfillment and are described as having the following characteristics:

■ The experience tends to be seen as a whole unit detached from usefulness, expediency, and purpose, and characterized by a disorientation in time and space.

■ The experience is completely absorbing.

■ One's perceptions may be ego-transcending, self-forgetful, impersonal, and detached.

■ The experience is felt as a self-validating, self-justifying moment that carries its own intrinsic value.

■ The emotional reaction in the peak experience is one of wonder, awe, reverence, humility, and surrender, accompanied by loss of fear, anxiety, inhibition, and restraint. There are feelings of pure gratification, elation, and joy, as well as perceptions of being integrated, spontaneous, and expressive.

■ While in this state, one feels at the peak of his or her powers, fully functioning, and without restraint and waste of effort.

According to Sachs (1984), the literature has described the runner's high using 27 adjectives or phrases, which include euphoria, gracefulness, spirituality, moving without effort, and glimpsing perfection. Sachs (1984) tentatively defined the runner's high as "a euphoric sensation experienced during running, usually unexpected, in which the runner feels a heightened sense of well-being, enhanced appreciation of nature, and transcendence of barriers of time and space" (p. 274).

There have been several published descriptions of the runner's high experiences. Mandell's (1981) account is probably one of the better known recollections, but our favorite is that of Mike Spino (1971, p. 222) who was one of the first to describe the phenomenon. An excerpt of his description follows:

My first step I felt lighter and looser than ever before. My shirt clung to me, and I felt like a skeleton flying down a wind tunnel. My times at the mile and two miles were so fast that I almost felt like I was cheating, or had taken unfair advantage. It was like getting a new body that no one else had heard about. My mind was so crystal clear that I could have held a conversation. The only sensation was the rhythm and the beat; all perfectly natural, all and everything part of everything else. Marty told me later that he could feel the

power I was radiating. He said I was frightening. . . . In the last half mile something happened which may have occurred only one or two times before or since. Furiously I ran; time lost all semblance of meaning. Distance, time, motion were all one. There were myself, the cement, a vague feeling of legs, and the coming dusk. I tore on. . . . I could have run and run. Perhaps I had experienced a physiological change, but whatever, it was magic. I came to the side of the road and cried tears of joy and sorrow. Joy at being alive; sorrow for a vague feeling of temporalness, and a knowledge of the impossibility of giving this experience to anyone.

Not all runners have experienced this state. Sachs (1984) cited four studies that showed as few as 9% to as many as 78% of runners who reported experiencing a sense of euphoria during runs. Even those who had experienced the phenomenon achieved it on an average of only 29.4% of the time. Runners have differing opinions as to what enables this experience to happen. Some cite the absence of problems, lack of concern with pace, time, or other things requiring concentration, while others suggest that optimal environmental and climatic conditions are necessary for the feeling to occur (Sachs, 1984).

The mechanisms used to explain the phenomenon are also subject to speculation. Morgan (1985a) identified three hypotheses as possible explanations for exercise-induced elation. The first maintains that distraction from stressful stimuli is responsible for the improved affect associated with exercise rather than exercise per se. A second explanation of exercise elation was termed the *monamine hypothesis* (Morgan, 1985a). Some evidence from animal experiments suggests that neurotransmitters such as norepinephrine and serotonin—both monamines—increase with exercise, but whether these are the source of the runner's high is still open to question. The endorphin hypothesis offers a third explanation (Morgan, 1985a). Endorphins are morphine-like compounds produced by the brain and pituitary gland that can reduce the sensation of pain and produce a sense of euphoria. These endogenous compounds, the most important of which is beta-endorphin, are released during somatic or psychological stress (Morgan, 1985b). Research with animals and humans has produced some evidence that plasma levels of endorphins are increased with exercise. Although this research cannot be considered conclusive, it continues to be a potentially fruitful area of investigation.

Another intriguing explanation of the runner's high has been attributed to a placebo effect, which also has been found to increase the secretion of endorphins (Hinton & Taylor, 1986). The placebo effect has been observed with certain individuals who have been told to expect analgesic effects from a placebo drug. These authors suggest that the increased endorphin release arising from subjective expectancies leads to the runner's high phenomenon. More specifically, it was hypothesized that because runners have become aware of the possibility of a runner's high, their expectancies may allow this to occur via a placebo response mechanism.

Suffice it to say that although the runner's high phenomenon may seem real for some runners, the concept remains elusive, subject to speculation, and lacking in scientific verifiability. As Morgan (1985a) pointed out, there have been no systematic attempts to validate psychometrically the occurrence of altered states of consciousness resulting from exercise. It is hoped that researchers will push beyond the introspective reports of these experiences and establish cause and effect. Knowing the key factors in producing the runner's high would enable the practitioner to direct the client's efforts toward achieving this desirable outcome.

Research on the Effects of Exercise on Mood States

Studies of mood as related to various forms of exercise have used the Profile of Mood States (POMS) almost exclusively. The POMS is a 65-item scale that yields six mood scores: tension/anxiety, depression/dejection, anger/hostility, vigor/activity, fatigue/inertia, and confusion/bewilderment (McNair, Lorr, & Droppleman, 1971). The POMS has been used mainly to measure changes in mood over time. In most of the research described in the following pages, some form of exercise has been used as an intervention or independent variable, and mood as the dependent variable. Mood scores are taken before and after the exercise intervention. With the exception of "vigor/activity," the moods measured by the POMS are negative. Therefore, when scale scores are profiled, a desirable configuration resembles a pyramid or "iceberg" as it is described by Morgan (1980). An example of this profile is shown in Figure 3.1. In this example, mood states of swimmers improved over the course of a semester compared with no significant improvements among control subjects (Berger & Owen, 1983).

Running has been a popular topic for mood researchers. A study of the acute effects of running for a minimum of 1 hour resulted in the significant lowering of "tension/anxiety" and "anger/hostility" (Markoff, Ryan, & Young, 1982). Other researchers found the effects of ultramarathon distances of 50 and 100 miles to have a significant effect on all POMS factors except anger (Tharion, Strowman, & Rauch, 1988). One study using the Previous Week form of the POMS compared marathon runners, joggers, and a control group of nonexercisers (Wilson, Morley, & Bird, 1980). In general, marathoners had better mood scores than joggers, who in turn had better scores than the nonexercising group. A comparison of the POMS scores of 348 marathoners with those of a group of 856 college students revealed significant differences favoring the runners in all items except anger. There was no difference in the latter item between groups (Gondola & Tuckman, 1982). It was suggested that perhaps average marathoners get as much psychological benefit from their training as more accomplished runners. Similar results were reported in a recent study that compared POMS scores of elite and non-elite runners (Frazier, 1988) and in a comparison of beginning and advanced runners (Dyer & Crouch, 1988).

Other forms of exercise also acutely affect mood states. A study that compared the effects of walking vigorously to walking in a slow, shuffling manner found significant differences in depression, vigor, and fatigue in favor of the brisk walkers (Snodgrass, Higgins, & Todisco, 1986). A comparison of jogging and aerobic dance with weight lifting and inactivity found that the two aerobic activities induced more positive moods after a semester of training (Dyer & Crouch, 1988). As we saw in Figure 3.1, swimming has also been observed to produce favorable mood effects (Berger & Owen, 1983). It is interesting to note that in this study, swimmers at beginning and intermediate skill levels experienced the same benefits.

The acute effects of exercise and hobby activities on mood states were the subject of a study comparing participants in two YMCA fitness classes with members of classes in painting, automechanics, photography, typing, and nutrition (Lichtman & Poser, 1983). Using the POMS, post-class scores were significantly lower on four of the six subscales for the exercise groups and on two of the subscales for the hobby class participants. Both types of activity lowered "tension/anxiety" and "depression/dejection" scores, but only exercise classes reduced the "anger/hostility" and "fatigue/inertia" scores. A comparison between running and massage

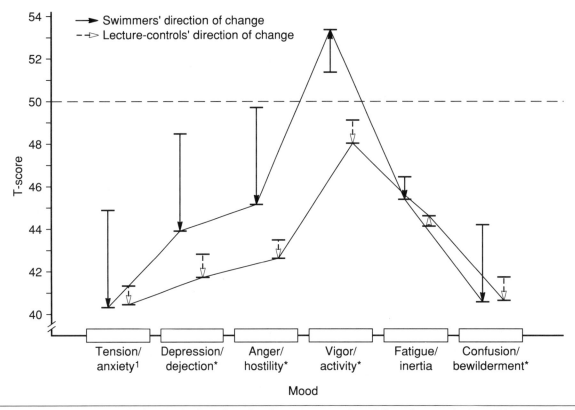

Figure 3.1 Mean *T* scores before and after class for the swimmers (*n* = 58) and controls (*n* = 42) on the Profile of Mood States. Swimmers' postexercise scores closely resemble Morgan's "iceberg" profile which reportedly identifies world class athletes.

[a] Pre- and postclass mood changes for swimmers were significantly greater than that for the controls at the 0.05 level. *p < 0.06.

From "Mood Alterations with Swimming—Swimmers Really Do Feel Better" by B.G. Berger and D.R. Owen, 1983, *Psychosomatic Medicine*, **45**(5), p. 429. Copyright © 1983 by the Psychosomatic Society. Reprinted by permission.

showed both to increase positive mood states and decrease negative mood states (Weinberg, Jackson, & Kolodny, 1988).

Unfortunately, most of the studies on mood have been cross-sectional, nonexperimental, or quasi-experimental studies using intact, convenient groups rather than randomizing subjects and employing other desirable controls. Comparatively few mood studies have overcome these design weaknesses. One of the better experimental studies compared a group of youthful offenders who were randomly assigned to either a special program of fitness training and counseling or a regular rehabilitation program (Hilyer et al., 1982). The exercise program resulted in several physiological and psychological benefits including lower tension and anger, higher levels of vigor, as well as major improvements in fitness. Two other controlled studies found that exercise produced significant improvements in mood (Fremont & Craighead, 1987; Steptoe, Edwards, Moses, & Mathews, 1989).

Although many mood studies have supported the exercise-mood connection, some researchers have failed to observe this relationship. In a study of 14 sedentary males, Hughes, Casal, and Leon (1986) failed to find any differences in POMS total mood or subscale scores that could be accounted for by the exercise program consisting of treadmill walking and stair-climbing. The authors suggested that exercise alone may not be enough to produce psychological benefits, but that there must also be either initial psychopathology, socialization as part of the exercise program, or a training effect.

Another controlled experiment that included exercise and mood-related variables also found no differences between experimental and control groups (King, Taylor, Haskell, & DeBusk, 1989). This study involved 120 healthy adults who were assigned to either a home-based aerobic program or a nonexercising, assessment-only control condition. Adherence to the exercise program exceeded 75%, but though expected changes in physical capacity were observed for the 6-month training period, no changes were observed in mood-related variables. However, mood variables in this study were assessed not by the POMS as in the previously cited studies but by a Likert rating scale.

A longitudinal study that used a national probability sample—a statistical sample representative of the U.S. population—of adults found that running had no significant effect on mood and severity of emotional problems (Agnew & Levin, 1987). Running was found to have a slight positive effect on perceived health, which was explained by the supposition that people who believe their health is good are more likely to run. It was suggested that previous studies, particularly cross-sectional studies, have tended to exaggerate the relationship between running and psychological outcomes by using subjects who are participating in well-coordinated and rigorous exercise programs. These authors believe such programs bear little resemblance to exercise patterns in the real world. It was also suggested that exercise may have a more limited effect on individuals of normal physical and psychological health.

Exercise intensity is a factor that may be of particular relevance in the study of mood. A study comparing mood scores of fit and unfit subjects found that high-intensity exercise caused increased tension and fatigue in both groups (Steptoe & Cox, 1988). Positive mood changes were observed only following low-intensity exercise. Similar results were observed in a follow-up study (Steptoe & Bolton, 1988). Morgan, Costill, Flynn, Raglin, and O'Connor (1988) observed mood disturbances and depression in competitive swimmers who were exposed to an intensive 10-day regimen. Monitoring of mood states during intense training was suggested as a means of preventing training staleness.

Although most of the studies reviewed indicate that exercise produces favorable changes in mood, it would be premature to conclude that there is a cause-effect relationship. Moreover, the mechanisms that would explain such an effect are nothing more than speculations. Many questions have yet to be answered, such as what characteristics of exercise might affect mood? Does intensity or length of exercise make a difference? To what extent is mood change during exercise related to the characteristics of the setting, particularly the social setting? How do people's expectations that exercise will make them "feel better" affect mood? These are but a few of the questions that must be addressed by well-designed, controlled studies before we can confidently state that exercise is a

factor in mood change. In the meantime, the exercise practitioner may adopt a position of cautious optimism while awaiting further research.

DEPRESSION

Considerable research has been done on the efficacy of exercise in the treatment of anxiety and depression, two of the more common mental health problems. The potential role of exercise in the prevention and treatment of each of these will now be considered.

Depression is a major mental health problem in the United States. An estimated 5% to 10% of the population suffer from this malady. Among those who suffer, a significant number commit suicide (Taylor, Sallis, & Needle's, 1985). Women are affected at a rate of 2 to 6 times that of men (Sime, 1984). It has been suggested that women are more susceptible to depression because of hormonal differences or social influences.

Beyond the mood swings and "down" feelings everyone experiences on occasion, depression usually involves symptoms that last a month or more (Dishman, 1986). Clinical depression is characterized by feelings of despair, sadness, hopelessness, low self-esteem, and pessimism. Symptoms range from minor fatigue, irritability, indecisiveness, and social withdrawal to suicidal feelings (Sime, 1984). *Reactive depression* is caused by life events while *endogenous depression* is of unknown origin. Treatment of depression is determined in part by its severity. Mild depression may subside quickly without intervention, while moderate depression may be spontaneously remitted within 6 months. Psychotherapy is often effective in the treatment of mild and moderate depression, although it is usually supplemented by antidepressant medications. Drug therapy is used to treat most cases of severe depression. Often, drastic measures such as electroconvulsive therapy are necessary. Because antidepressive drugs and "shock" therapy usually have undesirable side effects, exercise is an appealing alternative for some depressed patients (Dishman, 1986).

Exercise and Depression Research

Despite considerable research, the effects of exercise on depression are still being debated. Although it is widely believed that exercise has antidepressant effects, much of the research that supports this is debatable. Several reviews of the exercise-depression literature during the last decade have yielded mixed conclusions. Eight studies reviewed by Folkins and Sime (1981) all reported significant improvement in mood states as a result of exercise. This was particularly the case when the level of depression was higher than normal before exercise training. Of concern, however, was that only four of the studies reviewed observed an increase in fitness concomitant with an antidepressant effect. Weinstein and Meyers' (1983) review, citing "a small body of poorly designed research," concluded that the available literature failed to support the position that running plays a significant role in modulating affect change. A subsequent review agreed that the early research suffered from conceptual and methodological problems but that more recent research provided grounds for guarded optimism regarding the therapeutic effects of exercise (Simons, Epstein, McGowan, Kupfer, & Robertson, 1985). Referring to exercise therapy as a promising area of depression research, these authors called for more well-designed studies.

In view of the fact that depression often accompanies myocardial infarction, the effects of exercise are of considerable interest to patients and practitioners in cardiac rehabilitation programs. Few studies have addressed the problem, and results have been mixed. Taylor, Sallis, and Needle's (1985) review found only one uncontrolled study that showed significant improvement in depression among postmyocardial infarction patients and four studies that showed no exercise effect.

Despite the serious weaknesses in the design and methodology of much of the exercise-depression research, more recent research may hold some promise. A recent meta-analysis that reviewed 261 studies related to exercise and depression, 79 of which met the criteria for inclusion, concluded that exercise significantly decreased depression (McCullagh, North, & Mood, 1988). Exercise was also found to be an effective antidepressant for all age groups and to decrease depression equally for both initially depressed and nondepressed (i.e., low-depressed) subjects. In a subsequent analysis, it was observed that exercise reduced depression for all populations regardless of the purpose of exercise or aerobic fitness level (North & McCullagh, 1988). Larger decreases in depression were associated with longer exercise programs and more exercise sessions.

In one of the most frequently cited experimental studies of exercise and depression, depressed subjects were assigned to either a running treatment group or to one of two psychotherapy treatments (Greist, Klein, Eischens, & Faris, 1978). Six

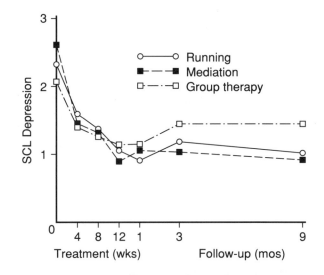

Figure 3.2 SCL depression scores by treatment condition (those who completed treatment only).

From "A Comparative Outcome Study of Group Psychotherapy Versus Exercise Treatment for Depression" by M.H. Klein, J.H. Greist, A.S. Gurman, R.A. Neimeyer, D.P. Lesser, N.J. Bushnell, and R.E. Smith, 1985, *International Journal of Mental Health*, **13**, p. 167. Reprinted by permission of M.E. Sharpe, Inc., Armonk, New York, 10504.

out of eight patients who ran improved within 3 weeks. One patient ran for 16 weeks before improving and another did not improve at all despite consistent adherence to the running program. In a related study, running therapy was compared with meditation-relaxation and group therapy (Klein et al., 1985). As shown in Figure 3.2, each of the treatments improved depression scores as measured by the Symptom Checklist. The subjects had maintained these improvements at a 9-month follow-up. The authors suggested that running could be added to the array of viable treatment options for depressed clients. A similar conclusion was reached in a study of the effects of aerobic exercise on clinical depression among four women (Doyne, Chambless, & Beutler, 1983). Using a multiple baseline design and controlling for the effects of expectancy, all four subjects lowered depression levels. The results showed that exercise can be a viable, cost-effective treatment for depression that, when programmed correctly, has no negative side effects and has the added benefit of improved physical health.

Two controlled studies found several types of exercise to be effective. An experiment that compared running and weight training with a control group found both forms of exercise to significantly reduce depression, while the subjects in the control group experienced no changes

(Doyne et al., 1987). These results contradicted the hypothesis that exercise must improve cardiovascular fitness to treat depression. In one of the better designed studies of exercise and depression, 47 depressed college women were randomly assigned to a rhythmic aerobics class, a relaxation placebo group, or a no-treatment control group (McCann & Holmes, 1984). Subjects in the aerobic group showed significantly reduced depression scores and greater improvements in aerobic fitness compared to the other two groups. Interestingly, the exercise treatment achieved its greatest effect primarily within the first 5 weeks.

Explanations of the Exercise Effect

Although there is no definitive explanation as to why exercise seems to have a positive effect on depression, there are several plausible hypotheses. Sime (1984) has summarized some of these possible explanations:

■ The increased blood flow and oxygenation accompanying exercise may have a beneficial effect on the central nervous system.

■ Exercise is known to increase norepinephrine while low levels of norepinephrine are associated with depression.

■ The development of a sense of mastery and self-control through regular exercise may help patients improve depressed states.

■ Improvements in body image and self-concept often associated with exercise are believed to be factors in preventing or ameliorating depression.

Another hypothesized mechanism is the "pyrogen" effect of exercise, which relates to the temporary increase in body temperature brought about by intensive exercise (Martinsen, 1990). Dishman (1986) has offered several other possible explanations for the antidepressant properties of exercise: feelings of achievement, feelings of self-control or competence, symptom relief or distraction, substitution of good habits for bad ones, development of patience, and consciousness alterations. These benefits are thought to apply only to nonpsychotic depression, particularly when it is primary (lasting for a month or more) and reactive (precipitated by life events). Exercise may also reduce depression that accompanies illness or disability by rehabilitating the disorder (for example, in cardiac rehabilitation) and restoring self-confidence for physical exertion and the resumption of normal life (Dishman, 1986).

Techniques for Increasing the Antidepressant Effects of Exercise

Because many who suffer from depression do not seek professional help, the potential usefulness of exercise may be enhanced by consciously trying to obtain mental health outcomes (Dishman, 1986). The following suggestions have been offered as ways to optimize the antidepressant effects of running (Sime, 1984):

■ Encourage people to run with someone who is supportive.

■ Provide novice runners with extrinsic rewards at the beginning of a program.

■ Teach novices to notice the short-term pleasures of exercise such as tension relief and the enjoyment of the outdoors.

■ Teach novices also to anticipate the long-term benefits of continued exercise involvement.

Berger (1984) has some additional suggestions. About 20 minutes of running appears to be the shortest time that would decrease depression, while running longer than 60 minutes may be less therapeutic. Secondly, keeping a running log provides the client with a source of motivation, immediate reinforcement, a chronicle of progress over time, a record of compliance, and an opportunity to note moods and other qualitative aspects of the run. A third suggestion is to make running fun. Fun may be enhanced by experimenting with location and time of day, using a radio or cassette player, or using some other means to occupy attention while running. Fourth, encourage clients to explore feelings of mastery of the body. For many people, feeling physically strong, powerful, and competent is a new and exciting experience. Finally, clients should be taught to set realistic, attainable goals and to raise goals gradually.

These principles are thought to prevent depression as well as to treat it. In an era when good health and prevention are emphasized, an approach that shifts the responsibility from the health-care provider to the individual is commendable and worth the additional efforts needed to foster it (Sime, 1984).

ANXIETY

Worry and anxiety are part of modern existence. For most people, it is not the occasional stressful experience or major life event, but rather daily hassles that tend to disrupt equanimity and even affect physical and mental health.

Understanding Anxiety

Anxiety differs from worry in that the source of anxiety is not specific. According to Rollo May (1977), anxiety involves a diffuse apprehension of some vague threat that is characterized by feelings of uncertainty and helplessness. Furthermore, anxiety can be seen as a threat to one's "essence" of personality, self-esteem, and self-worth. May (1977, p. 205) then defined *anxiety* as "the apprehension cued off by a threat to some value that the individual holds essential to his existence as a personality."

A common definition of *anxiety* in psychology is that of "a palpable but transitory emotional state or condition characterized by feelings and apprehension and heightened autonomic nervous system activity" (Spielberger, 1972, p. 24). The components of anxiety are thought to include the awareness of powerlessness in the face of threat, feelings of impending danger, a state of tense alertness, apprehensive self-absorption, and doubts about one's actions to counter the threat (Jablenski, 1985).

Behavioral manifestations of anxiety may range from extreme excitement or hyperactivity to a state of stupor (Jablenski, 1985). High levels of sympathetic nervous system activity and psychosomatic complaints such as fear, nervousness, irritability, nausea, fatigue, and muscular pain are common symptoms. Even minor episodes of anxiety are often associated with decreased work effectiveness, absenteeism, increased health-care costs, and personal unhappiness (Sime, 1984).

State-Trait Anxiety

The distinction between *state anxiety* and *trait anxiety* is important in understanding the experiential and behavioral effects of anxiety. *State anxiety* (A-State) is a transitory emotional state characterized by perceived feelings of tension and apprehension and heightened nervous system activity. State anxiety may vary in intensity and fluctuate over time. It involves an emotional reaction that occurs at a particular moment in time and at a particular level of intensity (Spielberger, Gorsuch, & Lushene, 1970). A-States are triggered by known causes and usually last a short time. State anxiety brought about by self-doubts and worry concerning a specific impending threat are accompanied by symptoms such as elevated heart rate, muscle tension,

visceral motility, and inability to concentrate (Dishman, 1986).

Trait anxiety (A-Trait) refers to relatively stable individual differences in anxiety proneness. Stated differently, individuals who are high in A-Trait typically respond to situations perceived as threatening with elevated levels of state anxiety. Trait anxiety refers to a predisposition to respond to stressful situations in an individually characteristic way. It is assumed that individuals who are high in A-Trait will manifest symptoms of A-State more readily due to a tendency to perceive a wider range of stimuli as threatening. High A-trait people are extremely sensitive to any situation that might threaten self-esteem (Spielberger et al., 1970). A theoretical model of the components and relationships of trait and state anxiety is shown in Figure 3.3.

To predictably respond to a wide range of events with feelings of tension, worry, nervousness, or apprehension indicates a high level of A-Trait. A-Trait is usually cognitively learned through exposure to threats, negative evaluations, or failure, and tends to be generalized to many situations. Cognitively learned anxieties frequently involve apprehension about performing important but uncertain tasks that are often compared to some standard of excellence by oneself or, particularly, by significant others (Dishman, 1986).

Effects of Exercise on Anxiety

Numerous studies over the past 20 years have explored the effects of exercise on both state and trait anxiety. Unfortunately many of these studies have had serious design weaknesses that limit their usefulness in explaining the relationship between exercise and anxiety. In practically all of the uncontrolled studies we reviewed, acute and chronic exercise were found to be associated with lower levels of anxiety after exercise. The studies we will now present are all controlled. We shall first consider the effects of acute exercise and then discuss long-term or chronic exercise effects.

Acute Effects

Several studies have observed that acute exercise reduces anxiety. Driscoll (1976) combined physical exertion and positive imaging to successfully lower test anxiety of college students. The treatment procedure used positive images after anxiety-causing scenes to instill positive feelings, and used an exercise task of running in place to help compete with and lower anxiety arousal. A comparison of

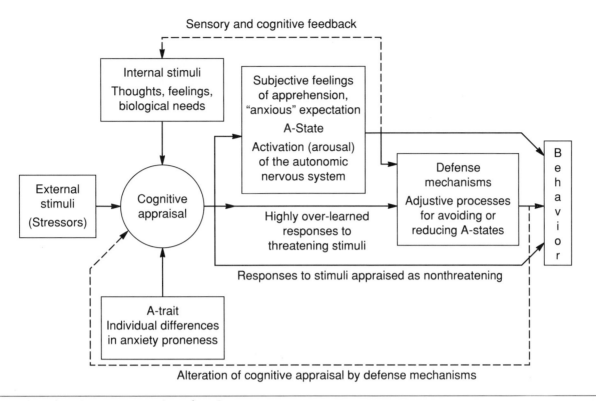

Figure 3.3 A trait-state conception of anxiety.

From "Theory and Research on Anxiety" by C.D. Speilberger. In *Anxiety and Behavior* (p.17) by C.D. Speilberger, 1966, New York: Academic Press. Reprinted by permission.

the effects of walking on a treadmill for 20 minutes at 70% of maximal heart rate, meditation, and resting quietly found that all three methods effectively lowered state anxiety scores (Bahrke & Morgan, 1978). To explain the rather surprising finding that resting quietly reduced anxiety, the researchers suggested that it is possibly the diversional effects of exercise, biofeedback, meditation, and other stress reduction methodologies rather than the physiological changes that account for the reduction in anxiety. In an extension of the previous study (Bahrke, 1981), an experimental group walked on a treadmill for 20 minutes at 75% of maximal heart rate and a control group sat quietly in a rocking chair with the option of light reading. Again there were no differences in the groups. Both techniques lowered anxiety but the decreases were not significant. In contrast to the earlier study (Bahrke & Morgan, 1978), the state anxiety of highly anxious subjects was not reduced.

A subsequent series of controlled studies compared the ability of exercise and quiet rest to reduce state anxiety and lower blood pressure (Raglin & Morgan, 1987). The first study used men with normal blood pressure, and the second employed men whose high blood pressure was pharmocologically controlled. In both studies the subjects alternately exercised in their own manner and level of intensity and rested quietly for 40 minutes in a sound chamber. The first study noted a significant reduction in state anxiety after exercising but not after resting. The second study showed no state anxiety differences between treatments. Concerning effects on blood pressure, the researchers observed no quantitative differences between the treatments, however, they noted qualitative differences that showed a stronger and longer-lasting effect after exercising.

Chronic Effects

Several studies have focused on the question of whether exercise over long periods of time is associated with reduced anxiety. In one such study, middle-aged police officers and fire fighters who exercised 3 times per week for 12 weeks significantly lowered anxiety levels while also improving fitness (Folkins, 1976). Similar results were observed in a study of youthful offenders (Hilyer et al., 1982). An experimental group that participated in a vigorous fitness program for 20 weeks with counseling improved significantly, both psychologically and physiologically. State and trait anxiety scores at the end of the training were lower for the fitness group as compared to the control subjects.

Considerably more research is needed to determine the effects of long-term exercise on anxiety. At present, the scarcity of controlled, systematic research on this topic prohibits definitive conclusions. However, medical, psychological, and exercise scientists generally agree that long-term exercise is usually associated with reductions in trait anxiety (Morgan & Goldston, 1987).

Exercise and Anxiety Reduction in Patients With Mental Disorders

The studies that have explored the use of exercise as a means of lowering anxiety levels with patients suffering from mental disorders have generally supported exercise interventions. Lion (1978), using a 2-month-long walk-jog program, observed significantly lower anxiety levels with psychiatric outpatients as compared to a placebo control group. A study that compared the psychological benefits of walking and jogging on a group of people hospitalized for neurosis showed that both forms of exercise markedly reduced anxiety after an 8-week treatment period as well as at a 6-month follow-up (Sexton, Maere, & Dahl, 1989). Joggers had greater aerobic gains but received no greater psychological benefits. The researchers found no relationship between aerobic gain and the reduction of anxiety at the end of treatment, although at follow-up subjects with higher aerobic fitness had lower levels of anxiety.

Patients suffering from anxiety disorders who received either intensive aerobic training (70% of maximum heart rate) or a program consisting of strength, flexibility, and relaxation exercises, benefited equally in the reduction of anxiety (Martinsen, Hoffart, & Solberg, 1989). Despite significant gains in aerobic capacity observed only in the former group, both groups achieved similar and significant reductions in anxiety. Because the level of aerobic fitness appeared to be unrelated to the reduction of anxiety, it was suggested that distraction from anxiety-provoking stimuli, enhanced self-efficacy, and experiences of mastery are the keys to lowering anxiety.

In a study of a group of people experiencing dysphoric moods, Fremont and Craighead (1987) compared the anxiety-reducing effects of running, cognitive therapy, and a treatment that combined running and cognitive therapy for 10 weeks. All three treatment groups lowered their anxiety levels significantly. The researchers suggested that for some patients exercise may be a viable alternative to other traditional treatments of dysphoric moods. Furthermore, the cost-effectiveness of exercise makes it a desirable alternative.

Of the few studies that failed to find exercise to be effective, a study of male psychiatric outpatients randomly assigned to a running treatment, a corrective therapy treatment, or a control group found no significant differences in anxiety among the groups (Hannaford, Harrell, & Cox, 1988). The running treatment did, however, lower anxiety slightly but not significantly.

In terms of plausible rationale for the inclusion of exercise in the treatment of anxiety, treatment has typically employed psychotherapy, behavioral therapy, and drug therapy. Exercise appears to share some of the stress-reducing properties found in these therapies as well as coping behaviors, such as biofeedback, hypnosis, meditation, and progressive relaxation (Dishman, 1986). Exercise may help manage anxiety by regulating the sympathetic tone of the autonomic nervous system, which distracts people from anxiety-provoking thoughts, and by helping people to interpret arousal symptoms with less concern (Dishman, 1986). Furthermore, because only one in four people who suffer from anxiety seeks professional treatment, exercise may be an effective option for controlling some forms of anxiety in some people (Dishman, 1986).

Gender Differences

Relatively few anxiety studies have looked at gender differences in exercise effects. A study of college students (Wood, 1977) found exercise to be less effective in reducing anxiety for women than for men. This finding could be particularly meaningful because anxiety is more common among women. However, results from more definitive studies have shown that the psychological responses to exercise are similar among men and women (Sime, 1984). Either way, this topic needs further research.

Cognitive Versus Somatic Anxiety

A distinction is often made between *cognitive* and *somatic* symptoms of anxiety. *Cognitive* elements of anxiety include worry, lack of concentration, and insomnia, and *somatic* elements include nervousness, tension, nausea, headache, palmar sweating, and a rapid pulse rate at rest (Sime, 1984). Sime has suggested a systematic relationship between the type of symptoms experienced, cognitive or somatic, and the sources of relief, either exercise or relaxation. For example, people who exercise vigorously report less somatic and more cognitive anxiety, while people who meditate report more somatic and less cognitive anxiety (Schwartz, Davidson, & Goleman, 1978). However, a recent study failed to replicate this finding (Steptoe & Kearsley, 1990). Employing 340 subjects, these researchers found no links between exercise and lower somatic anxiety or between meditation and reduced cognitive anxiety. We shall have to await further developments in this potentially important line of investigation.

Exercise Considerations

Although we still do not know enough about the anxiety-reducing effects of different types and intensities of exercise, we can make some generalizations. Exercise should be of at least moderate intensity (> 60% of maximum heart rate) and sustained for at least 20 minutes (Raglin & Morgan, 1987). According to Sime (1984), to effectively reduce anxiety, exercise must elicit sustained heavy breathing without causing exhaustion and should last from 20 minutes up to an hour or more. In addition, people should exercise at least 3 days a week and possibly more, depending on the anxiety symptoms (Sime, 1984). It should be pointed out that low-intensity exercise such as walking should not be excluded from further consideration (Raglin & Morgan, 1987). We would extend this recommendation to weight training, aerobic dance, and flexibility exercises until there is research to the contrary.

STRESS AND TENSION

Few psychological terms are used as frequently as *stress*. Indeed, volumes have been written on stress over the past 2 decades, both in popular and scientific literature. Although the impact of stress on people's lives is still not entirely clear, it appears to be a major factor in mental and physical health, interpersonal relationships, and careers. Being "stressed out" or "burned out" in one or more areas of life is all too common. The effects of stress on human functioning are of great interest not only to the physician, psychologist, and sociologist, but also to exercise and other health professionals. Stress is a universal human phenomenon often causing intense feelings of distress that are tremendously important to behavior and health (Lazarus, 1966). A partial listing of diseases associated with chronic stress is shown in Table 3.2.

Table 3.2   Some Diseases of Adaptation

Alcoholism	Hemorrhoids
Allergies	High blood pressure
Angina	Hyperactivity
Anxiety	Kidney stones
Arrhythmia	Krohns disease
Arthritis	Learning problems
Bronchitis	Menstrual distress
Caffeinism	Migraine
Colitis	Nail biting
Depression	Nicotine addiction
Diarrhea	Nightmares
Diverticulitis	Prostrate problems
Drug abuse	Schizophrenia
Dyslexia	Senility
Fatigue	Sex problems
Gout	Sleep problems
Headache	Stroke
Heart disease	Ulcers

From "Exercise, Body Chemistry, and Stress" by E.S. Rosenbluth, 1986, *Emotional First Aid*, 2(1), p. 35. Reprinted by permission.

The Nature and Terminology of Stress

Widely differing definitions of *stress* abound. According to Lazarus (1966), the province of stress is most clearly demarcated when we are dealing with extremes of biological and psychological disturbance brought about by unusually threatening or demanding life conditions. Lazarus used the term *stress* generically to represent a whole topical area, including the stress stimulus, the stress reaction, as well as the intervening processes. Conceived in this way, *stress* functions as a general label, like *motivation* or *cognition*, to define a complex, amorphous, interdisciplinary area of study (Lazarus, 1966).

The interpretation of stress that we shall use assumes that stress involves internal or external demands placed on an individual (stressor), an appraisal of the demands and the adequacy of one's ability to cope with them, and the stress response (Matheny, Aycock, Pugh, Curlette, & Cannella, 1986). The stress process begins when demands are made on an individual. Demands may be self-generated or may come from outside. Self-generated demands are related to self-imposed standards for behavior. Outside demands may come from such mundane sources as a traffic jam or a spilled drink, or from other more important sources such as major life events and intense interpersonal exchanges.

How one interprets a potential threat determines whether or not a stress reaction occurs. There are extreme differences in how people react to the same stimuli. What one person interprets as a threat may be taken in stride by another person. People tend to develop characteristic ways of assessing demands and coping with stressors. This individual style has been associated with stress-prone aspects of personality as in the Type A or coronary-prone personality or the supersensitive, anxious-reactive personality. The appraisal process, then, determines whether or not a demand will become a stressor. If personal resources are perceived to equal or exceed the perceived demand, then a stress response is unlikely, while situations perceived as being beyond personal resources are viewed as threats or stressors. A stress response, then, is triggered when there is a gap between perceived demands and perceived resources (Matheny et al., 1986).

The Stress Response

The stress response has psychological, behavioral, and physiological symptoms. Psychologically, a person may exhibit increased irritability and anxiety, decreased concentration, and narrowed perception. Behaviorally, some common symptoms are restlessness, tremors, loss of sleep, and a decrease in speech fluency. Physiological symptoms are those associated with the "fight or flight" or "alarm" reaction, which include dilation of pupils, increased heart rate and blood pressure, increased muscle tension, rush of blood to muscles and the brain, and an increased production of catecholamines and corticosteroids. If the alarm reaction is elicited frequently enough, a variety of psychophysiological maladies may result, such as ulcers, coronary artery disease, cerebral vascular accidents, migraine headaches, and backaches (Matheny et al., 1986).

Coping With Stress

Most individuals try to cope with stress as best they can. Coping involves efforts to prevent, eliminate, or weaken stressors, or at least to tolerate their effects in the least hurtful manner (Matheny et al., 1986). It should be noted that attempts at coping may be either healthy or unhealthy, conscious or unconscious. Matheny and colleagues (1986) identified 12 categories of coping behaviors that ranged from the more familiar techniques of cognitive restructuring, problem-solving, and

tension reduction to the less familiar techniques of stress monitoring, avoidance and withdrawal, and suppression and denial. These authors also identified five coping resources that, if present, are thought to strength a person's general resistance to stressors. They are social support, functional beliefs and values, confidence and control, self-esteem, and wellness. Wellness refers to overall good health, including physical fitness, weight control, a high level of energy, and the absence of smoking and excessive alcohol consumption. A model of stress coping developed by Matheny and colleagues (1986) has two major categories of coping strategies, either preventive coping or combative coping. Preventive coping uses techniques such as avoiding stressors when possible, adjusting the demands that we place on ourselves, and altering stress-inducing behaviors. Combative strategies for reducing stress include attacking stressors through problem solving or being assertive, learning to be more tolerant of stressors, and learning to lower arousal level through relaxation.

Preventing stress is a desirable goal. The development of prevention skills enables a person to avoid some stress-evoking stimuli, thereby evading the wear and tear that accompanies a stressful episode. When stress does occur, however, having the skills to combat it can lessen its effects. Effective ways to combat stress include relaxation techniques or cognitively redefining the situation so that the stressor does not seem so dreadful.

Research on Exercise and Stress

This model shows that exercise can play an important role in the coping model discussed previously. Because exercise is crucial to physical fitness, it is a factor in wellness and preventive coping. Exercise may also be an effective combative strategy because it can lower one's level of arousal. We shall now review the research on the relationship between exercise and stress.

Stress Reactivity

Numerous researchers have tried to determine whether exercise or fitness can effectively mitigate the effects of stress. In this section, we will address people's susceptibility to stress and the extensiveness of their stress reaction. We are particularly interested in the question of whether exercise and fitness play a role in lessening one's reactivity to acute, short-term stressors. Researchers in this area have typically employed physiological parameters, particularly blood pressure and heart rate, to quantify the effects of psychological stressors.

In an early review, Michael (1957) concluded that exercise conditions the stress adaptation mechanism, particularly the adrenocortical and autonomic processes, and provides a degree of protection by reducing the time necessary to elicit a stress response. In support of this conclusion, physically conditioned subjects were found to be less reactive to a cold presser stressor than were unconditioned subjects (Subhan, White, & Kane, 1987). Similarly, in a comparison of "high-fit" and "low-fit" subjects, the high-fit group had lower baseline levels of cardiovascular arousal and responded to psychological stressors less dramatically than the low-fit subjects (McGilley & Holmes, 1988). Figure 3.4 depicts the consistently lower systolic blood pressure and heart rate responses of the high-fit group.

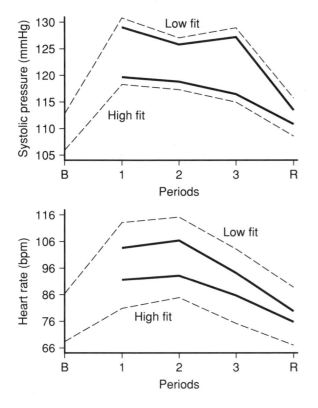

Figure 3.4 Systolic blood pressure and heart rate scores for the high-fit and low-fit subjects during the baseline (B) period, three stress periods, and recovery (R) period. Broken lines represent raw scores and solid lines represent residualized (adjusted for baseline differences) scores.

From "Aerobic Fitness and Response to Psychological Stress" by B.M. McGilley and D.S. Holmes, 1988, *Journal of Research and Personality,* **22**, p. 135. Reprinted by permission.

A comparison between aerobically trained and untrained subjects used various physiological indicators to measure responses to psychosocial stress (Sinyor, Schwartz, Peronnet, Brisson, & Seraganian, 1983). The trained subjects showed higher levels of norepinephrine and prolactin early in the stress period, as well as more rapid heart rate recovery and lower anxiety following exposure to stress. The results suggested that aerobically trained individuals may be capable of faster recovery both physiologically and emotionally. Keller and Seraganian (1984) reached a similar conclusion in two related studies that also explored the influence of aerobic fitness on autonomic reactivity to psychosocial stress. Both experiments monitored subjects' electrodermal responses to tasks designed to cause stress. Exercise participants showed faster recovery, which was thought to indicate more effective coping with emotional stress.

Several researchers, however, have not found exercise to reduce stress reactivity. In a study of sedentary smokers, Russell, Epstein, and Erickson (1983) found that exercise failed to reduce stress responses. The study compared exercise and smoking as coping responses to stress induced by a mental task, but neither effectively inhibited stress. Similarly, a study of 107 healthy Type-A male managers that compared aerobic exercise, weight training, and cognitive-behavioral stress management found only the latter to significantly mitigate behavioral reactivity to laboratory stressors (Roskies et al., 1986). Physiological reactivity was not reduced by any of the three techniques. These results led the authors to question the ability of behavioral treatments to modify physiological reactivity as well as the ability of existing measures to accurately assess changes in stress reactivity.

In the most extensive consideration of this topic to date, a meta-analysis of 34 studies showed that, regardless of the type of physiological and psychological measure used, aerobically fit subjects showed a reduced psychosocial stress response (Crews & Landers, 1987). A tentative explanation for this finding was that exercise acts either as a coping strategy that reduces the physiological response to stress, or it serves as an "inoculator" to foster a more effective response to psychosocial stress. Crews and Landers (1987) suggested that, because aerobic fitness is associated with improvements in cardiovascular function (such as reduced heart rate, lower blood pressure, increased stroke volume, and maximal oxygen uptake), perhaps aerobic exercise may decrease sympathetically mediated cardiovascular responses to psychosocial stress.

Exercise and Long-Term Stress

If it could be shown that exercise helps to "buffer" the effects of long-term stress, the implications would be enormous. For the individual, it would provide a convenient, safe, and inexpensive means of coping with stress, and give the exercise practitioner considerable leverage in the role of exercise advocate.

Exercise as a means of protecting health by decreasing the "organismic strain" resulting from stressful life events, such as divorce or a death in the family, has been explored with some success (Kobasa, Maddi, & Puccetti, 1982). A cross-sectional study of 4,628 men concluded that physical fitness may act as a buffer against stress by fortifying the body and increasing "hardiness" (Tucker, Cole, & Friedman, 1986). Comparable results were obtained in another major cross-sectional study of 4,351 people. The study found that people who were highly physically fit and who exercised tended to have a low level of somatic complaints and tension (Collingwood, Bernstein, Hubbard, & Blair, 1983).

More recently, Roth and Holmes (1985) investigated the relationship between stressful life events, physical fitness, and physical illness in a controlled study. They obtained life change histories of the past year from 112 subjects, who were then tested with a submaximal bicycle ergometer test. Subjects then kept records of all aspects of their physical health for 9 weeks and underwent psychological testing at the end of that period. As shown in Figure 3.5, high levels of stress during the preceding year were associated with poorer physical health, particularly for subjects with low levels of fitness. In contrast, life stress was found to have little impact on the physical health of fit subjects. The results showed that fitness moderates the stress-illness relationship. It was also suggested that improved fitness may diminish the effects of unavoidable stress. A longitudinal study of stress and well-being in adolescents (Brown & Siegel, 1988) corroborated these results. This study found that stressful life events had less impact on health as exercise levels increased.

An experiment with college students that compared exercise, the relaxation response, and group interaction with a no-treatment control group found that exercise and the relaxation response reduced short-term stress better than group support and that all three techniques were significantly better than no treatment at all (Berger, Friedman, & Eaton, 1988). Because researchers observed no long-term stress reduction benefits, they suggested

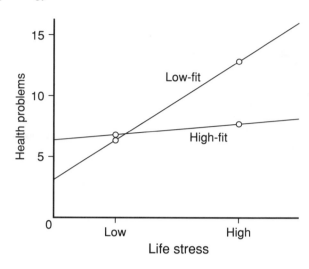

Figure 3.5 Regression lines predicting Health Record Form total severity scores from life stress and physical fitness.

From "Influence of Physical Fitness in Determining the Impact of Stressful Life Events on Physical and Psychological Health" by D.L. Roth and D.S. Holmes, 1985, *Psychosomatic Medicine*, **47**(2), p. 169. Reprinted by permission.

that regular exercise or relaxation is necessary to maintain reduced levels of stress.

A comparison of stress inoculation and jogging as stress-management interventions found both to be effective (Long, 1984). Figure 3.6 illustrates the effects of both treatments on trait and state anxiety and tension. A 15-month follow-up study revealed that both the jogging group and the stress-inoculation group had maintained reduced levels of anxiety and increased self-efficacy (Long, 1985). In two related studies, Long and Haney (1988a, 1988b) compared jogging with progressive relaxation using moderately stressed sedentary working women as subjects. Again both interventions significantly reduced stress symptoms and increased self-efficacy. These gains were also maintained at an 8-week follow-up. The second study was a 14-month follow-up. Both groups reported continued benefits of the previous intervention programs, and 64% claimed to be regularly using some structured form of exercise or relaxation.

Comparatively little research has addressed the use of exercise as an adjunct to other stress management techniques. One study compared stress-inoculation training (SIT), with and without an exercise component, with an unsupervised exercise program (Long, 1988). Although SIT with an exercise component was more effective than exercise alone in reducing anxiety and stress in school personnel, both treatments significantly improved preventive

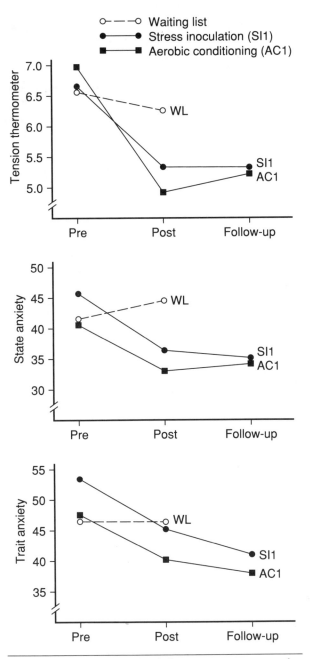

Figure 3.6 Mean ratings of change on measures of stress before and after treatment, and at 3-month follow-up.

From "Aerobic Conditioning and Stress Innoculation: A Comparison of Stress-Management Interventions" by B.C. Long, 1984, *Cognitive Therapy and Research*, **8**(5), p. 529. Reprinted by permission.

coping and lessened emotion-focused coping (i.e., ways of coping that regulate one's emotional reaction or make one feel better without changing the problem). SIT without an exercise component did not affect stress, anxiety, or coping ability. Long observed changes in stress and coping primarily

in subjects who were more sedentary and highly stressed at the beginning of the program. It should be noted that neither the SIT-plus-exercise nor the exercise group significantly improved fitness levels or involvement in physical activity. The unsupervised nature of the exercise programs was cited as the probable reason for this outcome.

Relatively few studies have failed to demonstrate the effectiveness of exercise in managing stress. However, one study in which highly stressed college students were assigned to aerobic exercise, relaxation, or a control group, did not find differences in self-reported measures of physical health following life stress (Roth & Holmes, 1987). Exercise was, however, found to be more effective than relaxation in reducing depression. The researchers suggested that, with regard to the influence of life stress on physical illness, aerobic fitness may serve more of a preventive role than a corrective one. As shown in an earlier study (Roth & Holmes, 1985), subjects who were already fit experienced fewer health problems following stress than subjects who were not. However, improvements in fitness were introduced after the onset of stressors, which may have been too late to cause a beneficial effect. Additional research is needed to clarify this question.

Assuming for the moment that exercise does have a mitigating effect on stress, the question of whether some forms of exercise are better than others has not been extensively addressed. DeVries (1981) recommended rhythmic activities such as walking, jogging, and cycling. Swimming has also been recommended to reduce stress (Berger & Owen, 1983). An uncontrolled study that compared swimming, body conditioning, Hatha yoga, and fencing for stress reduction and mood enhancement found that differences depended on the conditions under which the activity took place (Berger & Owen, 1988). The study maintained that for exercise to effectively reduce stress, it must be enjoyable and should have at least some of the following characteristics: aerobic, void of interpersonal competition, predictable, and repetitive. The more of these characteristics that are present, the more likely the activity is to reduce stress.

Exercise and Tension Reduction

Because muscle tension is a common symptom of stress, lessening tension may reduce the effects of stress. In a study of the immediate effects of exercise on resting muscle action potential, deVries (1968) observed a 58% reduction in muscular electrical activity after a bench-stepping task. Similarly, deVries found long-term reductions in muscle electrical activity of 25% in subjects who participated in 17 vigorous workouts.

In a comparison of the tranquilizing effects of exercise and meprobamate on 10 elderly subjects suffering from stress, deVries and Adams (1972) found that exercise at a heart rate of 100 beats per minute (bpm) significantly reduced muscle electrical activity. Neither meprobamate nor placebo treatments produced noticeable effects. Interestingly, exercise at an intensity of 120 bpm was slightly less effective than at 100 bpm. The researchers concluded that exercise was a more effective tranquilizer than meprobamate without the latter's undesirable side effects. Using exercise instead of tranquilizing drugs was especially recommended for the elderly to avoid further impairment of motor coordination and reaction time.

After reviewing the research literature, deVries (1981) cited several studies that supported the tranquilizing effect of exercise, but he concluded that additional corroborative research was still needed. However he did suggest that the tranquilizing effect of elevated body temperature caused by exercise may provide only an acute or immediate effect. DeVries also suggested that physical exercise of even low intensity facilitates proprioceptive stimuli, which are believed to be necessary for normal cortical function and therefore important to a state of relaxation. He recommended rhythmic exercise, such as walking, jogging, and cycling from 5 to 30 minutes at 30% to 60% of maximum heart rate. Highly intense exercise was found to be counterproductive in producing a tranquilizer effect.

SUMMARY

One of the major benefits of regular exercise is its effect on important psychological processes. This chapter has shown the relationships between exercise and mental health and affective processes. Exercise is associated with lowering anxiety, helping depression, and reducing stress and tension. Exercise can also favorably affect moods and perceptions of well-being and happiness. Although a causative link between exercise and improved mental health has yet to be established, psychological and physiological theories have been offered to explain the link.

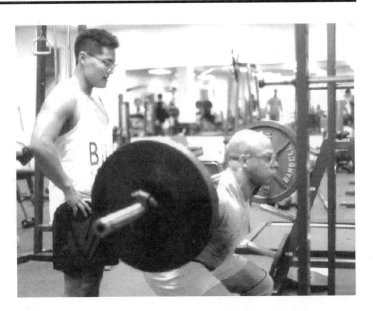

Chapter 4
Exercise, Fitness, and Personality

In the previous chapter we reviewed the effects of exercise on psychological processes that are generally short-lived. We shall now consider the more stable and enduring predispositions and characteristic behavioral patterns of *personality*. Personality has been a favorite topic among psychologists for years. It is therefore not surprising that the psychological literature contains many theories and investigative methods related to personality. In this chapter we will review and interpret the literature on personality and, where possible, generalize about the relationship between aspects of personality and exercise and fitness.

THE NATURE OF PERSONALITY

People differ in an infinite variety of ways—from their physical structure to their thoughts, feelings, and behavioral patterns (Brody, 1988). Personality

psychologists attempt to systematically describe these differences and to study their significance for understanding individuals. How personality psychologists go about this task, what they look for, and how they interpret their findings varies considerably. Scholars tend to define personality on the basis of their interpretation of a particular theoretical perspective and methodology. And, because personality theory has not developed anything resembling a consensus, there is as yet no classic or even widely accepted definition of personality.

For years psychologists disagreed about whether consistencies of behavior, usually referred to as *traits*, or situational factors were the primary determinants of behavior. However, a point of synthesis has now been reached whereby most psychologists consider both to be important (Dienstbier, 1984). For our purposes, we have adopted an interactionist position that views personality traits as the products of both inherited dispositions and learning gained through interaction with the

59

environment (Dienstbier, 1984). Although we acknowledge that situational factors are important influences on behavior, we shall direct our attention almost exclusively to the specific characteristics, or traits, of personality associated with long-term involvement in exercise and other forms of physical activity.

We are particularly interested in exploring the question of whether regular exercise over a prolonged time may change aspects of one's personality. We are also concerned with whether certain personality characteristics predispose one to become involved in physical activity. With regard to the first question, we may be setting ourselves up for disappointment by thinking that exercise may lead to changes in personality. As mentioned before, personality dimensions are quite stable and are therefore likely to change very slowly, if at all. According to Dienstbier (1984), expectations for significant changes in personality dimensions from short-term exercise programs should be minimal. The fact that much of the research has centered on exercise programs of approximately 10 to 12 weeks may account for many of the inconsistencies in the results and the failure to find changes in personality caused by exercise.

What might reasonably be expected of the relationship between physical fitness and personality? Before the flood of personality studies in the 1960s and 1970s, Raymond B. Cattell, an eminent trait psychologist, speculated about a relationship between fitness and personality (Cattell, 1960). Cattell hypothesized that a high level of fitness would reduce anxiety and neuroticism and would facilitate aggressive and extrovert adjustments. He also proposed that people likely to do well in intense physical training possess the traits of stability and low anxiety. Cattell called for research to explore relationships between personality and fitness without the element of competition, and to test and retest personality using experimental and control groups with the former undergoing an extended period of training.

If personality changes do occur as a result of extensive involvement in physical activity, how might these changes be explained? Dienstbier (1984) identified four potential mediators of personality change. The first of these is associated with physiological changes concomitant with regular training. Since the physiological systems that sustain prolonged physical effort are also involved in emotional arousal, it is reasonable to expect some changes in temperament and mood after extended training. The second possible mediator of personality changes is related to one's perceptions of physical changes accompanying exercise. The reduction in weight and body fat, increased energy level, and more youthful appearance often result in an improved body image that contributes significantly to a positive self-concept. It is generally accepted that a positive self-concept, or high self-esteem, correlates with psychological health. A related aspect of perception of physical change has to do with the increased sense of one's ability to master challenges and attain goals, which are the outgrowth of some dramatic improvements in performance after a few months of training. One's beliefs about self-determination and internal control are likely to be influenced positively by success in exercise endeavors. A third possible mediator of personality change centers on the lifestyle changes that often accompany commitment to training. It is not unusual for people to change their eating and sleeping habits as well as other behaviors to benefit their training. Of course changes in lifestyle will likely have a profound effect on relationships with other people and how one is perceived by others. The final mediator of personality change has to do with one's expectations for change. The more one believes that personality changes will occur with training, the more likely they are to occur. Changes in personality attributable to the placebo effect is a confounding variable that is seldom acknowledged or controlled in exercise and personality research.

RESEARCH FINDINGS REGARDING EXERCISE, FITNESS, AND PERSONALITY

There have been several reviews of the literature on personality and exercise. Folkins and Sime's (1981) assessment concluded that there was no evidence to support a claim of global changes in personality following physical fitness training. However, a more recent and more comprehensive review, despite finding serious methodological deficiencies in the research, noted a trend showing the positive effect of exercise on personality (Doan & Scherman, 1987). Which of these is the more accurate assessment? Can some accommodation of both of these positions be found? We shall return to these questions after a look at some representative research. We have grouped the research according to the personality instrument used.

The 16 Personality Factor Questionnaire (16PF)

The 16PF (Cattell & Eber, 1964) has without a doubt been the preferred instrument for researchers interested in the relationship between exercise and personality. Unfortunately, most of the studies using the 16PF have design weaknesses that limit the usefulness of the data. In addition, as Folkins and Sime (1981) pointed out, few of the personality factors in the 16PF are expected to change following short-term intervention, which calls the use of this instrument into question for studies of short duration. Nevertheless, because it has been the overwhelming instrument of choice, we shall review studies that have employed it. We should note that several of the 16PF dimensions comprise a second-order factor of "emotionality," which probably is influenced by exercise (Dienstbier, 1984). Second-order factors are broader patterns under which the more numerous primary personality factors are organized (Cattell, 1960).

The 16PF contains 16 primary personality dimensions derived through factor analysis (Cattell & Eber, 1964). A summary of the factors and their opposites follows:

A. Warm, sociable/aloof, stiff

B. Intelligent, bright/unintelligent, dull

C. Emotionally stable, mature/emotional, immature

E. Dominant, ascendant/submissive, mild

F. Surgent, enthusiastic/sober, glum

G. Conscientious, persistent/casual, undependable

H. Adventurous, outgoing/shy, timid

I. Sensitive, intuitive/tough, realistic

L. Suspicious, jealous/accepting, adaptable

M. Unconventional, self-absorbed/practical, conventional

N. Shrewd, sophisticated/naive, unpretentious

O. Timid, insecure/confident, self-secure

Q1. Radical, experimenting/conservative, moralizing

Q2. Self-sufficient, resourceful/group dependent, conventional

Q3. Controlled, willful/uncontrolled, lax

Q4. Tense, excitable/composed, phlegmatic

In addition to these 16 primary factors, two second-order scores may be derived by combining certain primary factors. A second-order factor of "anxiety" may be computed by combining scores on factors C, H, L, O, Q3, and Q4. Similarly, a second-order factor of "extroversion-introversion"

may be derived from scores on factors A, E, F, H, and Q2.

After reviewing five studies that used the 16PF in a before-after format, Dienstbier (1984) observed that exercise participants became more placid and relaxed. He also found some evidence that exercise resulted in lower emotional reactivity. He speculated that exercise, specifically running, may stimulate the sympathetic nervous system and associated glandular responses, and that the resulting increase in physiological capacity may be the major cause of reduced emotional tension and decreased anxiety (Dienstbier, 1984).

Doan and Scherman's (1987) research review presented a more comprehensive analysis of physical fitness and personality. Classifying studies based on their level of design sophistication, these researchers found that five of the six least sophisticated studies that used the 16PF showed improvement in personality dimensions. At a higher level of research design, only two of five studies observed changes in personality following exercise programs. Doan and Scherman (1987) noted only one true experimental study that used the 16PF. This study, which employed the junior-senior high school version of the instrument found no change in personality following a program of aerobic exercises.

A comparison of world class runners with a large group of less talented runners revealed only one factor in which the groups differed significantly—the world class runners were more "happy-go-lucky" (Nieman & George, 1987). As demonstrated in the profile shown in Figure 4.1, world class runners also were somewhat more practical minded and less self-sufficient than other runners.

A cross-sectional study of over 4,000 men and women conducted at the Cooper Clinic in Dallas found that people who had high levels of physical fitness and who exercised, tended to have few somatic complaints and low levels of tension (Collingwood et al., 1983). This study used the Clinical Analysis Questionnaire, which includes the 16PF. The 16PF was used with the Self-Rating Depression Scale in a nonexperimental study of men and women who participated in a program of aerobic and anaerobic exercise. The study found that personality changes were associated with improved aerobic, but not anaerobic, fitness (Jasnoski, Holmes, & Banks, 1988). The researchers also found that the exercise program had a more pronounced effect on the personalities of women. Most notably, the women realized significant changes in happiness, security, and control concomitant with changes in aerobic fitness, while the men showed significant changes only in stability.

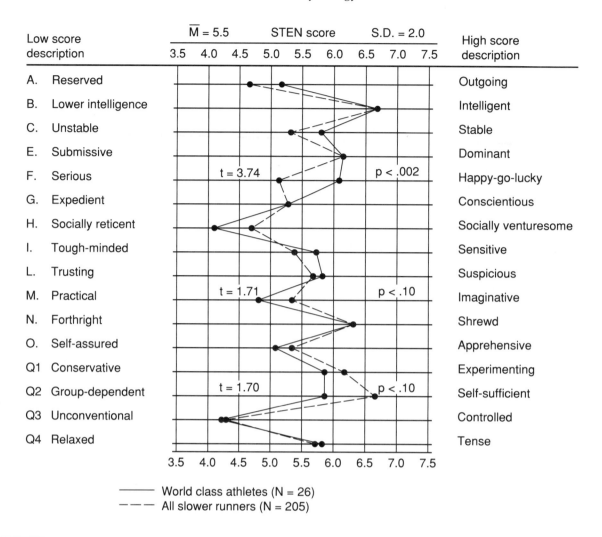

Figure 4.1   Comparison of means: World class vs. all slower runners.

From "Personality Traits That Correlate With Success in Distance Running" by D.C. Neiman and D.M. George, 1987, *Journal of Sports Medicine,* **27**, p. 350. Reprinted by permission.

Unfortunately, little can be concluded about exercise and personality from the research using the 16PF. However, despite the lack of consistent results, it would be premature to disregard this instrument. With better research designs and more emphasis on the second-order factors, the use of the 16PF could yield some solid data. Morgan (1980), citing Kane's (1970) productive use of second-order factors in research with athletes, offered that not enough focus on second-order factors may cause the negative results that are often found in 16PF research. Perhaps a more sophisticated analysis of the data from 16PF research might also yield new insights into the relationships between personality and aspects of exercise and fitness.

The Minnesota Multiphasic Personality Inventory (MMPI)

The MMPI (Hathaway & McKinley, 1948), a comprehensive personality measure comprising 13 subscales, was developed primarily as a clinical tool to identify psychopathology. However, it has also been used extensively with normal adults for a variety of purposes, including exercise and fitness research. Unfortunately, consistent results have not been forthcoming. As early as the 1950s the MMPI was employed in a study of 256 entering male college students that compared aspects of personality and level of physical fitness (Weber, 1953). This correlational study found no relationships between four items of fitness and nine subscales of the MMPI. In contrast, a nonexperimental study of 65 college men participating in an aerobic conditioning program observed several correlations between changes in personality and improved fitness (Sharp & Reilley, 1975). Surprisingly, subjects who initially scored highest on the aerobic tests also made the most psychological gains, while subjects with the lowest initial aerobic scores improved more aerobically but gained less psychologically.

Two other studies also illustrate the inconsistent results from studies using the MMPI. A comparison of physically active and sedentary men found the active group to be less depressed and more extroverted (Lobstein, Mosbacher, & Ismail, 1983). Although depression was the strongest discriminator between the groups, narcissistic tendencies and enthusiasm were more pronounced among active subjects, and social introversion more prevalent among sedentary subjects. In contradiction to these findings, a study that compared female controls (sedentary women) with women who participated in a walk-jog program for 15 weeks observed no significant improvements in personality as measured by the MMPI (Penny & Rust, 1980). Specific physiological changes were not reported.

An investigation that used the MMPI to study the personality structure of ultramarathoners produced some interesting results (Folkins & Wieselberg-Bell, 1981). The subjects included 42 men and 4 women who participated in a 100-mile race over rugged terrain. All MMPI scale means were within the clinically normal range for the entire group, however there were some interesting differences between those who finished the race and those who dropped out. Finishers tended to score higher on the psychopathic deviance scale and on the depression and schizophrenia scales. High scores on psychopathic deviance are associated with lack of social conformity, which shows a degree of shallowness in relations with others. This observation seems to be consistent with the behavior of the successful ultramarathoner, who must spend a lot of time in training and away from significant others. It was suggested that tolerance for deviant experiences may be an asset for participants in endurance events of this sort. Runners who scored higher on the MMPI are perhaps better equipped to cope with the extreme psychological states that can occur during such a demanding race, such as paranoid and hallucinatory episodes and prolonged sensory deprivation. The researchers emphasized the speculative nature of their observations and the need for further study.

Several researchers have employed the MMPI in studies of cardiac patients, again with mixed results.

Naughton, Bruhn, and Lategola (1968) noted slight improvement in hypochondriasis (a morbid concern with one's health) and depression scores for cardiac patients who participated in a program of physical training. In a study of the effect of an exercise-based rehabilitation program on 44 depressed patients, Kavanagh, Shephard, Tuck, and Qureshi (1977) observed a significant decrease in depression scores over 4 years. Scores for hysteria, hypochondriasis, and neuroticism were reduced also. In another study of cardiac patients, a comparison between program dropouts and compliers revealed several significant group differences (Blumenthal et al., 1982). Dropouts scored higher on social introversion and anxiety, and lower on ego strength. Additionally, compliers had lower hypochondriasis and depression scores.

The Eysenck Personality Inventory (EPI)

The EPI and its predecessor, the Maudsley Personality Inventory (MPI), have been used in several studies on exercise and personality (Eysenck, 1959; Eysenck & Eysenck, 1964). Both instruments were designed to measure extroversion and neuroticism. A lie scale is included in each instrument to identify subjects who tend to answer in a socially desirable fashion.

Considered biological in nature, Eysenck's theory of personality assumes that individual differences in extroversion are related to nervous system functioning. Introverts are assumed to have a more active ascending reticular system than extroverts, and are therefore assumed to be chronically more aroused and more responsive to stimulation (Brody, 1988). If this theory is correct, extroverts should be able to tolerate pain better than introverts. Indeed, a preliminary study of distance runners found extroversion to be associated with better performances in a 1,500-meter run (Briggs, Sandstrom, & Nettleton, 1979).

Individual differences in neuroticism are assumed to be related to the functioning of what Eysenck calls the "visceral brain," consisting of the hippocampus, amygdala, cingulum, septum, and hypothalamus, which control the emotions (Brody, 1988). Neurotic individuals are believed to have hyperarousable visceral brain systems, which predispose them to respond to emotional events with greater intensity than people who are not neurotic (Brody, 1988). Eysenck's theories on extroversion and neuroticism have been used in several studies related to fitness and sports performance. In addition, Morgan (1985a) has incorporated these constructs of extroversion and neuroticism in studies of elite athletes as well as in his mental health model for success in sports.

Another study using Eysenckian theory and the MPI compared 11- to 13-year-old male swimmers and nonswimmers. The results showed significant differences in both extroversion and neuroticism (Whiting & Stembridge, 1965). Nonswimmers were found to be more introverted and neurotic than swimmers. The results were consistent with the Eysenckian theory that introverts are more prone to phobias and anxiety because of their conditionability (their tendency to condition easily to fear). The researchers surmised that early unpleasant experiences in the water had a more distressing and lasting effect on the introverted and neurotic subjects. Teachers of nonswimmers found greater awareness of personality factors helpful in teaching the persistent nonswimmer.

Using the MPI, Massie and Shephard (1971) found significant increases in extroversion and decreases in neuroticism among participants in a YMCA "low gear" fitness class. The researchers believed these findings were the result of the increased social contacts associated with the group setting and the greater sense of well-being engendered by involvement in the program. Higher extroversion and lower neuroticism scores have also been found to be related to muscular strength in a correlational study of college men (Tucker, 1983). These results were corroborated in a subsequent study (Tucker, 1984). Of particular interest in the follow-up study were the changes that resulted from strength training. Although subjects who were extroverted and low in neuroticism were stronger initially, subjects who were introverted and neurotic realized greater strength increases over the course of the 4-month program.

Even though the studies presented here are far from conclusive, an awareness of the potential for personality change, particularly in extroversion-introversion and neuroticism, could be helpful to the exercise and fitness practitioner in the future. If involvement in group programs can be shown to exert a positive influence on the personalities of the participants, exercise professionals can further strengthen the program's rationale and justification.

THE EFFECTS OF PERSONALITY TYPE ON EXERCISE AND FITNESS

There have been numerous attempts to classify people into broad personality types based on preconceived ideas about how certain characteristics or habits relate to behavior. For example, law enforcement personnel use specific profiles when trying to spot potential offenders. Classification schemes can also help medical personnel identify maladies. A physician knows that a specific group of symptoms, usually referred to as syndromes, may indicate a particular disease or disorder. Some of the attempts to predict future behaviors or the outcomes of certain behaviors based on personality characteristics have been successful. We shall now review several theoretical typologies relevant to exercise and fitness.

Type A

The Type A behavior pattern is of considerable interest and importance to the exercise professional. Two cardiologists, Meyer Friedman and Ray Rosenman, developed the notion of the link between emotional traits and heart disease by carefully observing patient behaviors for several years and questioning the patients extensively about their lives (Friedman & Rosenman, 1974). They found that the Type A behavior pattern involved a chronic sense of time urgency, an excess of competitive drive, and an easily aroused hostility. The antithesis of the Type A behavior pattern was called Type B. Type B individuals do not exhibit the same degree of time urgency nor excessive competitiveness or free-floating hostility.

Originally, the most salient characteristic of Type A people was believed to be the habitual sense of time urgency or what Friedman and Rosenman (1974) referred to as "hurry sickness." Other important descriptors of the classic Type A person included the need to quantitatively accumulate material objects, a basic insecurity of status, an excess of aggression, impatience with others, and the tendency to try to do two or more things at once. Recent research refined the Type A construct, particularly with respect to the disease-producing elements. It is now suspected that the anger-hostility components may be the most significant disease-related characteristic, although some researchers believe that chronic and global cynicism may portend the greatest risk of cardiovascular disease (Girdano, Everly, & Dusek, 1990). Despite the disagreement on the exact mechanisms involved, few challenge the idea that individuals manifesting Type A behavior bear an increased risk of developing coronary heart disease (Roskies, 1983). One recent meta-analytic study did, however, question the existence of a coronary-prone personality and suggested instead the possibility of a "disease-prone" personality (Friedman & Booth-Kewley, 1987).

The results of almost 30 years of research have established links between Type A behavior and aspects of cardiovascular health. It has been demonstrated that the Type A behavior pattern is significantly more pronounced in subjects who already have heart disease. The vulnerability of Type A subjects to the development of cardiovascular disease has also been verified. Moreover, a cluster of coronary biochemical abnormalities in Type A people has been identified. Finally, the experimental inducement of Type A behavior followed by coronary symptoms has been successfully demonstrated in laboratory animals (Friedman & Rosenman, 1974).

Although the causes of Type A behavior have not been conclusively determined, considerable evidence points to the sociocultural environment as the likely origin (Girdano et al., 1990). Parental expectations and high standards of performance coupled with the cultural values of hard work and achievement are thought to be important influences on Type A development. Paradoxically, many of the behaviors rewarded by North American culture are the very behaviors that may foster the development of cardiovascular disease (Girdano et al., 1990). As Roskies (1983) pointed out, many healthy Type A individuals are likely to be ambivalent about changing behaviors that are prized by society. Furthermore, there is little social pressure to undertake treatment for Type A behaviors.

Exercise and the Type A Behavior Pattern

Efforts to modify Type A behavior through a variety of treatment programs have met with mixed success. Of interest to us are investigations that have used exercise as the intervention procedure. Several researchers have reported preliminary support for the notion of aerobic exercise as a way to reduce Type A behavior (Blumenthal, Williams, Williams, & Wallace, 1980; Jasnoski, Cordray, Houston, & Osness, 1987; Jasnoski & Holmes, 1981). Design limitations or methodological problems in these studies prohibit the conclusion that exercise is effective in modifying Type A behaviors, but the results are encouraging. However, two well-designed experimental studies have produced conflicting results. The first investigation compared the effectiveness of aerobic exercise, weight training, and cognitive-behavioral stress management in modifying behavioral and cardiovascular reactivity of healthy Type A people to psychosocial stressors (Roskies et al., 1986). Both exercise treatments were significantly less effective

than the cognitive-behavioral intervention in reducing behavioral reactivity. None of the three treatment groups significantly reduced physiological reactivity, as measured by heart rate and blood pressure, to stressful laboratory tasks. These results led the researchers to question the ability of behavioral treatments in general to modify physiological arousal and the ability of existing measures to accurately assess changes. They also questioned the relevance of physiological reactivity as an outcome measure in treatment programs for Type A people.

Overcoming many of the methodological problems of previous studies, Blumenthal and associates (1988) compared Type A subjects randomly assigned to an aerobics treatment group or to a strength and flexibility group. After a 12-week program, researchers found that participation in both groups was associated with reductions in overt behavioral manifestations of Type A mannerisms, but the group that received aerobic training was clearly more successful in reducing cardiovascular reactivity to mental stress. These results seemed to support the use of aerobic exercise as a means of reducing cardiovascular risk among healthy Type A people.

Although it would be premature to conclude that exercise effectively reduces the cardiovascular risks associated with Type A behavior, results such as these are certainly encouraging. However, corroborating research is necessary, as well as studies of how reactivity is reduced.

Internal Versus External Control of Reinforcement

Over the past 25 years the concept of reinforcement control has been applied to many forms of behavior. Rotter (1966) developed the idea of reinforcement control to distinguish between people based on whether they attribute reinforcement to their actions or to outside forces. When people perceive reinforcement as the result of luck, chance, fate, or as controlled by others, they believe in external control. When they believe that reinforcement is contingent on their own behavior or on some relatively permanent personal characteristic, they believe in internal control (Rotter, 1966).

An individual learns to differentiate events that are causally related to preceding events from those that are not. It is hypothesized that when a reinforcement is perceived to be contingent on one's own behavior, the occurrence of that behavior will increase the expectancy for that reinforcement. On the other hand, if a reinforcement is perceived as unrelated to one's actions, its occurrence will not increase expectancy for that reinforcement. A person's experiences of various reinforcements is therefore important in determining the degree to which they would attribute reinforcement to their own actions (Rotter, 1966).

In the early research, evidence was presented that supported the hypothesis that people who have a strong belief in their own destiny are likely to behave in the following ways:

■ Be more alert to aspects of the environment that will provide useful information for future behaviors.

■ Take steps to improve one's environmental condition.

■ Place greater value on reinforcement for skill or achievement and be generally more concerned with ability.

■ Resist attempts to influence one's behavior (Rotter, 1966).

Although the locus-of-control construct has been applied to many forms of behavior, health-related behaviors have been of particular interest to researchers. In a review of literature on this topic, Strickland (1978) found support for the position that "internals" tend to engage in precautionary health measures through appropriate remedial strategies more than "externals" when a disease or disorder occurs. There are also indications that the development of an internal locus of control could lead to improved health practices for those who are inclined to believe that life events are beyond their control. However, Strickland cautioned against assuming that internal beliefs are always helpful. Attempts at mastery are most appropriate when events are actually controllable. When internals persist in actions that bring no relief, they may actually make matters worse. Strickland proposed that people learn to specify the reality of their life situation, their possible responses, and the potential for controlling reinforcement.

Another major finding of this review was that congruence of expectancies and situations appears to enhance behavior change. It was suggested that health professionals would be more effective if treatments were tailored to individual expectancies. Externals seem to respond better to conditions in which structure is imposed from outside, while internals prefer situations that permit them to assume responsibility and work independently (Strickland, 1978).

Exercise and Locus of Control

The theory of locus of control could be of considerable importance to exercise and fitness. One would presume that a person with an internal locus of control would be more likely to adopt exercise as a regular practice and would also tend to adhere to a fitness program better than an external person. It would also seem likely that internals would be better able to benefit from individual exercise programs while externals would do better with a highly structured and closely supervised group program. However, the existing research presents a somewhat muddled picture of the relationship between exercise and locus of control. When Slenker, Price, and O'Connell (1985) reviewed the literature, they found six studies that showed a relationship between exercise and internal locus of control and six that did not. The diversity of inventories used in these studies and the array of dependent variables studied were cited as major factors in the disparity of results. With this in mind, we shall discuss the rather modest amount of research on exercise and fitness that has tried to determine locus of control.

Two early studies used Rotter's (1966) general measure of internal-external control termed the I-E Scale. In one study, junior high basketball players had significantly higher scores on internal control than gymnasts and nonparticipants (Lynn, Phelan, & Kiker, 1969). In the second study, Sonstroem and Walker (1973) compared locus of control and attitudes toward physical activity. They found that college men who were internal had more favorable attitudes toward physical activity, had significantly higher fitness scores, and reported significantly more voluntary involvement in exercise than others in the sample. The locus of control of children ages 6 to 14 who participated in an 8-week fitness camp changed significantly, becoming less external and more internal at the end of the program (Duke, Johnson, & Nowicki, 1977). This study used the Children's Internal-External Control Scale (Nowicki & Strickland, 1973).

Following Rotter's (1975) suggestion that measures related to specific behavioral situations would be more predictive for those behaviors than general measures such as the I-E Scale, several instruments have been developed for exercise and fitness behaviors. The Health Locus of Control Scale (HLOC), a popular specific measure, has been used in many studies of health-related behaviors (Wallston, Wallston, Kaplan, & Maides, 1976). The HLOC is an 11-item scale conceived as a unidimensional measure of beliefs regarding the extent to which health is determined by behavior. One of the earlier studies to use the HLOC scale failed to find support for the theoretical expectations regarding HLOC scores and exercise adherence (Dishman & Gettman, 1980). The researchers did find, however, that subjects with low health and fitness scores and an external locus of control were significantly less likely to adhere to a program than subjects with an internal locus and high scores on health and fitness. A recent cross-sectional study that used the HLOC explored the relationship between locus of control and participation in a broad range of physical activities among more than 1,000 college students (Carlson & Petti, 1989). Participation in activities requiring high caloric expenditure was found to be more frequent among subjects with an internal locus of control, while low caloric expenditure activities were associated with an external locus.

A subsequent revision of the HLOC, called the Multidimensional Health Locus of Control Scale (MHLOC), was developed to accommodate a theoretical elaboration that had recast control of reinforcement as a multifactored phenomenon (Wallston, Wallston, & DeVellis, 1978). The revised format included a subscale for internal health locus of control and two subscales related to external control (powerful others and chance). Unfortunately, exercise research using the MHLOC has failed to produce consistent results (Adamson & Wade, 1986; Laffrey & Isenberg, 1983; O'Connell & Price, 1982; Slenker et al., 1985).

In recent years, at least three locus of control scales specific to exercise have been developed. Noland and Feldman (1984, 1985) developed the Exercise Locus of Control (EXLOC) to assess perceived control over one's own exercise behavior. They included scales for internal control, and in addition to scales for the external control of chance and powerful others, they developed a third external scale for environment that incorporated factors related to weather and exercise equipment. In a study using EXLOC with a group of 64 women, only scores on the environment scale were significantly related to exercise behaviors, which indicated that those who believed that the weather and other environmental factors controlled their exercise behaviors tended to exercise less (Noland & Feldman, 1984).

A follow-up study of 434 women revealed important age differences in EXLOC scores (Noland & Feldman, 1985). For women between the ages of 24 and 45, none of the four subscales was related to exercise. For subjects ages 46 to 65, exercise was positively correlated with internal control and negatively correlated with chance and powerful others. In contrast to the earlier study, environmental factors were not related to the exercise behaviors of either group.

A second exercise-specific measure, called the Exercise Objectives Locus of Control Scale (EOLOC), consisted of three subscales representing internal control, chance, and powerful others. McCready and Long (1985) used the scale to study the exercise behaviors of 61 women. Based on the relationship between exercise adherence and scores on EOLOC, locus of control variables were not predictive of program attendance. A second study that used the EOLOC found only a weak relationship between locus of control and exercise initiation (Long & Haney, 1986).

Whitehead and Corbin (1988) introduced another multidimensional measure of locus of control for physical fitness behaviors called the Fitness Locus of Control (FITLOC). Although we could find no research that used this instrument in studies of exercise or fitness behaviors, FITLOC is based on sound rationale and the preliminary reliability and validity studies indicate good potential. We hope that extensive research will result from this development.

Although the utility of the locus of control construct in studies of exercise and fitness may seem rather dubious, we would caution against summarily dismissing it. As better measures are developed and the research using the measure becomes more sophisticated, perhaps locus of control will be found to be of value in predicting exercise involvement. In addition, future complex multidimensional theoretical models of exercise behaviors may find that locus of control interacts with other factors to influence adherence or other exercise behaviors. We hope that research efforts will continue to incorporate this construct. We shall then see more definitively the extent of its usefulness to the exercise practitioner.

Personality Hardiness

One of the more promising lines of research in the study of the stress-illness relationship is one that considers the role of personality as a mediator of the illness-producing effects of stress (Gentry & Kobasa, 1979). Kobasa (1979) conceptualized "hardiness" as a personality style that enables one to withstand or effectively cope with potentially stressful situations with minimal debilitating effects. *Hardiness* consists of three traits: a sense of personal control over external events; a sense of involvement, commitment, and purpose in daily life; and flexibility in adapting to unexpected changes by perceiving such changes as challenges or opportunities for further growth (Gentry & Kobasa, 1979). Gentry and Kobasa believe that the combination of these characteristics mitigates the potentially unhealthy effects of stress and prevents the organismic strain that often leads to physical illness. The relationship between physical illness and the frequency and severity of stressful life events has been demonstrated by several researchers and is illustrated in Figure 4.2.

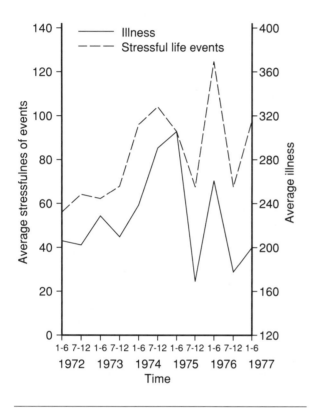

Figure 4.2 Stressful life events and illness over time.

From ''Hardiness and Health: A Prospective Study'' by S.C. Kobasa, S.R. Maddi, and S. Kahn, 1982, *Journal of Personality and Social Psychology,* **42**(1), p. 173. Copyright 1982 by the American Psychological Association. Reprinted by permission.

Initial studies have been generally supportive of the hardiness construct. Kobasa (1979) found high-stress, low-illness executives to exhibit more of the characteristics of hardiness than high-stress, high-illness executives. In an extension of this research, 259 executives were studied for 2 years (Kobasa, Maddi, & Kahn, 1982). High-stress, low-hardiness executives reported twice as much illness as high-stress, high-hardiness executives, and over 3 times as much illness as low-stress executives.

Exercise and Hardiness

Some research has focused on exercise in connection with hardiness and its ability to mitigate the illness-producing effects of stress. Hardiness empowers a person to transform a stressful event by gaining information about the event, acting decisively with regard to it, and learning from the process. Exercise, on the other hand, is thought not to alter stressful events themselves, but to reduce the mental and physical strain that stress produces (Kobasa, Maddi, & Puccetti, 1982). A model of the factors and relationships believed to be important to the stress-illness relationship are shown in Figure 4.3. In this model, personality variables and social support influence the choice of coping styles, which ultimately affect strain and illness outcomes (Gentry & Kobasa, 1979). The model also accounts for other nonpsychosocial susceptibility and resistance factors, specifically constitutional predisposition (family medical history, patterns of coping with stress, and physical and psychological resiliency) and regular physical exercise.

We found two studies that have addressed the hardiness-exercise relationship. In a study involving 137 male business executives, hardiness and exercise were found to interact with stressful events to decrease illness (Kobasa, Maddi, & Puccetti, 1982). Subjects who scored high in both hardiness and exercise remained healthier than those who scored high in only one or the other component. These results seemed to support the notion that personality hardiness and exercise in combination are more effective in preserving health than either one is alone. A later study of 85 business executives extended the resistance resources to include social support with hardiness and exercise (Kobasa, Maddi, Puccetti, & Zola, 1985). Results again emphasized the importance of multiple resistance resources. The more resistance resources available, the less likely one was to become ill. In terms of relative effectiveness, hardiness provided the greatest protection against illness. Although social support and exercise provided some protection from illness, their effects were small compared to the contribution of hardiness.

Although the results of these studies are preliminary, the future for this line of inquiry looks promising. The identification of other resistance resources and the extent to which they help individuals stay healthy should be a priority of future research. Although the contribution of exercise appears to be relatively small, it is nonetheless important to the overall reduction of the unhealthy effects of stress. We should note that the two studies just cited used an inexact technique to

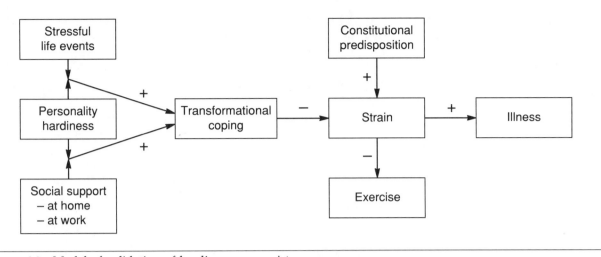

Figure 4.3 Model of validation of hardiness as a resistance resource.

From "Social and Psychological Resources Mediating Stress Illness Relationships in Humans" by W.D. Gentry and S.C. Kobasa. In *Compliance in Healthcare* (p. 111) by R.B. Haynes, D.W. Taylor, and D.L. Sackett (Eds.), 1979, Baltimore: Johns Hopkins University Press. Reprinted by permission.

arrive at an exercise score. Perhaps a more sophisticated method for quantifying exercise would be more instructive of the role it plays in the stress-illness relationship.

Running Addiction

In the past decade there has been a great deal written about running addiction. Although the emphasis is on addiction to running, one would presume that similar forms of addiction could develop with other forms of aerobic exercise, such as swimming or bicycling. Although there is some disagreement about how best to describe an inordinate affinity for and involvement in running, "addiction" is the word most often used in the running and sport psychology literature. However, the phenomenon has also been described as a "compulsion," "dependence," "obsession," and as a "healthy habit" (Sachs & Pargman, 1984). It should be noted that some authors and researchers employ the term "dependence" rather than addiction to avoid some semantic difficulties associated with the latter. These terms are also frequently used interchangeably, which is a practice we shall adopt.

Running addiction is defined as a psychological and/or physiological addiction to regular running that is characterized by withdrawal symptoms after 24 to 36 hours without running (Sachs, 1981). Morgan (1979) cited two basic characteristics of negative addiction. First, negatively addicted runners believe that they need exercise to cope and that they cannot live without running daily. Second, if

deprived of exercise, these runners will experience withdrawal symptoms. Withdrawal symptoms often include anxiety, restlessness, guilt, irritability, tension, and discomfort as well as apathy, sluggishness, lack of appetite, sleeplessness, and headaches. Withdrawal symptoms are brought on when a planned run is missed; they are usually not experienced on an expected off day or rest day. Corroboration of the latter point was recently provided in an investigation of 31 competitive runners that studied the withdrawal effects of taking a regular Sunday break from training (Crossman, Jamieson, & Henderson, 1987).

The presence of withdrawal symptoms is considered crucial in determining the existence and the degree of addiction (Sachs & Pargman, 1984). The study of withdrawal effects has been somewhat difficult because few regular runners are willing to give up a workout in the name of research (Sachs, 1981). A study in which one group of runners that missed a regular workout was compared with another group that ran as usual found that the group did not run had higher depression scores and higher galvanic skin response scores (Thaxton, 1982). These results showed that even slight variations in training may have negative effects on regular runners.

There has been considerable discussion as to whether or not exercise, and running in particular, can actually become addictive or whether perceptions or withdrawal are due to one's expectations or a placebo effect. Sachs and Pargman (1984) suggested that addiction is a process rather than a condition, and therefore is not an all-or-none state.

From this perspective, addiction is an extension of ordinary behavior or ordinary behavior taken to the point of dependence, compulsion, or pathology. Addiction is therefore considered to result from a high degree of involvement with a substance or an activity, rather than a result of the drug or activity itself (Sachs & Pargman, 1984). When viewed this way, one can see that exercise can indeed be addictive.

Positive Addiction

An influential point of view presented several years ago saw running addiction as a positive, rather than a negative, phenomenon. This notion was popularized by William Glasser (1976) in his book, *Positive Addiction*. Glasser maintained that exercise improves psychological and physical strength, and that running is the hardest but surest way to achieve a positive addiction (Glasser, 1976). Glasser identified several criteria for attaining a positive addiction:

■ The activity must be something one chooses to do.

■ It must have some value to the person.

■ It must be something the person can become proficient in and can do on his or her own.

■ The activity must have sufficient worth for a person to devote about an hour a day to it.

■ The activity must have an inherent value for the person to persevere long enough to become positively addicted.

Once the positive addiction is established, failure to continue is marked by withdrawal symptoms such as pain, discomfort, anxiety, or guilt (Glasser, 1976). Even if one meets all of the criteria for a positive addiction, not everyone is able to achieve this state. To become addicted, one needs to practice the activity several times each week for as much as an hour each time. It may, however, take up to a year to attain the addictive state, if it is attained at all (Glasser, 1976).

One study found that college students who exercised regularly tended to fit an addictive personality profile (Kagan & Squires, 1985). The more the subjects exercised the more they fit an addictive profile. Men who exercised the most, scored higher on rigidity and compulsiveness, while women who exercised the most seemed to be noncompulsive but hard-driving. Both men and women who ran as their primary form of exercise had addiction scores that equaled or exceeded the cutoff score for alcohol addiction.

Regular exercise was apparently used most heavily by students who were most likely to experience high levels of stress. It was speculated that exercise provided a form of release for these subjects. The researchers concluded that, in terms of personality characteristics, individuals can become addicted to regular exercise.

How pervasive is exercise addiction among regular runners? A study of 345 runners found that most runners experienced deprivation sensations when they were unable to run (Robbins & Joseph, 1985). Over 50% of respondents reported feelings of restlessness, irritability, frustration, guilt, and fatigue. In a study of 459 Australian marathoners, subjects reported an even higher level of discomfort when a planned run was missed (Summers, Machin, & Sargent, 1983). In this study, 83% of the marathoners experienced these sensations. Although men and women reported similar levels of running commitment, the women perceived themselves to be more addicted to running and to experience more withdrawal symptoms than the men did. In another study of over 300 runners who were attempting their first marathon, 48% claimed to have experienced a runner's high, which is considered a prerequisite for running addiction (Summers, Sargent, Levey, & Murray, 1982). However, only 24% reported achieving a runner's high during the marathon in which they were being studied. About half of the subjects reported withdrawal symptoms when training was interrupted. The researchers computed an addiction score based on questionnaire items. They found that 17.4% were highly addicted to running and that 46% were moderately addicted. In contrast, research with 20 elite swimmers who were studied after 2 days and 5 days away from training failed to provide evidence of withdrawal (Crossman et al., 1987). Despite self-reports of being addicted to swimming, subjects showed no significant changes in mood or anxiety during the layoff period.

Negative Addiction

Although addiction to running is generally positive and desirable, it is not without a potentially negative side. For a minority of runners who are positively addicted, running may gradually move from being important and central to being controlling and dominating.

Morgan (1979) has described the symptoms associated with negative addiction as needing daily exercise to cope and believing that one cannot live without running every day, experiencing withdrawal symptoms after a layoff, and continuing to exercise when it causes vocational, social, and even medical problems. The last symptom is probably the most telling with respect to a negative exercise addiction. Hard-core addicts persist in running despite tendinitis, stress fractures, and medical advice to the contrary, often to the point that overuse injuries become crippling. They also tend to give their daily runs higher priority than job, family, or friends. Placing running first often puts the other aspects of the runner's life at risk. The need to devote 3 to 4 hours a day to running leaves little time for a spouse, children, or friends. The addict's career is also likely to suffer.

A study that investigated the conflict between runners and their spouses found significant problems such as neglect, loss of shared interests and friends, fatigue, and neglect of work to be consistently related to commitment to running (Robbins & Joseph, 1980). This study also revealed that 42% of highly committed runners had reappraised a relationship because of their involvement in running.

Can exercise addicts recognize their dependent state? Some may be aware of an inordinate amount of time and effort devoted to running and may even be conscious of some deterioration in other aspects of their lives. Like most other "junkies" however, most feel that they are in control. The exercise-dependent person may therefore need help coming to terms with their problem. Some addicted runners may require therapy, while others can profit from an educational approach. The exercise practitioner should provide information about exercise addiction, particularly symptoms of the condition, and be available to talk with clients about this problem. The information contained in Table 4.1 would be valuable to a person struggling with this problem.

Through his clinical experience, Morgan (1979) noted that serious runners tend to turn inward and begin to adopt unconventional priorities when they reach about 100 miles a week.

Of course, the point at which running becomes addictive varies widely with the individual. A good indication that one's involvement with running may be getting out of hand is the need for ever-increasing dosages of running. Similar to "junkies" who develop tolerances for their drug habits, the running addict requires more frequent, more intense, and longer runs to experience a runner's high (Morgan, 1979).

There are few theoretical perspectives to help us understand this phenomenon. One helpful model is a typology of commitment to running developed by Joseph and Robbins (1981) that identifies four levels of involvement:

Table 4.1   Proposed Diagnostic Criteria for "Exercise Dependence"

(A) Narrowing of repertoire leading to a stereotyped pattern of exercise with a regular schedule once or more daily

(B) Salience with the individual giving increasing priority over other activities to maintaining the pattern of exercise

(C) Increased tolerance to the amount of exercise performed over the years

(D) Withdrawal symptoms related to a disorder of mood following the cessation of the exercise schedule

(E) Relief or avoidance of withdrawal symptoms by further exercise

(F) Subjective awareness of a compulsion to exercise

(G) Rapid reinstatement of the previous pattern of exercise and withdrawal symptoms after a period of abstinence

Associated features

(H) Either the individual continues to exercise despite a serious physical disorder known to be caused, aggravated, or prolonged by exercise and is advised as such by a health professional, or the individual has arguments or difficulties with his partner, family, friends, or occupation

(I) Self-inflicted loss of weight by dieting as a means toward improving performance

From "Exercise Dependence" by M.W. DeCoverly Veale, 1987, *British Journal of Addiction*, **82**, p. 736. Reprinted by permission.

Type I
Running as the most important commitment
Runs 40 miles or more each week and meets some of the following criteria: keeps a log, runs intervals, races at least monthly, reads running literature weekly, more than 50% of friends are runners.

Type II
Running as a crucial commitment
Runs from 11 to 40 miles a week and meets some of the following criteria: doesn't taper during winter or bad weather, races occasionally, runs intervals, maintains a log, reads less than weekly, fewer than 50% of friends are runners.

Type III
Running as a hobby
Runs from 11 to 40 miles a week, but doesn't exhibit as many of the associated behaviors such as racing frequently, keeping a log, or running intervals.

Type IV

The occasional runner

Usually runs less than twice a week, runs less than 11 miles per week, tapers in winter and bad weather.

Pargman (1980) presented another helpful conceptualization. He believed that exercise involvement can be located on a continuum according to the nature and strength of one's motivation. Addiction/dependence (A-D) would represent one end of the continuum and commitment/dedication (C-D), the other. This model hypothesizes that A-D runners tend to participate with less psychological awareness and intellectual understanding about their running and tend to emphasize perceived exhilaration and joy and focus less on motivational or causal factors. A-D runners experience withdrawal symptoms when a need to run is not satisfied. In contrast, C-D runners participate on a more rational and pragmatic basis. Rather than running for the emotional or euphoric feelings, C-D runners understand their reasons for running. Whether it is to lose weight or lower blood pressure, C-D runners are reinforced by successfully achieving their running goals. Rather than loving the running experience and looking forward to it, C-D runners accept and integrate the run into their normal routine.

It is possible for a person to shift position on the continuum. Conceivably a C-D person may come to appreciate the emotional outcomes to the point that instrumental objectives assume less importance and the running experience itself becomes more central.

Explanations of the mechanisms involved in the process of exercise addiction are similar to those used to explain the runner's high phenomenon. These explanations refer to the role of neurotransmitters and endorphins. Other tentative explanations also have interesting possibilities. Robbins and Joseph's (1985) behaviorally based explanation offered two possibilities for withdrawal symptoms. The first is a therapeutic explanation that centers on the use of running as a means of coping with problems and escaping daily tensions, or as a means of modifying dysphoric moods or psychophysiological distress. When running is not available, individuals who depend on it for these reasons are likely to experience deprivation distress. A second behavioral explanation, called a mastery hypothesis, is related to the possible dependence of some runners on the daily reinforcement of competence and self-worth that running provides. Running may be so central to the identity of some runners that they experience distress when forced to miss a workout.

A physiological explanation has recently been offered that hypothesizes that exercise dependence is related to sympathetic arousal (Thompson & Blanton, 1987). Thompson and Blanton suggested that exercise dependence is mediated by adaptive reductions in sympathetic output during exercise, which is a result of the increased efficiency of energy use associated with exercise training. Because of the lowered sympathetic output, a person must engage in ever-increasing levels of exercise to produce pre-training levels of physiological arousal during and immediately following the task. Figure 4.4 shows a model that illustrates the cycle of exercise dependence. This explanation supports the position that exercise dependence is related to the arousal-producing properties of catecholamines.

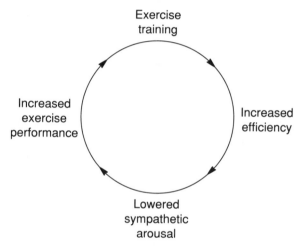

Figure 4.4 The cycle of exercise dependence.

From "Energy Conservation and Exercise Dependence: A Sympathetic Arousal Hypothesis" by J.K. Thompson and P. Blanton, 1987, *Medicine and Science in Sports and Exercise*, **19**(2), p. 96. Copyright © 1987 by the Endocrine Society. Reprinted by permission.

Despite the debate over whether exercise addiction is a true addiction or a well-established habit, a person can engage in regular activity that will result in mental and physical health if it is not taken to extremes. By encouraging and supporting the efforts of our clients while cautioning and monitoring against excesses, the exercise professional may play a crucial role in the client's long-term exercise involvement (Sachs, 1981).

One view of addiction assumes that something cannot be both healthy and addictive. Peele (1981) believed that a true addiction impairs one's functioning. This author advised people to look beyond the short-term gratification of an activity to its overall effect. To determine if the activity is harmful requires an analysis of its impact on other parts of one's life. Exercise, like other activities, can reach a point of diminishing returns. How much exercise does one actually need to realize cardiovascular benefits? How much exercise can a person tolerate before experiencing orthopedic difficulties? How much time can a person devote to exercise without interfering with home, family, or career? These are questions that must be answered individually, but one must be aware of the tradeoffs. Knowing the tradeoffs and evaluating the impact of the activity on the other aspects of one's life are the best guarantees that one will not become addicted (Peele, 1981).

PERSONALITY DISORDERS ASSOCIATED WITH EXERCISE

In this section we discuss two pathological conditions that have been identified as potential problems associated with chronic exercise.

Compulsive Exercise and Anorexia Nervosa

Several clinical reports have linked compulsive running with anorexia nervosa. Norval (1980) dubbed four female patients "running anorexics." These patients were originally seen because of complaints of amenorrhea. Each of the patients was described as an intensive jogger who took part in long-distance races and trained with male runners. All were described as having approximately 80% of normal body weight, but none reported problems with diet or eating-related difficulties. Other clinical reports have found more explicit ties between compulsive running and anorexia (Chalmers, Catalan, Day, & Fairburn, 1985; Waldstreicher, 1985).

Yates (1987) has summarized the research on the connection between running and eating disorders. In fact, most of the research on the possible connection between running and anorexia has been spawned by the research of Yates, Leehey, and Shisslak (1983) who, after interviewing 60 obligatory runners (i.e., runners who were addicted or highly committed), issued a preliminary, highly conjectural report. The report noted that the character, style, and background of obligatory runners were similar to that of anorexia nervosa patients.

Two major differences were also noted: Most anorexics were women while most obligatory runners were men; secondly, most cases of anorexia begin in adolescence, whereas most instances of obligatory running occur in the 3rd to 5th decade of life.

Among the parallels identified were similar family background, socioeconomic circumstances, and personality characteristics. The anorexic woman was described as having been a model child with a hazy sense of self and dependent on the opinions and judgments of others. Anorexic symptoms often occurred during a period of change, and the pursuit of thinness provided an identity, a sense of control, and the opportunity to master a difficult goal.

The qualities identified in compulsive runners that parallel anorexics included an interest in hard work and high achievement. They were also uncomfortable with anger and tended to inhibit the direct expression of emotion. Commitment to running seemed to occur at a time of heightened anxiety, depression, and identity diffusion. By assuming the identity of a runner, they realized a sense of self, a feeling of control over internal and external circumstances, and the ability to master a difficult goal. It was also suggested that both groups may represent a single mode of behavior, characterized by "grim asceticism" and the avoidance of passive, receptive pleasures. Psychological characteristics that may be shared by both groups are introversion and a tendency toward social isolation, as well as compliant and self-effacing behavior (Yates, Leehey, & Shisslak, 1983).

This report elicited a number of research studies and articles that refuted many of its points. A study that tested the hypothesis that the two groups shared common personality traits compared 43 obligatory runners with 24 anorexic patients using the MMPI (Blumenthal, O'Toole, & Chang, 1984). Results indicated that, in general, obligatory runners fell within the normal range of behavior while anorexics did not. The researchers therefore concluded that obligatory runners do not suffer from the same degree of psychopathology as anorexia nervosa patients. In a follow-up article, Blumenthal, Rose, and Chang (1985) commented that a psychopathological or disease model of habitual running was misleading and perjorative. They presented a tentative alternative model that was based on the belief that habitual running is a coping strategy for the regulation of emotion. The basic assumption of the proposed model is that running serves to enhance positive emotions and reduce negative emotions. The habitual runner comes to rely on running as a method of emotional management.

Other researchers have also failed to find support for a connection between running and anorexia nervosa. In a study of 136 male and 64 female runners, Goldfarb and Plante (1984) found no relationship between fear of fat, a central characteristic of anorexia nervosa, and running involvement. They did, however, observe runners to have high obsessive-compulsive and anxious tendencies, which are characteristic of anorexia. It was suggested that perhaps obligatory running and anorexia share an underlying obsessive-compulsive disorder. Overall the data showed that runners represent diverse personalities and are capable of training and competing without signs of psychopathology. A study that compared 31 high-mileage, 18 low-mileage, and 18 nonrunners found similar results (Wheeler, Wall, Belcastro, Conger, & Cumming, 1986). The runners displayed no evidence of psychopathology nor any abnormalities characteristic of anorexia patients. Two additional studies (Knight, Schocken, Powers, Feld, & Smith, 1987; Weight & Noakes, 1987) also found nothing to support the hypothesis of Yates and colleagues (1983).

Although there appears to be little support for a direct connection between habitual running and anorexia, the exercise professional should be alert to clients who show signs of impairing their health and normal occupational and social functioning as a result of exercise. Excessive weight loss in runners may be attributable not to a psychological problem but rather to an overzealous desire to minimize body fat to reach optimal performance levels (Smith, 1980). In most instances, the prognosis for reversing this trend is excellent, especially if the runner is counseled appropriately. The role of the exercise professional in such situations would be to provide the necessary factual information and, perhaps, to analyze the body composition so that the person could see the implications of their current level of exercise. If a client fails to respond appropriately after receiving this type of information, the practitioner should recommend that the person's physician be brought in.

The Athlete's Neurosis

What happens when an "exercise addict" breaks a leg or a person who has lived a very active life for many years suddenly loses the capacity to continue that lifestyle? Or how do physically active people respond to the inevitable decline in physical prowess attributable to aging? Although people respond in highly individual ways to such eventualities, there are some reports of serious psychological problems attributable to loss of one's physical capabilities.

A clinical investigation of 72 neurotic men identified a sizable number who appeared to overvalue health and fitness and who displayed inordinate pride in their previous sickness-free lives (Little, 1969). Characteristic of this group was pride in their excess of physical stamina, strength, and skill. For athletic neurotics, the precipitating factor in the neurotic breakdown was most often a direct threat to their physical well-being in the form of illness or injury. Neurotic symptoms were observed to occur almost immediately following injury. In the case of illness preceding neurosis, both the symptoms of the illness and the additional neurotic symptoms tended to be perpetuated and exaggerated. The neurotic disorders suffered by the athletic subjects (mainly anxiety and reactive depression) were clinically indistinguishable from those seen in nonathletic patients. However, the athletic group reported greater hypochondriacal somatic symptoms and panic attacks. Athletic neurotics, in contrast to nonathletic patients, were virtually void of neurotic markers in their lives before the appearance of the illness or injury. The majority had enjoyed satisfactory personal relationships, were generally outgoing and sociable, and had histories of excellent health.

Little (1969) reported that the incidence of athletic neurosis approximated 40% of new cases of neurotic syndrome. The source of the neurosis in these cases was attributed to the shock of a serious threat to an overvalued and waning physical prowess. The people who are most vulnerable to athlete's neurosis are those who have overvalued physical prowess, which creates a preneurotic vulnerability (Little, 1979). People in such a state of specific vulnerability are thought to be relatively resistant to nonrelevant stressors, but collapse into serious maladjustment when the inevitable stressor finally occurs. Prevention of athlete's neurosis includes a change in attitude and behavior and the broadening of interests before the onset of a debilitating episode. Although the treatment of athlete's neurosis is beyond the capability of the exercise practitioner, some help may be provided to susceptible clients in the way of prevention. For example, the practitioner could encourage the development of other interests and recreational skills that require less physical prowess.

THE SELF-CONCEPT

A major part of an individual's personality can often be inferred from how that person behaves toward oneself. Consistent patterns of self-deprecation or self-aggrandizement are readily apparent, even to casual observers. How people perceive, evaluate, and behave toward themselves is related to self-concept. In this section we will review the theory and research related to self-concept and exercise.

The *self-concept* has been defined and interpreted in many ways. It has been described as the "totality of the individual's thoughts and feelings with reference to himself as object" (Rosenberg, 1979, p. 7). To Combs (1971), *self-concept* refers to those aspects of the perceptual field to which we refer when we say "I" or "me," that is, the organization of perceptions about self that represents who one is. According to this interpretation, self-concept is composed of thousands of perceptions of varying clarity, precision, and importance relating to oneself: who one is, what one stands for, where one lives, what one likes or dislikes, and so on. The self-concept can be viewed as an organization of ideas, an abstraction, or a pattern of perceptions that represent the essence of one's being (Combs, 1971).

Marsh and Shavelson (1985) contended that self-perceptions are formed through experience with and interpretations of one's environment. Self-perceptions are influenced especially by the evaluations of significant others, reinforcements, and attributions for one's own behavior. They described several other features that are considered critical to the understanding of self-concept, including the notion that it is multifaceted—made up of categories such as social self-concept and physical self-concept. Another key element of this conceptualization assumes a hierarchical structure. The overall, or general, self-concept is derived from self-perceptions in all major categories, which in turn are influenced by important subcomponents. The general self-concept is also assumed to be stable. As one descends the hierarchy, self-concept depends increasingly on specific situations and becomes less stable. Change in general self-concept would require many situational experiences that are inconsistent with one's general self-concept. Yet another important characteristic of self-concept is its evaluative character. People judge themselves against absolute standards, such as an Olympic champion who has a seemingly perfect figure, and relative standards, such as peers. People also judge themselves with respect to perceived evaluations of significant others.

Research on Exercise, Fitness, and Self-Concept

Many studies have explored the relationships between exercise and self-concept. Unfortunately much of the research can again be faulted either for design inadequacies or methodological weaknesses. Sonstroem (1984) identified several deficiencies in the research literature, including incomplete and vague research reports, the use of unvalidated or inadequate self-concept measurement scales, inferences of causality from correlational studies, studies that fail to employ control groups, the use of inappropriate statistics, and faulty interpretation of results.

Despite these shortcomings, attempts to prove the potential for exercise and fitness to improve self-concept are not a lost cause. Exercise and fitness programs have excellent potential for promoting self-acceptance and improving one's sense of physical competence (Sonstroem & Morgan, 1989). However, one of the greatest needs at the moment appears to be better scholarship and well-planned, theoretically-based research.

Several reviews of the research have explored the relationship between exercise and self-concept. Folkins and Sime (1981) generally confirmed the assumption that fitness training improves self-concept. This review reported on several experimental studies that found positive changes in self-concept as a result of exercise programs. The researchers suggested that changes in self-concept might be associated with the perception of improved fitness rather than with actual changes in physical fitness.

An extensive review of the research that focused on children's programs (Gruber, 1986) found that changes in self-concept were associated with participation in directed play or physical education programs. Using a voting procedure as well as meta-analysis, Gruber analyzed 84 studies, including 27 controlled experimental studies, and concluded that participation in organized programs of physical activity contributed to the development of self-esteem in elementary school children. Another very important conclusion was that physical fitness activities were superior to other components of an elementary school physical education program in developing self-concept.

Sonstroem's (1984) thorough review of self-concept research classified studies into categories based on their sophistication of the experimental design. In the least rigorous design category, the preexperimental category, Sonstroem reviewed six studies that collectively reported a preponderance of positive results. However, due to the methodological shortcomings of these studies, results should be viewed with skepticism. Among the seven studies classified as quasi-experimental, Sonstroem again found remarkably consistent findings of enhanced self-concept after engaging in exercise programs. In the most rigorous of the research categories, Sonstroem found only four studies that used true experimental designs. All of these studies reported positive changes in self-concept following fitness training. However, even these studies were open to criticism. None of these studies could demonstrate that changes in self-concept were produced by changes in physical fitness. Sonstroem nevertheless concluded that exercise programs seem to be associated with significant increases in self-esteem, and that increases are more pronounced for subjects who are initially lower in self-esteem.

If changes in self-concept do occur as a result of participation in a fitness program, to what do we attribute the change? We have already seen that changes in physical fitness have not yet been directly linked to the changes in self-concept. In Table 4.2, Sonstroem (1984) suggests several possible agents of self-concept change. This is a list of hypothesized agents only and Sonstroem stresses the need for further research.

Another major concern in self-concept research centers on the weaknesses of self-report measures. The lower portion of Table 4.2 identifies some possible influences on self-concept scores. These agents are rarely addressed in fitness and exercise research. Sonstroem concluded his review by making several recommendations for future research.

New Developments in Exercise and Self-Concept Research

Until recently, practically all of the research on physical fitness training and self-concept has used global measures of self-concept. Now more exercise studies are using new multidimensional self-concept measures. A study of the effects of a physically and mentally demanding 26-day Outward Bound experience on 361 participants demonstrated that short-term changes in self-concept may occur and be maintained over time (Marsh, Richards, & Barnes, 1986). Using the Self Description Questionnaire III (SDQ III), which measures 13 facets of self-concept, the dimensions of physical ability and appearance improved significantly over the course of the program, and the gains in both were maintained at an 18-month follow-up.

The SDQ III was also used in a study that compared female athletes and nonathletes for self-concept differences (Marsh & Jackson, 1986). The study found that female athletes had a higher self-concept of physical ability than nonathletes, but there were no differences between the groups with regard to

Table 4.2 Possible Agents for Self-Esteem Change in Exercise Programs

Program agents
  Increase in physical fitness
  Goal achievement
  Feelings of somatic well-being
  Sense of competence, master, or control
  Adoption of associated health behaviors
  Social experiences
  Experimental attention
  Reinforcement of significant others
Score agents
  Self-presentation strategies
  Defensiveness
  Social desirability
  Perceived task demands
  Expectancy, suggestion
  Perceived leader or group pressures

From "Exercise and Self-Esteem" by R.J. Sonstroem. In *Exercise and Sport Sciences Reviews Vol. 12* (p. 139) by R.L. Terjung (Ed.), 1984, New York: Macmillan. Used by permission of Macmillan Publishing Company.

self-concept of physical appearance. Female athletes had much higher self-concepts of physical ability and placed a higher value on this dimension than nonathletes. No other self-concept differences were significant, although athletes were slightly higher on general self-concept than nonathletes. This pattern of results was consistent with studies on high school and young adult groups.

A study that compared SDQ III scores of female high school students in a cooperative fitness group with those in a competitive group found cooperation to be more effective in improving self-concept of physical ability (Marsh & Peart, 1988). Although both groups realized significant fitness gains, self-concept scores for physical ability in the competitive group declined over the course of the 6-week program, while they improved for the cooperative group. The researchers suggested that the competitive program forced participants to compare their physical abilities with the most physically able to a much greater degree than in the cooperative group. Moreover, in a setting with few winners and many losers, the average level of self-concept is likely to decline.

The recent publication of a new self-concept instrument specific to the physical domain should be of considerable interest to exercise researchers and practitioners (Fox & Corbin, 1989). This instrument, titled the Physical Self-Perception Profile, assumes a multidimensional, hierarchical structure for the physical self, which is presumed to

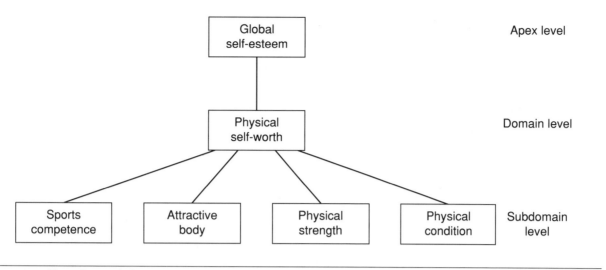

Figure 4.5 Hypothesized three-tier hierarchical organization of self-perceptions.

From "The Physical Self-Perception Profile: Development and Preliminary Validation" by K.R. Fox and C.B. Corbin, 1989, *Journal of Sport and Exercise Psychology,* **11**, p. 414. Copyright 1989 by Human Kinetics Publishers, Inc.. Reprinted by permission.

be an important aspect of global self-esteem. As shown in Figure 4.5, the components of "physical self-worth" include sports competence, body attractiveness, physical strength, and physical condition. Preliminary research results have generally supported theoretical expectations. Physical self-worth seems to function as the generalized outcome of perceptions in the four subdomains of the physical self. Physical self-worth also has been shown to be a mediator of the relationship between each of the subdomains and global self-esteem.

Another recent development of considerable interest is a suggested model and recommended methodology for investigating self-concept changes resulting from exercise (Sonstroem & Morgan, 1989). The proposed model, shown in Figure 4.6, is hierarchically arranged with specific physical self-efficacy judgments at the base and global self-esteem at the apex. Changes in lower level elements are assumed to be instrumental to changes in higher order self-conceptions. The model depicts a horizontal dimension that represents testing done before and after an intervention program. Although the suggested model is considered tentative, it appears to be an excellent beginning toward building a better understanding of physical dimensions as they relate to global self-concept.

TRENDS IN EXERCISE AND PERSONALITY RESEARCH

With the exception of the new surge in research on self-concept, there has been a very obvious decline in exercise and personality research in recent years, particularly in research that uses standard instruments such as the MMPI, 16PF, EPI, and similar personality measurements. This decline may be due to a loss of interest in the topic or to frustration caused by the inconsistent findings from among the myriad of studies already completed. The diminution of interest certainly cannot be attributed to having learned all we need to know about the topic. For example, we still do not know with any certainty if regular exercise participation results in personality change or if certain personality types are attracted to specific types of activity.

However, the general trend toward a weakening of interest does not appear to extend to all aspects of the exercise-personality relationship. Interest is still quite strong in some of the special topical areas such as hardiness, Type A behavior, and especially self-concept. It could very well be that there is interest in these areas because of the better theory available.

An interesting new development is a theoretical system that proposes that exercise and personality are integrally linked. Proponents of this system believe that personality can be deliberately changed through a form of exercise chosen specifically for a particular person (Gavin, 1988). Through self-assessment, a profile is developed for the dimensions of psychosocial characteristics, body strengths and weaknesses, and movement. The psychosocial characteristics include sociability, spontaneity, self-discipline, aggressiveness, competitiveness, concentration, and risk tolerance. The

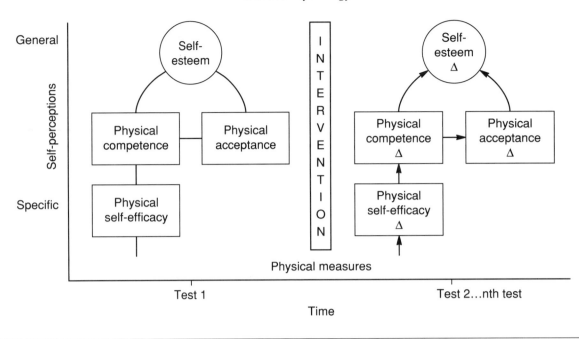

Figure 4.6 Proposed model for examining exercise and self-esteem interactions.

From "Exercise and Self-Esteem: Rationale and Model" by R.J. Sonstroem and W.P. Morgan, 1988, *Medicine and Science in Sport and Exercise,* **21**(3), p. 333. Copyright © 1988 by the Endocrine Society. Reprinted by permission.

body assessment rates strength, flexibility, and shape, and analyzes characteristic attitudes and symbolic meanings of various areas of the body. The movement assessment rates preferences regarding force, control, linearity, speed, and extension.

After a person's profile has been developed, 12 popular sports and fitness activities are classified based on their contribution to the psychosocial, physical, and movement dimensions. With this approach, people are supposedly able to choose activities that can help them move toward a desirable personality change. The system has many interesting possibilities for research as well as for practical application. Unfortunately, there is no published research that we can find that addresses any portion of the theory, so we are unable to judge its merits other than by intuition. We would hope that research is forthcoming. Such a model would be a valuable aid to exercise practitioners in helping clients to select appropriate activities.

SUMMARY

The relationship between exercise and personality has been a favorite topic of researchers for approximately 3 decades. However, despite the extensive research, few generalizations can be made with confidence about the effects of exercise or improved physical fitness on personality. A major reason for the lingering ambiguity is the lack of a theoretical model to explain the relationships between personality variables and exercise. The paucity of controlled experimental research is another factor that hinders understanding. Although findings are far from conclusive, regular exercise and improved physical fitness seem to be associated with emotional stability, self-assurance, extroversion, and low levels of neuroticism. Whether or not exercise effectively reduces the emotional reactivity associated with Type A behavior is still a matter of debate, as is the question of the relationship between exercise and locus of control. Addiction to aerobic exercise, usually running, is characterized by unpleasant withdrawal symptoms if workouts are missed. Exercise addiction may have positive or negative consequences, and clients should be cautioned to balance exercise with other aspects of their lives. Recent developments in self-concept theory and research show the physical dimension to be an important component of global self-esteem. Participation in exercise programs has consistently been associated with increases in self-esteem in children and adults.

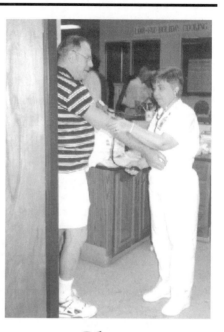

Chapter 5
Theoretical Models of Exercise Behaviors

Reflective of the infancy of exercise psychology, the current theoretical explanations of exercise are best described as tentative and limited. So far, few efforts have been made to develop theories unique to exercise, although some researchers have attempted to adapt existing psychological theories to explain and predict exercise behaviors. The complexity of these models ranges from very simple to the elaborate and detailed. We will review some of the more promising theories and the research they have spawned.

A knowledge of theory can help exercise practitioners understand the key elements associated with initiating and maintaining exercise behaviors. It can also help them evaluate changes in behavior that occur as a result of a planned intervention. Perhaps a brief introduction to the nature and

functions of theory would be helpful before we discuss specific theories.

A theory is a set of conventions created to represent significant aspects of human behavior. To develop a theory to explain certain behaviors, assumptions must be made about the nature of those behaviors (Wrightsman, 1972). In setting forth a theory, the relevant assumptions are systematically linked to each other and a set of empirical definitions are provided. There are rules that govern the systematic interaction between the assumptions and associated concepts (Hall & Lindzey, 1978). Put differently, a theory presents a set of interrelated constructs, definitions, and propositions that form a systematic view of phenomena by specifying relationships among variables (Kerlinger, 1973).

Theories have several important functions. By providing a unified set of constructs and relationships, theory enables one to organize and interpret large pieces of information and to incorporate known empirical findings in a logically consistent and reasonably simple framework (Wrightsman, 1972). Secondly, theory leads to the expansion of knowledge by spurring research. The usefulness of a theory is determined by its verifiability, or its capacity to generate predictions that can be confirmed, and its comprehensiveness. Ideally, a theory should lead to accurate predictions of certain empirical events (Hall & Lindzey, 1978).

For exercise practitioners, theory is most useful when it enables them to predict certain behaviors and provide guidance in planning interventions. For example, a theory of exercise adherence would identify and describe the factors relevant to adherence. This knowledge would then enable the practitioner not only to plan programs effectively, but also to predict which clients are most likely to drop out. Armed with this information, the practitioner could then plan suitable interventions.

A notion about how certain phenomena relate does not constitute a theory. The term *theory* should be reserved for more extensive and elaborate systems of ideas (Bannister & Francella, 1971). In apparent recognition of this principle, many authors and researchers do not call their conceptualizations *theories*, but *theoretical models*, which implies something less than a true theory. This is not to imply that theoretical models are not useful, but they should be considered as preliminary or tentative theories that are subject to elaboration and refinement.

PSYCHOLOGICAL MODEL FOR PHYSICAL ACTIVITY PARTICIPATION

One of the rare theoretical models to address participation in physical activity was developed by Sonstroem and colleagues (Neale, Sonstroem, & Metz, 1969; Sonstroem, 1974, 1976, 1978). Sonstroem's research using the Physical Estimation and Attraction Scales (PEAS) is based on a paradigm that explains the relationship between involvement in physical activity and self-esteem (Sonstroem, 1978). This paradigm, although represented as tentative and incomplete, is one of the few models involving fitness that allows the testing of hypotheses. Moreover, the PEAS is useful in measuring attitude change. Sonstroem's theoretical model is an attempt to identify mechanisms of participation in physical activity

and the psychological benefits derived from one's involvement (Sonstroem & Kampper, 1980). Figure 5.1 summarizes the major elements of the model.

Stated simply, it is assumed that involvement in physical activity increases physical ability, which raises one's physical self-estimation and leads to higher levels of overall self-esteem. Because people with high self-esteem take pride in their bodies, they continue to exercise, thereby maintaining or increasing fitness. Additional physical activity leads to increased perceptions of physical ability and heightened self-esteem, which results in even greater attraction to physical activity, and the cycle continues. According to the model, physical estimation (EST) and attraction (ATTR) exert mediating influences in relationships between physical fitness, physical activity, and self-esteem. As we shall see, there are parallels between this model and self-efficacy theory.

In developing the EST scale, the researchers assumed that perceptions of physical ability were a subcategory of global self-esteem and believed that physical estimation played a mediating role between physical ability and self-esteem. Although early research failed to find significant relationships between physical fitness and global self-esteem, both physical fitness and self-esteem were positively associated with EST scores, which supported the notion of physical estimation as a mediating variable (Sonstroem, 1976, 1978). As seen in the model, self-esteem may influence physical estimation, and physical estimation may influence self-esteem. It was also believed that physical estimation, rather than physical fitness or self-esteem,

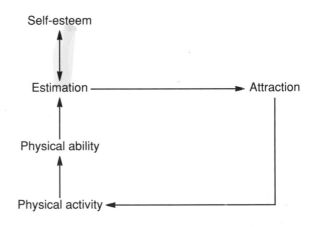

Figure 5.1 Psychological model for physical activity.

From "Physical Estimation and Attraction Scales: Rationale and Research" by R.J. Sonstroem, 1978, *Medicine and Science in Sport and Exercise*, **10**(2), p. 101. Copyright © 1978 by the American College of Sports Medicine. Reprinted by permission.

influenced a person's attraction to, or interest in, physical activity.

Early research using the PEAS to test the theoretical model concluded that although physical ability was not directly related to global self-esteem, perceptions of physical ability as measured by EST was significantly related to self-esteem (Sonstroem, 1976). Secondly, perceptions of physical ability were related to interest in physical activity as well as to the actual level of physical performance. A third conclusion was that favorable perceptions of physical ability are related to an absence of maladjustment, neuroticism, and personality disorder. Finally, interest in vigorous physical activity corresponded with actual level of physical activity (Sonstroem, 1978).

A subsequent study (Sonstroem & Kampper, 1980) attempted to improve the predictive ability of the theoretical model by adding the locus of control construct. This study, which involved male adolescents, found both the PEAS and the psychological model to be effective in predicting initial exercise involvement, but of no value in predicting exercise adherence. The general locus of control measure failed to enhance the ability of the model to predict exercise behavior. The authors suggested that if attitude scales were more specifically related to the populations and behaviors being studied, they might be more effective in predicting exercise involvement.

Both the model and the PEAS were based on data obtained primarily from male adolescents. Fox, Corbin, and Couldry (1985) were the first to test the entire model with college-age men and women. This study found that the Attraction (ATTR) scale contributed to the model for the men but not for the women. Physical estimation did, however, emerge as a key factor in the relationships between self-esteem, fitness, and involvement in physical activity for both the men and the women. Somewhat surprisingly, EST scores were more highly correlated with self-esteem for women than for men (.53 for women and .30 for men). The researchers speculated that this finding may reflect the recent increase in interest among women in sport and exercise, as well as the greater emphasis now being placed on women having a strong, fit body.

Although this study supported the model overall, it was recommended that future research use scales that are more specifically related to individual perceptions of the importance of physical activity and scales designed to measure attraction to specific categories of activity, rather than a general attraction. It was also suggested that perceived

physical ability as measured by EST may in fact be a two-dimensional construct represented by perceived health-related fitness and perceived ability in sports. If this is the case, specific measures of each would probably be more helpful in predicting involvement in physical activity.

An extensive study of the psychometric properties of the PEAS yielded several findings with interesting implications for using the scales with adults (Safrit, Wood, & Dishman, 1985). One particularly useful finding was that the instrument could be shortened without weakening it psychometrically. Moreover, 12 items on the EST scale were found to be appropriate for both men and women, permitting gender comparisons on physical self-estimation. The ATTR scale, however, was not found to be effective in appraising attitude toward participation in physical activity. The study also found that the attraction factor was stronger for women than for men, which led to the suggestion that separate ATTR scales be used for men and women.

Although researchers have pointed out several aspects of the theoretical model and the associated instrument that require future research, the results are generally encouraging with respect to their ability to explain involvement in physical activity. Especially noteworthy is the apparent durability of the physical estimation component, which has held up well in several studies (Safrit et al., 1985).

In a critique of the psychological model for physical activity participation, Sonstroem (1988) acknowledged the ineffectiveness of the model in predicting exercise adherence. This lack of predictive power was attributed to several factors. First of all, interest in or attraction to exercise and believing oneself to be capable of exercise may not be sufficient to sustain exercise. A second weak spot in the predictive utility of the model is contained in the PEAS items, particularly those that comprise the ATTR scale. Because they were developed for young men, many of the items have little relevance to the exercise behaviors of adults. Finally, recent interpretations of attitude theory tend to discount the ability of broad attitudes toward an object (such as exercise) to predict subsequent behavior. It should be noted, however, that the ATTR scale has, in several instances, successfully predicted initial attraction to exercise.

The psychological model for physical activity participation may have some limited value for the exercise practitioner. The model may help in understanding the relationship between physical activity and self-esteem. It may also help in planning interventions. If practitioners were to use this model as a guide to enhance clients' self-esteem or encourage continued participation, they would focus on the physical activity and physical ability levels of the model. The practitioner would make every effort to get a client off to a good start, and then closely monitor gains and emphasize these improvements to the client. We would then expect this awareness of increased physical abilities to raise physical estimation and ultimately overall self-esteem. Heightened physical abilities and increased physical estimation would be expected to encourage continued participation in physical activity. Although these suggestions for intervention are speculative, this use of the model would provide a way to test the effectiveness of such interventions.

The ATTR scale may also be of some value in predicting potential program candidates, but neither scale is likely to provide useful information about exercise adherence.

THE HEALTH BELIEF MODEL

The health belief model (HBM) has been one of the most enduring theoretical models associated with preventive health behaviors. Considered a psychosocial model, it was developed to help predict compliance with preventive health recommendations. The model has been described as a "value-expectancy" model. In other words, behavior is predicted based on the value one places on an outcome and on one's expectation that a given behavior will lead to that outcome. It is assumed that people will not comply with preventive health recommendations unless they have minimum levels of motivation and relevant information, perceive themselves as potentially vulnerable and the condition as threatening, believe in the efficacy of the intervention, and anticipate few difficulties in taking the recommended action (Becker & Maiman, 1975).

Rosenstock (1974), credited with the early work on the model, determined that the model should include a large component of motivation and individual perception, a theoretical orientation to explain a range of health problems, and a focus on current dynamics confronting the individual rather than on a history of past experience.

The model, summarized in Figure 5.2, contains three major elements. First, a person's readiness to take action is determined by their perceived susceptibility to a particular illness and by their perceptions of the severity of the consequences.

The second element involves an internal or external stimulus, that triggers the appropriate health behavior. Demographic, psychological, and social factors, although seen as having some potential effects on one's motivations and perceptions, are not viewed as direct causes of compliance. The third element in the model consists of a person's evaluation of the advocated health behavior in terms of its perceived benefits versus perceived barriers (physical, psychological, financial, and otherwise) (Becker & Maiman, 1975).

The HBM has been the subject of considerable research in recent years. Janz and Becker (1984) reviewed 46 studies on a variety of preventive health behaviors and sick role behaviors. This review, which included 18 prospective and 28 retrospective studies, found substantial empirical support. The "perceived barriers" element was found to be the most useful theoretical dimension across study designs and behaviors. "Perceived susceptibility" contributed most in studies of preventive health behaviors, while "perceived benefits" was of most value in understanding sick role behaviors. "Perceived severity" was found to be weakly associated with perceived health barriers, but strongly associated with sick role behaviors. The efficacy of various interventions for modifying model dimensions is virtually unknown due to very little experimental research. This is, however, viewed as a potentially profitable focus for future research. Moreover, the lack of standardized measures for model components impairs the interpretation of results and limits comparisons of findings across research studies.

Despite current limitations, several researchers have used the HBM in studies of exercise behaviors. In one of the earlier studies, Tirrell and Hart (1980) explored the relationship between beliefs and knowledge about health and subsequent exercise compliance among coronary bypass patients. The perception of barriers was most strongly related to compliance, followed by perceived susceptibility. A composite of the HBM yielded a low positive correlation with combined compliance measures, but no relationship was found between demographic factors and compliance. Lindsay-Reid and Osborn (1980), studying the effects of predisposition factors derived from the HBM and age on the exercise behaviors of fire fighters, unexpectedly found that perceptions of susceptibility to heart disease and to general illnesses were negatively associated with exercise participation. Subjects with lower perceived susceptibility were more likely to begin exercising than those with high susceptibility. The authors suggested that motivation and

Individual perceptions   Modifying factors   Likelihood of action

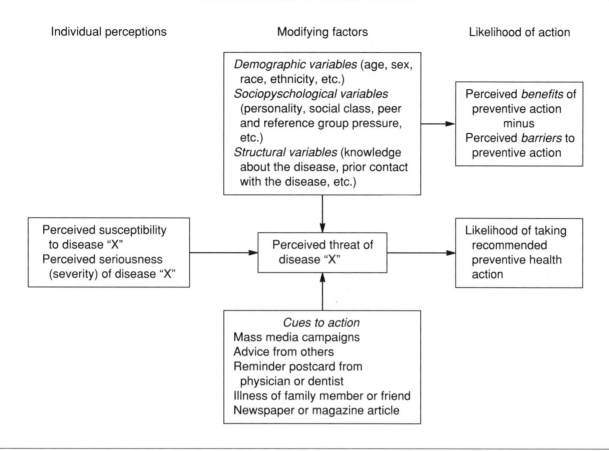

Figure 5.2 The health belief model as predictor of preventive health behavior.

From "Patient Perceptions and Compliance" by M.H. Becker, J.P. Kirsch, D.P. Hafner, R.H. Drachman, and D.W. Taylor. In *Compliance in Health Care* (p. 79) by R.B. Haynes, D.W. Taylor, and D.L. Sackett (Eds.), 1979, Baltimore: Johns Hopkins University Press. Reprinted by permission.

readiness to comply may function differently for various preventive measures. If this is so, the dimensions of the HBM may need to be refined.

In perhaps the most comprehensive study of the HBM and exercise behavior, Slenker, Price, Roberts, and Jurs (1984) demonstrated support for a revised version of the model. Again, "perceived barriers" to action was the best predictor, explaining 40% of the variance in jogging behavior. Other variables including health motivation, benefits of jogging, perceived complexity of jogging, perceived severity and susceptibility to disease, and cues to action accounted for 56% of the variance in jogging behavior. The researchers pointed out that all the variables that affect exercise behaviors can potentially be modified through education. This finding has practical implications for the exercise practitioner. Perhaps most important is the need to educate clients in solving problems associated with perceived barriers to exercise. Exercise leaders should suggest ways to deal with time problems, family and work responsibilities,

and other barriers. Programs should also provide support in the form of baby-sitting services and convenient class scheduling.

In a study that compared obese and nonobese adolescents with respect to dieting and exercise behaviors, cues to exercise (e.g., exposure to exercise equipment or seeing a friend exercise) and social approval of dieting were the best predictors of exercise behaviors of obese subjects, although these variables explained only 23% of the variance (O'Connell, Price, Roberts, Jurs, & McKinley, 1985). None of the HBM variables predicted the exercise behaviors of the nonobese adolescents. Although this study failed to support the HBM, the model itself may not have been the problem. The researchers cited age as a possible factor limiting the utility of the model. Moreover, the validity and reliability of the study's questionnaire items to measure model variables were not proven.

Although the HBM has promise for explaining and predicting exercise behaviors, much remains to be done before the practitioner can use this model as a guide to behavior change. Considerable research needs to be done to check the validity and reliability of the instruments used to measure the various dimensions of the model. Perhaps an even more serious question is whether exercise is substantively different from other preventive health behaviors. If, as Sonstroem (1988) suggested, the HBM was developed essentially to predict a single instance of one specific behavior, it may be unrealistic to expect the model to predict exercise behaviors because exercise encompasses a variety of behaviors carried on over time. Another limitation that Sonstroem pointed out is the model's emphasis on illness avoidance. As we have seen, people exercise for a variety of reasons, not just for health. The present model does not account for this diversity of motives. However, a great many adults do begin exercise programs for health reasons and the HBM may prove useful in working with this large segment of clients.

Despite its present limitations, we believe the HBM has promise for answering important questions about exercise. A theory is supposed to stimulate questions, foster research, and open itself up for criticism and refinement. The HBM has done all of this and will probably continue to do so.

THE EXERCISE BEHAVIOR MODEL

To more fully explain exercise behavior, Noland and Feldman (1984) modified the health belief model to form the exercise behavior model (EBM). The EBM is a comprehensive theoretical model intended to identify and integrate factors that are likely to affect one's decision to participate in regular exercise. The model, shown in Figure 5.3, is quite similar to the HBM with only one significant departure. Instead of the major theoretical element of "perceived susceptibility/seriousness of disease," the EBM uses an element called "predispositions." This element hypothesizes four predispositions that influence readiness for exercise: (1) perceived locus of control for exercise, (2) attitude toward physical activity, (3) self-concept, and (4) exercise-related values such as health, appearance, and physical fitness. The model assumes that people are ready to exercise if they have an internal locus of control for exercise, a positive attitude toward physical activity, a positive self-concept, and positive values for health, physical appearance, and physical fitness.

Like the HBM, the EBM presents modifying factors under the headings of "cues to action"

and "general" factors. The latter heading includes structural variables, such as experience with and knowledge about exercise, and physical variables, such as health status and physical fitness. According to the model, the likelihood of taking action would depend on the individual's assessment of the benefits of exercise versus perceived barriers to involvement. If barriers are perceived as greater than the benefits, it is assumed that the person will not participate regardless of favorable predisposition or modifying factors that support exercise.

In early research using the model, Noland and Feldman (1984) studied the relationship between predisposing factors and the exercise behaviors of 64 female students. Only attitudes toward physical activity and the environment subscale of exercise locus of control correlated with exercise behavior. A significant correlation was reported between exercise and the combined scores on attitudes toward physical activity, exercise locus of control, and physical fitness. A much larger study involving 271 women ages 25 to 65 also confirmed aspects of the EBM model (Noland & Feldman, 1985). Subjects were divided into age categories of younger (25-45) and older (46-65) to analyze the data. The variables accounted for 38% of variance in exercise behavior for the older group and 17% for the younger group. Consistent with the earlier study, attitude toward physical activity was the best predictor of exercise behavior for both groups. "Barriers to exercise" was significant only for the younger subjects, while exercise locus of control variables were significant only for the older women.

Although these studies did not test the complete exercise behavior model, the model may have potential for explaining some of the complexities of exercise behavior. Much more research, however, will be needed to determine whether the model can provide useful insights for the practitioner.

THEORY OF REASONED ACTION

The theory of reasoned action has amassed considerable support in a variety of experimental and naturalistic settings in recent years. Described by its originators (Ajzen & Fishbein, 1980; Fishbein & Ajzen, 1975) as a means of predicting and understanding behavior, the theory assumes that people are usually rational and make systematic use of the information available to them. The theory also maintains that people consider the implications of their behaviors before deciding to engage in

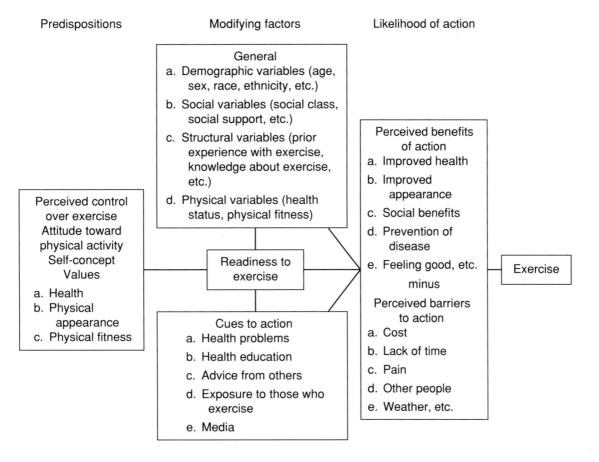

Predispositions   Modifying factors   Likelihood of action

Figure 5.3 Exercise behavior model.

From "Factors Related to the Leisure Exercise Behavior of 'Returning' Women College Students" by M.P. Noland and R.H. Feldman. This article is reprinted with permission from *Health Education*, **15**(2), 1984, p. 35. *Health Education* is a publication of the American Alliance for Health, Physical Education, Recreation and Dance, 1900 Association Drive, Reston, VA 22091.

them—thus the title, theory of "reasoned action" (Ajzen & Fishbein, 1980).

The theory's basic assumption is that most social behaviors are voluntarily controlled and that intention is the immediate determinant of behavior (Ajzen & Fishbein, 1980). Barring unforeseen events, people are expected to behave in accordance with their intentions. Because intentions tend to change with time and circumstances, the shorter the interval between the measurement of intention and the observation of the behavior, the greater the correlation between intention and actual behavior (Ajzen, 1985).

As shown in Figure 5.4, behavioral intentions are the product of two basic determinants: attitude toward the behavior and social norms. Attitude towards a behavior is based on a person's positive or negative evaluation of performing the behavior. This approach to the study of attitudes represents a major departure from more traditional attitude studies that center on a person's attitudes toward

an object, a person, an institution, and so on. The second determinant of intention, social norms, has to do with how a person perceives social pressures to perform or not to perform a specific behavior. People tend to engage in a given behavior when they evaluate it positively and believe that others think they should perform it (Ajzen, 1985). The relative importance of attitude and social norms is thought to vary depending on the situation, the individual, and the behavior in question. In using the theory to predict behavioral intention, empirically derived weights are assigned to each of these variables.

Although the factors of attitude and social norms sufficiently explain some behaviors, to fully understand behavioral intention one must understand why people hold certain attitudes and perceive certain subjective norms. The theory of reasoned action assumes that attitude toward a behavior is determined by salient beliefs about the behavior that link the behavior with some valued outcome

Reasoned Action

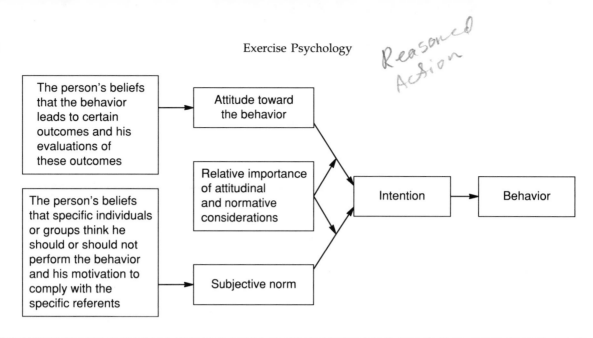

Figure 5.4 Factors determining a person's behavior. Arrows indicate the direction of influence.

Reprinted from "A Theory of Reasoned Action: Some Applications and Implications" by M. Fishbein, in *1979 Nebraska Symposium on Motivation Vol. 27* (p.69) by H.E. Howe and M.M. Page (Eds.), by permission of University of Nebraska Press. Copyright © 1980 by the University of Nebraska Press.

or attribute. A person who believes that a particular behavior will generally lead to positive outcomes will tend to hold a favorable attitude toward performing the behavior. The term *behavioral beliefs* refers to the beliefs associated with one's attitude toward a specific behavior.

Subjective norms are based on a person's beliefs about how important individuals or groups think he should behave. These are termed *normative beliefs*. Subjective norms may exert pressure to behave in a certain way despite one's attitude toward a particular behavior.

The theory explains behavior through successive steps. A person's beliefs about exercise and what they perceive important others believe about it determine their attitudes toward exercise and their perceptions of social norms regarding exercise. Subsequently, attitudes and subjective norms significantly influence one's intention to exercise. Finally, a person's intent to exercise determines the actual exercise behavior.

Unlike many behavioral theories, the theory of reasoned action does not directly incorporate demographic elements, personality characteristics, social roles, intelligence, and other traditional variables. Such factors, termed *external variables*, are recognized as potentially important, but only to the extent that they influence a person's beliefs, attitudes, or perceptions of norms. Although the effects of external variables may enhance the understanding of a specific behavior, the theory of reasoned action is primarily concerned with the

factors that intervene between external factors and behavior (Ajzen & Fishbein, 1980).

Application of the Model to Exercise

In a study that compared joggers and nonexercisers, Riddle (1980) found substantial support for the theory. A correlation of .82 was observed between behavioral intention and actual jogging behavior. Also consistent with the theory, behavioral intention was successfully predicted by the combination of the attitude factor and the normative factor. However, the attitude factor was a much stronger predictor than the normative factor, as reflected by the standardized regression coefficients of .643 and .157, respectively. The study also found strong positive correlations between the two predictors of behavioral intention and their subcomponents. Perhaps the most useful finding was the differences in beliefs about the consequences of regular jogging between joggers and nonexercisers. Joggers as a group had much stronger beliefs about the consequences of jogging and stronger evaluations of those consequences than nonexercisers. A suggested strategy, therefore, for changing behavior would be to try to change people's beliefs about the behavior. To entice nonexercisers to become involved, the exercise practitioner might try to convince them of the positive consequences of regular exercise and persuade them to evaluate these consequences favorably. In addition, beliefs that disregard the negative consequences of exercise should be strengthened.

Sonstroem (1982) applied the theory of reasoned action in a study of participants in a college faculty fitness program. Despite the small sample size, he found some support for the model with a low positive correlation between behavioral intention and attendance over 12 weeks. The study also found differences between habitual exercisers and nonexercisers with respect to beliefs about exercise, which corroborated the work of Riddle (1980). Subjects with good attendance believed that program participation made them feel better mentally, and they generally discounted the negative ideas that participation was too demanding, too time-consuming, too tiring, or otherwise unpleasant. The study reinforced the point that beliefs are modifiable and, therefore, an important avenue for improving exercise participation.

Pender and Pender (1986) also demonstrated limited support for the theory. Although they found that attitudes and subjective norms influenced intentions to exercise, these variables accounted for only 5.5% of the variance in exercise intention. When body weight was considered along with the model variables, the researchers were able to account for 15% of the variance. People who were at or close to their recommended weight were more likely to indicate intentions to exercise during the following week than overweight or underweight people. In contrast to other studies, subjective norms were found to exert a stronger influence on intentions to exercise than attitude, although correlations between these variables and intention were comparatively low.

Although the studies cited so far have generally supported the theory of reasoned action, an investigation that used the theory to assess the impact of fitness testing and individual counseling on exercise intentions did not find the theory very helpful in predicting intentions (Godin, Cox, & Shephard, 1983). Only attitude was significant in predicting intention to exercise. Although the addition of an external factor (current physical activity habits) increased the successful predictions of exercise intentions, the researchers concluded the theory required modification before it could reasonably explain exercise behavior.

Another test of the theory also demonstrated limited support. A study of adult male and female partners found that attitude was the only variable predictive of intention to exercise for both sexes (Godin & Shephard, 1985). Several external variables, such as prior exercise experience, age, educational level, socioeconomic status, and spouse's intention, improved the prediction of intention to exercise somewhat for men but very little for women.

A study designed to identify the cognitive profile of people who intend to exercise but do not follow through found little difference between that group and people who do follow through on their intention to exercise (Godin, Shephard, & Colantino, 1986). The two groups differed significantly in only two beliefs about exercise: Inactive intenders were more likely to believe that exercise would be too tiring and too time-consuming. The authors suggested that health promotion programmers strive to counter the belief that exercise is exhausting. They also suggested that time management be emphasized when promoting physical activity to sedentary clients who have expressed an intention to exercise. With regard to the theoretical model, they recommended that additional cognitive variables and social and environmental factors be explored.

A study of students in grades 7 to 9 yielded results that contradicted the proposition that intention is the immediate determinant of behavior (Godin & Shephard, 1986). Personal attributes, particularly attitudes and exercise habits, as well as the interaction between prior experience and current exercise habits contributed significantly to the prediction of exercise intentions.

A study of university employees also found that attitude and current exercise habits influence intention to exercise (Godin et al., 1987). Information on exercise behaviors obtained 3 weeks after exercise intentions were recorded showed proximal exercise to be the result of habit. Distal exercise behavior, assessed at 2 months, was explained by a combination of intention and proximal behavior. The authors observed that the inclusion of habit improved the prediction of intention to exercise. With regard to the theoretical model, attitude was again important in determining intention to exercise, but subjective norms did not influence intention.

It would appear that the theory of reasoned action, as originally conceptualized, is only of modest value as a predictor of exercise behavior. The assumption that behavioral intention can account for actual exercise behaviors has not been sufficiently demonstrated. Moreover, the assumed determinants of intention, attitude toward behavior, and social norms, have not predicted behavioral intention with any consistency. It would probably be premature, however, to disregard the theory. Some fault may lie with the research that has used the model. For example, none of the studies reviewed explained exactly how the relative weightings for subjective norm and attitude were obtained or how measures of behavioral intention were developed. We have also seen that the predictive power of the theory can be enhanced with the addition of certain external variables. Perhaps future research will identify additional variables, reconfigure the model, or use some combination of these strategies to yield more accurate predictions of exercise behavior.

THEORY OF PLANNED BEHAVIOR

One of the authors (Ajzen, 1985) of the theory of reasoned action extended the theory by introducing the concept of *control* as a factor in predicting behavior. *Control* is concerned with the extent to which nonvolitional internal and external factors interfere with one's attempt to perform a behavior. The theory of planned behavior postulates that the strength of an attempt to perform a behavior interacts with one's degree of control to determine the likelihood of the behavior occurring.

It is assumed that the harder one tries and the greater one's control over interfering internal and external factors, the greater the likelihood of obtaining the behavioral goal. Deficiencies in skills, abilities, knowledge, and adequate planning are internal factors that can interfere with control. External factors include time, opportunity, and the dependence of the behavior on the cooperation of other people. To accurately predict behavior over which people have only limited control, one must not only assess behavioral intention but also estimate perceived control over the behavior of interest (Ajzen & Madden, 1986). The theory of planned behavior predicts that the more resources and opportunities individuals believe they have, and the fewer obstacles they anticipate, the greater their perceived control over the behavior. The hypothesized relationship of the control factor with the other components of the theory is shown in Figure 5.5. As indicated in the figure, the three conceptually independent variables of attitude, subjective norm, and perceived behavioral control interact simultaneously to determine behavioral intention. If exercise were the behavior in question, we would assume that the more favorable the attitude and subjective norm toward exercise, and the greater the person's perceived control over factors affecting exercise participation, the stronger his or her intention to exercise would be.

Early research has provided encouraging support for the theory. In two experiments designed to test the model, Ajzen and Madden (1986) demonstrated the theory of planned behavior to be superior to the theory of reasoned action with respect to class attendance and earning an "A" grade. The researchers found that perceived behavioral control influenced behavioral intention, which was independent of attitude, subjective norm, and prior behavior. In addition, results suggested that perceived control can significantly influence behavioral motivation—that is, the more control one has over attaining a goal, the stronger one's intention to try to achieve it. In another early test of the theory, Schifter and Ajzen (1985) found it to be very successful in predicting intentions to lose weight and moderately successful in predicting actual weight loss.

At a very preliminary stage, the theory of planned behavior shows promise for explaining and predicting exercise behaviors. Although to our knowledge it has not yet been used in a study of exercise, the model accommodates one of the more difficult problems associated with exercise adherence—that is, the common barriers to regular exercise participation. It is quite possible that research with this model that accounts for control factors, particularly external factors, will be much more accurate in predicting exercise adherence than other approaches reviewed thus far.

SELF-EFFICACY

An important theoretical framework that emphasizes cognitive processes in the acquisition and retention of new behavior patterns is the social cognitive theory of Bandura (1977a, 1982, 1986). Social cognitive theory presents a model of causation in which environmental events, personal factors, and behavior operate as interacting determinants. This interaction, called *reciprocal causation*, is thought to improve personal control and self-direction (Bandura, 1986). Social cognitive theory identifies self-efficacy as one of several possible mechanisms of behavioral change. Self-efficacy is believed to act in concert with other mechanisms in the regulation of behavior (Bandura, 1986).

According to social cognitive theory, self-efficacy involves more than the possession of knowledge and skills. It also includes the perception that one is capable of performing effectively. Bandura (1986, p. 391) defines *perceived self-efficacy* as a judgment of one's "capability to organize and

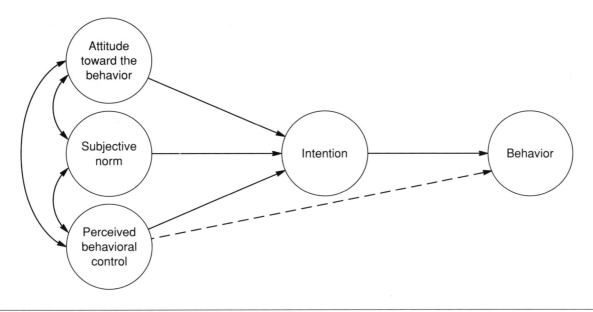

Figure 5.5   Theory of planned behavior: version 1 with solid arrow, version 2 with broken arrow.

From "Prediction of Goal Directed Behavior: Attitudes, Intentions, and Perceived Behavioral Control" by I. Ajzen and T. Madden, 1986, *Journal of Experimental Social Psychology*, **22**, p. 458. Reprinted by permission.

execute courses of action required to attain designated types of performances."

Perceived efficacy is believed to affect both the initiation and persistence of behavior. Self-efficacy judgments influence one's choice of activities and environmental settings. They also determine the amount of effort people will expend and how long they will persevere despite obstacles or aversive experiences. People tend to involve themselves in activities and behave with confidence, even in difficult situations, if they perceive the activities to be within their capability. On the other hand, people avoid situations that they perceive as beyond their ability to cope.

Expectations of personal efficacy are believed to be based on four factors: performance accomplishments, vicarious experience, verbal persuasion, and physiological states (Bandura, 1977a). Performance accomplishments, called *enactive mastery*, are thought to be a particularly influential source of efficacy. Bandura (1982) asserts that enactive mastery produces the highest, strongest, and most generalized increases in efficacy. In general, successes tend to raise expectations and failures tend to lower them. *Vicarious experience* involves judging one's probable success at a task based on observations of the behaviors of others. Seeing others perform threatening activities without adverse consequences may influence how people evaluate their own chances of success. *Verbal persuasion* is concerned with attempts to

influence efficacy beliefs by suggestion. Verbal persuasion works best if a person is also provided with performance aids. Physiological states resulting from emotional arousal may also influence perceived efficacy. Perceptions of anxiety or fear may be associated with impaired performance and lowered self-efficacy.

It is important to distinguish between efficacy expectations and outcome expectations. Perceived self-efficacy is a judgment of one's ability to perform a task, while an outcome expectation is a judgment of what the performance of the task will produce. An outcome is the consequence of an act (Bandura, 1986). This distinction is important with respect to health-promoting behaviors such as exercise. If people lack self-efficacy, they will probably behave ineffectually, even though they know what to do and how to do it (Bandura, 1986).

Self-efficacy research has been conducted on many forms of behavior. The enhancement of self-efficacy has been found to be an effective treatment of phobias. Perceived self-efficacy has also been found to predict changes in coping behaviors, stress reactions, physiological arousal, depression, pain tolerance, physical stamina, behavioral self-regulation, self-motivation, athletic attainments, and other forms of behavior. The success that has been achieved in the very divergent domains of behavior and the array of procedures used lend strong support to the position that self-efficacy operates as an important mechanism in human behavior (Bandura, 1986).

Self-Efficacy in Exercise and Fitness Programs

Self-efficacy has been applied quite extensively to the study of health behaviors. O'Leary's (1985) review of this literature supports the position that the effects of therapeutic interventions are mediated in part by changes in perceived self-efficacy. There is rapidly mounting evidence that self-efficacy plays a significant role in initiating and maintaining health behaviors such as smoking cessation, pain management, control of eating disorders, cardiac rehabilitation, and adherence to preventive health programs.

Several investigators have explored aspects of the theory's use in understanding and predicting exercise and fitness involvement. Weinberg, Gould, and Jackson (1979) found substantial support for the theory in an experimental study of muscular endurance under competitive conditions. In this study, high-efficacy subjects persisted longer in the task than low-efficacy subjects. In addition, high-efficacy subjects performed better after an initial failure, while low-efficacy subjects did poorer after experiencing failure in the first trial. This finding is consistent with self-efficacy theory. A subsequent study (Weinberg, Gould, Yukelson, & Jackson, 1981) corroborated the finding of a relationship between efficacy expectations and physical performance. This study also demonstrated that self-efficacy can be modified by providing information about performance accomplishments.

A study of participants in a university fitness program found adherence to be related to self-efficacy and outcome expectations (Desharnais et al., 1987). At the beginning of the program, potential dropouts were less confident of their ability to attend the program regularly and expressed higher expectations of program benefits than adherers. The combination of self-efficacy for program participation and expectation of outcome accounted for 12.5% of the variance between adherers and dropouts. It was suggested that adherence might be improved if potential dropouts' expectations of outcome were lowered and self-efficacy for program participation enhanced.

A study of postmyocardial infarction patients found self-efficacy judgments to be an important link between functional status and physical performance (Ewart, Taylor, Reese, & DeBusk, 1983). Self-efficacy estimates were predictive of treadmill test performance and were, in turn, modified by

the subjects' performance on the test. Self-efficacy judgments following treadmill testing were more accurate predictors of subsequent home exercise than was performance on the treadmill test. These results make a very strong case for exercise testing to increase self-efficacy of myocardial infarction patients. The study also found that counseling reinforced changes in self-efficacy brought about by exercise testing and facilitated the generalization of these changes to other physical activities.

Patients with chronic obstructive pulmonary disease who received an exercise prescription after treadmill testing along with exercise training successfully increased their home exercise behaviors (Kaplan, Atkins, & Reinsch, 1984). In this study, behavioral changes were mediated by changes in perceived efficacy for walking. Changes in efficacy expectations for other forms of exercise depended on their similarity to walking. These results supported Bandura's position that expectancies are specific and, therefore, cannot generalize to unrelated forms of exercise.

A study of patients with coronary artery disease that compared the self-efficacy expectations of a circuit weight training group with a volleyball group supported the specificity of self-efficacy (Ewart, Stewart, Gillian, & Keleman, 1986). Participation in circuit weight training produced greater changes in strength and endurance as well as increased self-efficacy for activities that were similar to the training tasks. Self-efficacy measures obtained during testing and training indicated that subjects did not alter self-efficacy for a new domain until they had performed a similar task. For example, only the circuit weight training subjects increased their perceived ability to perform tasks requiring significant arm or leg strength. In considering this finding, the researchers questioned the wisdom of prescribing only walking or jogging for postmyocardial infarction patients. Although walking and jogging may reduce cardiovascular risk, they may not increase patient confidence and help patients overcome fears of participating in a full range of daily activities. It was suggested that for maximum psychological and motivational impact, exercise programs should be designed to increase self-efficacy by exposing patients to a variety of activities with gradually increasing performance goals.

A recent study of college students compared social cognitive theory with the theory of reasoned action in predicting exercise behaviors (Dzewaltowski, 1989). Results showed social cognitive theory to be a better predictor. The theory of reasoned action explained only 5% of the variance in exercise behavior, while social cognitive theory accounted for 13.9%. Another significant finding showed that high self-efficacy subjects exercised more frequently than low self-efficacy subjects.

A test of the effectiveness of the cognitive appraisal processes contained in the latest version of the protection motivation theory (PMT) substantiated the importance of self-efficacy in predicting exercise involvement of college women (Wurtele & Maddux, 1987). Considered a model of health decision-making, PMT (Rogers,1983) included self-efficacy and response-efficacy dimensions as well as perceived vulnerability and severity of the threat as factors in determining intentions to adopt a particular health behavior. *Response efficacy* is the belief in the efficacy of a recommended coping response. Results of the Wurtele and Maddux study strongly supported the importance of perceived vulnerability to a health threat in increasing intent to exercise. Women who believed themselves to be at risk for heart and circulatory disease due to sedentary lifestyles indicated stronger intentions to adopt a recommended exercise program than those who perceived themselves to be less vulnerable. Moreover, self-efficacy for successfully starting an exercise program was the strongest predictor of exercise intentions. Of particular interest was the identification of a "precautionary strategy," which suggested that high–self-efficacy subjects may intend to adopt a recommended behavior even if they perceive the health threat to be minimal or their personal risk to be low. In other words, if the behavior is perceived as easy to perform, vulnerability and response efficacy can be relatively low and still prompt the initiation of the recommended behavior.

Despite the limited research that has applied social cognitive theory to studies of exercise, the theory shows promise for explaining exercise behaviors. The model seems particularly useful for studies of exercise motivation and adherence—two topics of considerable practical value to the exercise professional. One apparent difficulty in applying the model is that because self-efficacy estimates are highly behavior-specific, measures must be tailored to the behavioral domains of interest (Bandura, 1982). Nevertheless, as evidence of the model's validity increases, we will probably see more research that uses the theory.

SUMMARY

A theory is a means of organizing and presenting ideas and clarifying complex relationships. This chapter has presented several theoretical approaches to understanding exercise. Although most of these theories are based on psychological theories created to explain other behaviors, one theoretical model specifically developed to explain exercise and sport behaviors is the psychological model for physical activity participation. At present, the model and the associated scales have only limited value for the practitioner, however, the researcher may find the model suitable for elaboration. The health belief model and its derivative, the exercise behavior model, are also of limited value to the practitioner. Neither model has been sufficiently tested in exercise and fitness applications. Nevertheless, future research may lead to modifications that will improve the utility of these models. Based on the evidence to date, the theory of reasoned action, as originally conceived, is probably not very useful in explaining exercise behavior. Modifications of the theory, such as the theory of planned behavior, show promise but need further development. Self-efficacy theory, although not yet extensively used in the study of exercise and fitness behaviors, appears to have potential for the researcher as well as the practitioner, particularly in the important areas of exercise motivation and adherence.

Part II

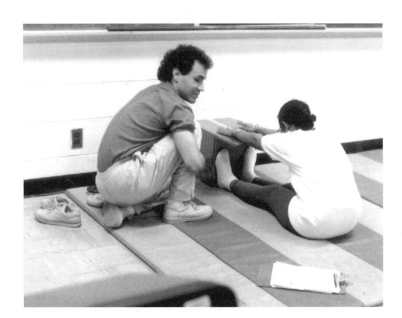

Applying Psychological Principles

Understanding the principles, theories, and foundational concepts of exercise is not enough. The exercise practitioner must also know how to convert that understanding into an operational prescription and treatment plan to bring about a successful behavioral change. Part II will use the framework developed in Part I to introduce learning principles in treatment application. Behavioral change concepts and techniques will be described through clinical application procedures and illustrated with scenarios for the exercise setting.

Chapter 6 explains how motivational techniques affect level of effort and intensity of exercise behaviors. We will describe proven techniques as well as techniques that show promise and apply them to exercise programs. Chapter 7 reviews the major learning principles that affect behavioral change. Each of these approaches is well established in the psychological arena and has begun to be applied in the fields of exercise and health promotion. Behavioral concepts and their applications will be related to exercise prescriptions and treatment plans. Chapter 8 introduces the foundations of counseling skills and discusses the role of counseling in exercise programs. Descriptions of basic theoretical foundations will also give the practitioner a conceptual framework from which to operate. Chapter 9 reviews the major principles of group dynamics including the role of the exercise practitioner as a group leader. Group communication, group conflict, problem solving, and decision making are variables that can all dramatically alter the direction and outcome of an exercise program. The effective management of these dynamics will be considered. Chapter 10 addresses exercise with special populations. The special populations that will be discussed include people involved in cardiac rehabilitation, the overweight, the elderly, children and youth, and people with physical disabilities.

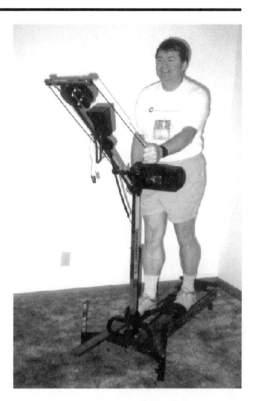

Chapter 6
Motivating Exercise Behaviors

To this point we have discussed two dimensions of motivation as they relate to exercise and fitness. Chapter 1 reviewed why motives initiate exercise behaviors, and chapter 2 considered adherence to exercise behaviors. To complete the triumvirate of motivation we shall now consider the remaining aspect, which relates to *intensity of behavior*. Intensity of behavior refers to the strength of a behavior, or the amount of effort expended in achieving a specific behavioral objective. This is usually the meaning that comes to the layperson's mind when hearing the term *motivation*. How much one works at a task, or how hard one tries to succeed at something, whether it be school, a job, sports, or even a fitness class, the amount of effort put forth is usually important to the outcome.

To even have a chapter that discusses techniques of motivation is to make a big assumption about the nature of motivation. Some psychologists believe the concept of motivation is an unnecessary construct because they perceive human beings as innately active and self-determining. According to this viewpoint, it is presumptuous to assume that an outside entity, such as another person, can influence or control an individual's behavior. We are not denying that much of human behavior is self-determined, however, we do believe that one person can at the very least influence the behavior of another.

A common leadership role is to influence the levels of effort of those under supervision. Indeed, the football coach who gives a rousing pep talk before the big game is trying to get the players "fired up" to compete with intensity. The sales manager who awards prizes and bonuses to produce more sales is attempting to elicit higher levels of performance from the sales force. In much the same fashion, the exercise practitioner most often tries to increase an individual's level of effort.

Generally speaking, there are considerable individual differences in the effort people expend in a given task. For example, if we were to observe a typical fitness class, some class members would be running around a track while others would be walking. Of those running, some would be running faster than others. Even two people running at the same speed would not necessarily be expending the same amount of effort due to differences in capacity. The challenge for the exercise leader is to help the person function at an optimal level of exercise intensity. As we have already seen, there is a narrow margin between an intensity level sufficient to produce a training effect and one so high that it results in cessation of exercise. The exercise leader must be skilled in helping the client identify and maintain the appropriate level of intensity for the duration of a workout. This chapter addresses the techniques that have proved helpful in eliciting changes in intensity levels of exercise behaviors.

Because no single theoretical approach to motivation has proven comprehensive enough to satisfy all areas of application, we have collected usable techniques from several sources, particularly from learning and cognitive theories for motivational strategies that have worked well in applied settings.

Although the purpose of this chapter is to review techniques that have been helpful in adjusting exercise clients' level of effort, we will somewhat broaden the concept of intensity to include more than effort considerations. We will also discuss intensity in relation to various techniques for developing enduring program interest, enthusiasm, and commitment. To accomplish these broader goals, we must go beyond a strict interpretation of exercise intensity.

We shall divide our discussion into two parts: The first will deal with techniques derived from more traditional theoretical approaches to motivation, and the second will present practical suggestions based on our own experience or on that of others. Our main concern is to give the exercise practitioner some practical ideas for client motivation.

INCENTIVES

In contrast to theories that conceive motivation as an internal force that drives a person toward a goal, incentive motivation theories are based on the assumption that external factors energize goal-directed behaviors. Incentives, in effect, "pull" the person toward a goal. *Incentives* have been defined as "external stimuli that influence behavior" (Chung, 1977, p. 59) or "goal objects which motivate us" (Petri, 1986, p. 163).

Following are some basic assumptions about the nature and functions of incentive motivation theory:

■ We work to accomplish goals that have characteristics that influence our behavior (Petri, 1986).

■ Incentives can be either positive or negative. Positive incentives are attractive and stimulate approach behaviors while negative incentives prompt avoidance behaviors (Petri, 1986).

■ Incentives energize behavior. Incentive motivation mediates between the stimulus characteristics of a goal and the responses directed toward it (Petri, 1986).

■ Incentives are relative rather than absolute. The value attached to a particular incentive may change as a function of time or circumstances (Petri, 1986). An incentive may appeal to one person but not to another (Chung, 1977).

■ The anticipation of reward is the effective determinant of behavior. Future incentives are effective because of one's anticipation of them (Beck, 1978).

■ Incentive motivation can be aroused whenever appropriate stimulus conditions are present (Beck, 1978).

■ By manipulating the potential consequences of incentives, one may influence the behavior of others (Chung, 1977).

Our definition of *incentive* is consistent with the more conventional interpretation: An incentive can be virtually anything that is external to the individual as long as it is something that a person wants strongly enough to initiate behaviors to obtain it. In everyday terms, incentives are typically thought of as material objects, such as trophies, awards, T-shirts, or even money. Psychological states may also function as incentives that stimulate behaviors. We shall now review some incentives that have potential for increasing exercise behaviors.

Tangible Incentives

The use of tangible incentives to promote involvement in exercise is universal. Trophies, plaques, award certificates, time off, T-shirts, pen sets, and other items have been effective motivators in many programs. Under the right circumstances, most people will respond to incentives of this sort. Another tangible incentive used less frequently is some kind of financial reward. Rushall and Pettinger (1969) found money to be an effective incentive to increase the work output of young swimmers. The use of financial incentives to stimulate exercise attendance has shown promise in promoting program involvement. One research study (Pollock, Foster, Salisbury, & Smith, 1982) found that when a participant was reimbursed for course fees if their attendance was good or if the participant and employer shared the fee, program attendance was better than when the participant paid the entire fee or the employer paid all of the fee and made no attendance demands.

Most authors, however, caution against the overuse of tangible incentives. One problem with this technique is the possibility that extrinsic factors will replace one's intrinsic interest in the activity itself. The greatest concern, however, is that involvement will end when the tangible incentives are no longer available or no longer effective. Probably the best strategy is to use tangible incentives early in the program to help establish behaviors and then gradually reduce their use as a person becomes more involved and the exercise becomes a habit. By that time the exercise itself should provide enough inherent satisfaction to maintain the behavior.

A second limitation in the use of tangible incentives has to do with the satiation factor, or when the object no longer holds reinforcement value. For example, a person who has a drawer full of T-shirts earned by running 10-K races is not likely to be motivated by a T-shirt to participate in a corporate fitness program. The use of a variety of incentives would probably help maintain the effectiveness of tangible incentives.

Psychological Incentives

Chapter 1 provided an extensive discussion of motives for exercise and fitness. All of the motives identified in that chapter could be considered incentives. The desires to improve health, be more attractive, socialize with others, and feel better, can provide the necessary impetus to become active or to stay active.

Alderman and Wood (1976) identified several incentives for involvement in sport, some of which have relevance for exercise and fitness. We shall summarize four of these incentives and briefly suggest how they might apply to exercise and fitness activities.

Independence

Incentives associated with opportunities to function without the help or criticism of others are *independence incentives*. Exercise provides ample opportunities to fulfill a need for independence. When walking, jogging, or biking alone one is in complete control. Decisions about how far to go, which route to take, how fast to go, how hard to work, what to think about, and when to quit are all determined by the individual alone. Few situations present the opportunities to be so completely unencumbered by social convention, rank, and other interpersonal considerations, as solitary exercise. Although most people prefer to exercise in groups, this may be one important reason why some choose to exercise alone.

Arousal

Incentives that have to do with excitement, stress, and interesting experiences, particularly in terms of novelty, uncertainty, complexity, and dissonance, are *arousal incentives*. Physical activity presents ample opportunities to satisfy a need for stimulation or arousal. Competing against a well-matched opponent in a tennis game, pitting one's abilities against a difficult environmental challenge, such as rock climbing, learning a new skill or developing even greater skills in an activity such as one of the martial arts, are examples of challenging and interesting physical activities.

Esteem

Incentives that center on opportunities for status, prestige, recognition, and social approval are *esteem incentives*. Esteem plays a potentially important role in fitness programs. Recognition from peers, other participants, and class leaders for progress in an exercise program is important in motivating future participation. Approval from significant others confirms that we are doing something worthwhile and important.

Excellence

The need to be good at something is basic to the *excellence incentive*. As White (1959) demonstrated, competence is an important human motive. Opportunities abound for a person to demonstrate excellence in fitness-related activities. Most clients should probably be encouraged to develop their own criteria for excellence rather than to meet some external standard for excellence.

The remaining psychological incentives that Alderman and Wood identified include affiliation, or social involvement; power, or the need to control others; and aggression, or the need to dominate or intimidate others. The last two incentives probably have little use in exercise programs, although they may be operative for some individuals.

We have intentionally omitted negative incentives from our discussion because we believe that the positive approach is better for most people. There are those, however, who may function effectively with negative incentives, for example, people who wish to avoid obesity. Some people may be sufficiently motivated by the threat of becoming fat to diet and exercise. Taken to the extreme, however, this incentive may lead to anorexic or bulimic behaviors. Poor muscle tone and fear of incapacity or death are other examples of negative incentives that may be effective for certain clients. As a general rule, however, fear, blame, ridicule, and other negative incentives are less effective than positive incentives in promoting exercise involvement.

INTRINSIC MOTIVATION

The concept of *intrinsic motivation*, which is central to Deci and Ryan's (1985) self-determination theory, provides yet another approach to motivating exercise behavior. Intrinsic motivation is thought to be a central energy source. The underlying premise is that people are born with a basic undifferentiated need to be competent and self-determining, which motivates their early development. Children spend large amounts of time learning, undertaking challenges, solving problems, and performing other activities for which there is no external reward. Adults spend comparatively less time involved in such activities. The rewards for these activities are inherent, that is, the activities are motivated by the spontaneous, internal experiences that accompany the behavior (Deci & Ryan, 1985).

The typical conceptualization of intrinsic motivation has been that an individual engages in activities for their own sake rather than for some extrinsic reward. Deci (1975) found this conceptualization too limiting and chose to define intrinsically motivated behaviors as behaviors in which a person engages to feel competent and self-determining.

Deci (1975) hypothesized two kinds of intrinsically motivated behaviors. The first type of intrinsically motivated behavior is to seek out challenge when faced with no stimulation. Going for a run or looking for a game of basketball are examples of seeking challenge through exercise. The second kind of intrinsic motivation involves conquering a challenge or reducing incongruity. Deci theorized that people feel competent and self-determining only when they can reduce incongruity or conquer challenge. Striving to improve a personal record in a road race is an example of this type of motivation. Because pleasurable stimulation results in personal satisfaction, people engage in the process of seeking and conquering challenges that are optimal for them.

Some people seem to lose intrinsic motivation as they get older. Deci believes this phenomenon is due to the undermining effects of rewards and controls. Receiving extrinsic rewards for a given activity tends to weaken intrinsic motivation. Working for rewards leads to a change in the source of reinforcement. If an individual receives internal rewards (e.g., satisfaction for achieving an exercise goal) and also receives external rewards for achievements, the individual may begin to expect external reinforcement and no longer respond to personal satisfaction as an incentive. If the rewards become the reason for the activity, people are inclined to respond only when rewards are available (Deci, 1977).

Rewards are assumed to have two facets: a controlling aspect and an informational aspect. The controlling aspect is believed to establish a cause-and-effect connection between a behavior and a reward, and the informational aspect informs people about their competence and self-determination at some activity. The informational aspect affects feelings of competence and self-determination. When the informational aspect of a situation is clear and positive, there is an increase in intrinsic motivation. When the controlling aspect of a reward is clear or when the informational aspect is negative, there is a decrease in intrinsic motivation (Deci, 1977).

Deci has speculated that the aim of the rewarder in giving rewards has an important impact on the receiver's interpretation of the reward. If the rewarder is perceived as manipulative, the rewards will probably be interpreted as controlling. The more authoritarian the rewarder, the more likely the rewards are to undermine intrinsic motivation. In contrast, if the rewarder is perceived as supportive and the rewards are viewed as providing performance feedback, the more likely the rewards are to be interpreted as informational, which enhances intrinsic motivation.

Deci and Ryan (1985) have offered four propositions that summarize the basic concepts and relationships of self-determination theory. We shall present these propositions and discuss their implications for physical activity:

Proposition I

External events related to behavior will affect a person's intrinsic motivation if the external events are perceived as causing the behavior.

■ Events that are perceived as externally controlled will undermine intrinsic motivation, whereas those that are perceived as internally controlled will enhance intrinsic motivation.

Implications

1. Exercise participants need to have a major role in program planning.

2. Participants need to feel a sense of ownership of their program.

3. If participants have some control in program development, they are more likely to have intrinsic motivation and long-term involvement.

Proposition II

If individuals participating in challenging activity believe that external events affect their level of competence, the external events will also affect their intrinsic motivation.

■ External events that promote perceived competence enhance intrinsic motivation; those events that diminish perceived competence decrease intrinsic motivation.

■ Feelings of competence are increased when individuals succeed or receive positive feedback, that is, if they have some sense of self-determination.

■ Feelings of incompetence are increased when individuals fail, receive negative feedback, or see no relationship between their behavior and the outcome, that is, it they have no sense of self-determination.

■ Increases in intrinsic motivation as a result of perceived competence, and decreases in intrinsic motivation as a result of feelings of incompetence, occur only if participants perceive themselves as responsible and in control.

Implications

1. Program activities and levels of complexity should include variety that is appropriate to the individual.

2. The exercise professional should help participants find their exercise "niche."

3. Participants should be given ample opportunities to succeed in program activities.

4. All tasks assigned should be seen as "doable" by the client.

5. The exercise leader should:

- provide positive feedback,
- encourage participants to support each other,
- structure activities for success, and
- discourage participants from comparing themselves to each other.

Proposition III

Events relevant to behavior have three potential aspects: (a) The informational aspect facilitates a sense of internal control and perceived competence, thus enhancing intrinsic motivation, (b) the controlling aspect facilitates a perceived external control, thus undermining intrinsic motivation and promoting extrinsic compliance or defiance, and (c) the amotivating aspect facilitates perceived incompetence, thus undermining intrinsic motivation and promoting amotivation.

■ The degree of influence held by these aspects will affect participants' perceptions of control, competence, and intrinsic motivation.

■ Choice and positive feedback tend to be informational.

■ Rewards, deadlines, and surveillance tend to be controlling.

■ Negative feedback tends to be amotivating.

Implications

1. Making a program client-centered and providing ample positive feedback facilitates perceived personal control, perceived competence, and intrinsic motivation.

2. Situations that require a person to give up autonomy, either to secure a reward or to meet imposed demands, are likely to undermine intrinsic motivation.

3. If rewards are used, they should be informational rather than controlling.

4. All forms of negative feedback, which result in feelings of incompetence, a decrease in intrinsic motivation, and lack of motivation for the activity should be minimized, if not eliminated.

Proposition IV

Events that are internally informative facilitate intrinsic motivation. Internal events perceived as controlling create pressure and undermine intrinsic motivation. Internal events that are amotivating reinforce feelings of incompetence and undermine intrinsic motivation.

■ Many influential events occur internally (e.g., needs, feelings, and expectations).

■ Being negatively controlled by oneself can be as detrimental to intrinsic motivation as being controlled by others.

■ However, information regulated internally enhances self-determination and intrinsic motivation.

Implications

1. The exercise leader should be alert to signs that participants are applying too much pressure and making unrealistic expectations for themselves.

2. The exercise leader must provide positive feedback and emphasize exercise enjoyment to promote intrinsic motivation.

Competition

How does competition affect intrinsic motivation? Because competitive activities are included in some programs, perhaps some insights from self-determination theory would prove helpful. Deci and Ryan (1985) have distinguished between two forms of competition. *Indirect competition* is when an individual or group competes against an impersonal standard such as one's previous best record or some kind of standard. The concept of indirect competition also includes competing with aspects of the environment, such as in mountain climbing, skiing, or canoeing. Indeed, components of indirect competition are found in all sports activities. *Direct competition* involves people struggling against each other to gain some advantage, and typically involves winning and losing.

Indirect competition may help people improve their competence in a task and thereby maintain or enhance intrinsic motivation. Success would be expected to increase intrinsic motivation because it carries with it information about competence. It is only when one's performance in indirect competition is pressured, either from external or internal sources, that it would be expected to decrease intrinsic motivation. In direct competition, the primary focus is often on winning rather than on performing well. This focus emphasizes an extrinsic orientation and subordinates an intrinsic one. Controlling and informational aspects are also operative in the competitive situation. When the focus is placed not so much on winning but on playing well, the detrimental effects of direct competition on intrinsic motivation are lessened (Deci & Ryan, 1985).

If competition is part of an exercise and fitness program, the exercise leader should emphasize indirect rather than direct forms of competition. The exercise leader can perhaps best serve the clients by encouraging them to compete against their own best record or against aspects of the environment. However, there may be interest in direct competition, especially among younger clients. If demand for direct competition is overwhelming, emphasis should be placed on participating, having fun, and playing well rather than on winning. There should also be less emphasis on league championships and extramural participation.

GOAL SETTING

Goal setting is a motivational technique that has effectively increased performance in several areas of application ranging from business and industry to education, sport, and, to a lesser extent, exercise. Goal setting has been described as a "limited" approach to motivation compared to more elaborate theoretical approaches such as drive theory or instinct theory, and is considered to fall within the broad domain of cognitive psychology (Locke, Shaw, Saari, & Latham, 1981).

Locke and associates (1981, p. 126) have defined a *goal* as "what an individual is trying to accomplish; it is the object or aim of an action." The term *goal* typically refers to "attaining a specific standard of proficiency on a task, usually within a specified time limit." The basic assumption underlying the extensive research reviewed by these authors was that goals serve as "immediate regulators of human action" (Locke et al., 1981, p. 126). Locke and colleagues concluded that the beneficial effect of goal setting on task performance is one of the most sound and replicable findings in the psychological literature. Ninety percent of the studies they reviewed, whether laboratory or field studies, showed positive or partially positive results for goal setting. In view of this fact, it is surprising that goal setting has received comparatively little attention as a technique to increase motivation for exercise.

The Functions of Goal Setting

Given that goal setting is an effective means of increasing motivation, how does the process work? There are at least four mechanisms by which goals affect task performance:

- By directing attention and action
- By mobilizing energy expenditure
- By prolonging effort over time
- By motivating a person to develop relevant strategies to attain goals (Locke et al., 1981)

We will now discuss how each of these principles might apply to exercise and fitness programs.

Directing Attention and Action

A metaphor for a person without goals is "a ship without a rudder." Goals provide direction for people's behaviors and keep them focused on what they should be concentrating on or attending to. As Mager (1968, p. 13) stated, "if you're not sure where you're going, you're liable to end up someplace else." Goals provide a cognitive map to guide the individual to the desirable end state. Without specific exercise and fitness goals, a person is likely to "drift," that is, casually go through the motions with little thought or effort directed toward improvement.

Mobilizing Energy Expenditure or Effort

This principle is central to intensity of behavior. What motivates people to work hard and put forth the necessary effort to experience a training effect? Without someone continually goading them or without specific objectives in mind, people are not likely to work at a level of intensity that yields significant outcomes. Goals have been shown to elicit higher levels of effort in areas other than exercise, and there is ample reason to believe that they would serve the same function in programs of exercise and fitness. If people have a specific goal to attain during a class period, they will no doubt work harder than they would if they had no specific outcomes in mind.

Prolonging Effort Over Time

As we have discussed at some length, one of the major concerns of the exercise professional is program adherence. The incorporation of goal setting into the exercise prescription promises to have a positive effect on the continuance of exercise behaviors. Properly set goals are not likely to be reached easily or quickly. A person, therefore, is required to expend effort over a prolonged period to attain the goal. Another advantage of goal setting is that it helps maintain interest. The process of reviewing, revising, or updating goals keeps people continually involved. Persistence of behaviors can therefore be enhanced through ongoing evaluation of progress toward a goal.

Motivation to Develop Strategies for Goal Attainment

A sedentary person who has set a personal goal of running a 10-K race in 50 minutes cannot meet this objective without devising a workable plan. How people go about realizing an objective involves many factors and decisions. In developing a plan of action, any number of potentially successful strategies could be adopted. The main point, however, is that when people have a definitive goal that they strongly desire to achieve, they will actively seek ways to reach that goal.

Goal Setting in Exercise and Fitness

Although research on the effectiveness of goal setting in increasing exercise behaviors is limited, goal setting undoubtedly has a great deal of potential as a practical motivational tool for the exercise professional. Nelson (1978) demonstrated that instructions to aim for a specific goal resulted in better performance on a muscular endurance task than instructions to merely "do your best." In this experiment, subjects who were given realistic normative information, fictitious normative information, or obtainable goals performed significantly better than the control group, which was simply told to do as many repetitions as possible. The results of this study were seen as supportive of the use of goals to elicit higher levels of performance.

A study on the influence of goal setting on reducing risk factors addressed the issue of whether collaboratively set goals are more productive than provider-set goals (Alexy, 1985). Goal setting was found to be effective in changing risk-related behaviors, however, there was no indication that client participation in goal setting was better than a directive approach to setting goals. In this study, aerobic exercise frequency and duration increased significantly over baseline for both experimental goal groups as well as for the control group, which did not receive goal-setting information. This result was explained as possibly due to the current cultural interest in exercise and the ready access to fitness facilities and information.

A study of junior high girls (Tu & Rothstein, 1979) looked at the effects of personality on goal setting and jogging performance. Students were typed as independency motive oriented (IMO) or dependency motive oriented (DMO) and assigned to two goal conditions, either teacher-imposed goals or subject-set goals. Results showed that IMO students performed better and improved more quickly when they set their own goals. In contrast, DMO subjects seemed to perform better under teacher-imposed goals. The authors concluded that an individual's personality should be considered when selecting motivational techniques for physical performance.

In probably the most significant research to date concerning the effects of different goal-setting approaches on exercise adherence, Martin and associates (1984) found flexible goals to be significantly better than fixed goals, and time-based goals better than distance-based goals, in promoting program attendance. Unexpectedly, subjects who had distal goals (set at 5-week intervals) adhered better than those who had proximal goals (set weekly).

Generalizations From Goal-Setting Research

Locke and Latham (1985) have made a significant contribution to sport psychology by suggesting applications. Many of these suggestions are applicable also to goal setting in exercise and fitness. Following is a summary of these suggestions:

■ *Specific goals are much more effective than general goals.* Ambiguous statements such as "do your best" do not tell a person what to do, when a task has been completed, or how well it has been done. In contrast, goals that are specific and quantitative

inform a person of exactly what needs to be done. For example, to tell someone working on the bench press to do three sets of 10 repetitions using 60% of maximum, provides a specific goal and, following execution of the exercise, provides feedback about how well the person has done.

■ *Difficult or challenging goals result in better performance than moderate or easy goals.* Assuming that a person has adequate ability, the higher the goal, the higher the performance. For a 45-year-old sedentary person trying to "get back in shape," a long-term goal of running a sub-40-minute 10-K race may very well be beyond their capabilities, but a 55-minute 10-K race might be an appropriate long-term goal. Goals should be realistic for an individual based on such factors as age, sex, present physical condition, and interests. For optimal effectiveness, goals should be both specific and challenging.

■ *Use short-term or intermediate goals to help attain difficult or long-term goals.* By setting manageable intermediate goals, a person can see incremental progress toward the long-range goal. A person who wants to lose 60 pounds is less likely to become discouraged if the task is broken down into manageable short-term goals.

■ *Goal setting is most effective when feedback is provided to point out progress.* Periodic evaluation lets a person know if their progress is on-track. Measurements of flexibility or percent body fat are examples of the periodic assessments that inform clients of progress toward their goals. This type of information is also instrumental in motivating further action.

Some fitness activities have built-in feedback. A person doing sit-ups knows how many repetitions he or she has done. Exercises on a weight machine provide the client with immediate knowledge of results, both in terms of number of repetitions and the amount of resistance being used. Although feedback on cardiovascular involvement in an aerobic activity is more difficult to ascertain, taking the time to get a pulse rate will provide this information. Feedback is only of value when used in relation to a goal. In this case, heart rate should be compared to one's target heart rate.

■ *To be effective, goals must be accepted by the client.* Goals that are important and meaningful to the client are more likely to result in a commitment to their attainment. Unlike businesses, fitness programs involve the participation of the client in the goal-setting process. As we have seen, the perception of program "ownership" is essential to continued involvement.

■ *The development of a strategy or plan of action facilitates goal attainment.* If a person has multiple goals, they must devote time to each. For example, if a person has goals to improve aspects of flexibility, strength, and cardiovascular fitness, each of these dimensions must receive ample attention. A plan in which a person decides to work on strength and flexibility for 2 days per week and cardiovascular fitness for 3 days illustrates this approach. Such a plan would also specifically spell out the muscle groups to be strengthened and the exercises to be done. This process would be repeated for each exercise goal.

The Goal-Setting Process

To use goal setting effectively, the exercise practitioner needs to be thoroughly familiar with the process. Locke and Latham (1985) identified the following steps for productive goal setting:

1. *Specify the objective or tasks to be done.* What does the client want to accomplish? Be sure that your client's program goals are stated in specific, quantifiable terms.

2. *Determine how progress toward the goal will be measured.* Fortunately, progress in the various dimensions of fitness can usually be measured easily. Time, resistance, repetitions, $\dot{V}O_2$max, and distance are the typical measures of progress.

3. *Specify the standard to be reached.* The specific degree of performance to be achieved should be indicated. Running 20 miles per week, earning 100 aerobics points a month, increasing performance on the sit-and-reach flexibility test by 3 inches in 6 weeks, and losing 2 pounds per week for 10 weeks are examples of specific degrees of performance. The standard to be reached is usually based on prior performance information. Because clients who are just beginning a program have no recent performance history, the exercise practitioner should participate in the goal setting.

4. *Specify the time period in which to reach the goal.* This step can be combined with step 3. Clients should be encouraged to set short-term, intermediate, and long-term goals.

5. *Prioritize goals.* When a client has multiple goals it is helpful to rank them. The purpose of this step is to direct appropriate attention and effort according to the degree of importance.

Because goals are based on past performance and judgments of future capabilities, goals may need to be modified from time to time. This is particularly true for intermediate and long-term goals. Faulty judgment or changes in circumstances may make goal adjustments desirable, especially if goals are to be motivational devices.

Goal setting should be a significant part of the exercise practitioner–client relationship. Despite the paucity of goal-setting research related to exercise, the process of setting, evaluating, and revising goals is probably one of the better means of maintaining exercise motivation.

BEHAVIORAL TECHNIQUES OF MOTIVATION

Several behavioral change concepts have been well researched in psychological studies of therapeutic process and outcome. Although these and other related concepts are sometimes applied to exercise, they are not usually treated as an integral part of a motivation and treatment plan. Following are descriptions of a few important and potentially effective techniques. Chapter 7 provides a more comprehensive review of behavioral change strategies applicable to motivation and the exercise setting.

Shaping

People often enter exercise programs with fairly ambitious goals. One effective approach to move clients toward these goals is called *shaping*. Sometimes referred to as the method of "successive approximation," shaping involves the development of new behaviors by the successive reinforcement of closer approximations to the target behavior (Martin & Pear, 1978). One begins with an existing behavior, that may only remotely resemble the desired behavior, and reinforces that partial representation of the target behavior. Then, through the process of reinforcing sequential and progressive steps, the behavior is gradually shaped toward the final behavior.

Instructors often use this technique without even being aware of it. In teaching people to swim, an instructor typically spends time getting the students accustomed to the water. This step alone may have to be broken down into smaller steps if a person is afraid of the water. When the students can put their faces in the water and take their feet off the bottom of the pool, then they are ready to learn a prone glide. The stroke is then shaped by adding a kick, an arm stroke, and finally rhythmic breathing and stroke coordination. With a progressive and systematic approach, a skill as complex as swimming can be learned. One cardiac rehabilitation program shaped health-related target behaviors by providing reinforcement for each quarter of a pound lost, each mile completed, and each instance of perfect attendance for a month (Hoepfel-Harris, 1980).

In exercise and fitness programs, most of the behaviors that need to be shaped have already been learned. For example, walking, running, and riding a bicycle have usually already been well learned. Shaping, then, needs to be applied only to duration, intensity, resistance, or repetitions. Starting a walking program, then gradually increasing distance, speed, or duration are typical first steps in shaping one's ability to run a 10-K race or even a marathon.

When new skills have to be acquired or existing behaviors modified, the following guidelines for shaping should be helpful (Martin & Pear, 1978):

1. *Select the terminal behavior.* The behavior should be precisely stated, for example, "to run a mile in 9 minutes or less."

2. *Select an appropriate reinforcer.* Reinforcers should be readily available, presented immediately, and used over and over. Use as many reinforcers as feasible.

3. *Develop a plan for shaping.* Begin by tentatively listing successive approximations of the terminal behavior. Select an initial behavior within the client's present capabilities and proceed in a logical sequence toward the terminal behavior.

4. *Implementation.* Begin by reinforcing the initial shaping step. If walking a lap around a track is the first step, reinforce the person for completing that task. A person who can consistently perform at the specified level is ready for the next approximation. Proceed in sufficiently small steps. Moving too quickly may cause the client to lose the previous approximation. If you have moved too fast or have taken too large a step, re-establish the previous approximation before proceeding. Moving too slowly is also undesirable.

5. *Be prepared to make changes along the way.* Because shaping plans are based on best guesses, adjustments may be necessary. Speed up, slow down, or retrace steps if the client is losing interest or not making progress. Direct observation and written records can be helpful in monitoring the clients' development and in "fine tuning" the program.

Using successive approximations not only makes new behaviors more accessible, but also maintains interest and motivation. The key to successful shaping is reinforcement at each step. Giving continuing reinforcement lessens the likelihood that the client will become bored or discouraged.

Presbie and Brown (1977) cited Cooper's aerobic training as a particularly valuable application of shaping procedures. The program, tailored for different ages and sexes, consists of graduated exercise goals that guide an individual in the gradual increase in exercise capacity. The point system provides a handy measure of progress and a good source of motivation. By setting reasonable point goals and reinforcing their accomplishment, a person can move forward in a systematic fashion.

Prompting

Another effective technique for establishing a behavior is the use of *prompts*. A prompt is any antecedent that helps initiate a behavior (Presbie & Brown, 1977). Prompts can be verbal, physical, or symbolic. A verbal prompt may be a simple statement such as "Okay, let's get going." Examples of physical prompts are supporting a person lightly as they swim and helping someone overcome a "sticking point" in the bench press. A symbolic prompt is a cue that reminds a person to begin a behavior. Laying out workout gear the night before or placing the exercycle in front of the television are examples. Although prompts are helpful in beginning new behaviors or in getting past difficult points, they should not be continued indefinitely. To encourage clients to become independent, prompts should be gradually removed—a process called *fading*. By using a prompt less and less over time, a client can gain increasing independence without a sudden withdrawal of support.

Activity Reinforcement

Another procedure that helps motivate exercise behaviors is sometimes referred to as the Premack principle or "Grandma's Rule" (Presbie & Brown, 1977). Just as "grandma" made us eat our vegetables before getting dessert, this behavior modifier makes people exhibit a lower preference activity before allowing them to do a higher preference activity (Presbie & Brown, 1977). For example, a fitness leader might require a group to complete an endurance training session before playing volleyball. Another example would be having to work out before reading the evening newspaper or making a weekend outing contingent on earning a designated number of aerobics points.

APPLIED MOTIVATIONAL TECHNIQUES

To this point, we have presented motivational techniques with clearly delineated psychological foundations. We shall now present motivational procedures that have been used successfully in fitness and exercise programs, although they may not have obvious psychological roots and may be based on various theoretical positions. We have also included some motivational techniques that have not to our knowledge been used in fitness and exercise programs, but that seem to have good potential.

Assuming Personal Responsibility for Fitness

Over the last 20 years, the general public has become much more aware of the active role they can play in improving their health. Many people are no longer willing to concede the responsibility for their health to physicians and other health-care professionals. A more contemporary approach makes people active and responsible participants in matters concerning their health in partnership with health-care professionals (Alderman, 1980). This principle has sound basis in psychological theory and research ranging from Rotter's (1966) theory of internal locus of control to De Charms' (1968) ideas about personal causation and Deci and Ryan's (1985) work with the concept of self-determination. A client's program and its ultimate outcome are the responsibility of the client. The exercise professional should serve as a facilitator by providing information, skills training, and support to help the client meet self-originated exercise and fitness goals. Whitehouse (1977) advocated opportunities for individual creativity and personal choice to develop a sense of self-investment and an incentive for participation. As we have seen, perceptions of control over one's program content are important to exercise program attendance (Thompson & Wankel, 1980).

Feedback on Progress

A person who commits considerable time, effort, and money to exercise probably has specific outcomes that he or she would like to realize. An important motivational technique that capitalizes on this inherent interest is to provide periodic feedback on dimensions of fitness that are not concomitant with one's regular workout. Franklin (1984) suggested that body composition measures, serum lipid evaluations, as well as submaximal exercise tests can be powerful motivators, especially if progress is noted. Franklin also pointed out the motivational potential of self-administered monitoring of pulse rate or body weight at weekly intervals.

Systems for monitoring progress on a workout-by-workout basis have also proved to have motivational benefits. Scherf and Franklin (1987) developed a data documentation system for use in a cardiac rehabilitation program in which participants record body weight, resting heart rate, exercise heart rate, laps walked, laps run, and total laps after each exercise session. This data is recorded on individual record forms that are easily accessible. Records are reviewed by staff members monthly and computations of total miles, average exercise heart rate, and attendance percentage are noted. The record cards are then returned to the participants with appropriate comments. Individuals who meet certain performance goals are recognized in a monthly award ceremony. By providing an ongoing awareness of progress, this system has been effective in promoting continued interest and enthusiasm needed to maintain long-term exercise participation.

Charting Attendance and Performance

Public recording of attendance and performance have also proven to be effective motivational techniques. Performance feedback can be made even more effective by converting the information to a graph or chart (Franklin, 1984; Presbie & Brown, 1977). A performance graph usually represents data in a form that is easily understood, usually depicting the performance dimension on the vertical axis and the temporal dimension on the horizontal axis. A major benefit of graphs is that one can tell at a glance what changes are occurring. A behavioral chart enables a person to note even small changes in performance, which may be important to maintain interest, especially as one reaches the point when increments of improvement become smaller and occur less frequently. For these reasons, the visual presentation of feedback is superior to verbal or tabular forms of performance feedback (Presbie & Brown, 1977).

Another benefit of public recording and sharing of behavioral information is its effect on future performance. The act of charting performance changes may serve as reinforcement or punishment in reaching target behaviors. Improvement in performance can be reinforcing, while lack of improvement or regression can prompt a person to change behaviors that may be detracting from performance. Recording and charting keep a person constantly informed, and often the increased cognitive awareness is all that is necessary to bring about changes in the target behavior.

A second source of possible reinforcement is the positive comments stimulated by the posting of performance data. If people know that their workout record is available for everyone to see, they are much more likely to strive for steady progress and work harder to achieve exercise goals than if no one else is privy to this information. Having ready access to information about an individual's progress facilitates interpersonal communication and enables the exercise leader and other class members to provide verbal praise and encouragement (Presbie & Brown, 1977). The effectiveness of recording attendance as well as the performance information of young swimmers was demonstrated by McKenzie and Rushall (1974). In this study, the public marking of attendance at practice was found to reduce absenteeism, tardiness, and leaving early. Additionally, the employment of a program board on which swimmers recorded completed work units significantly increased work output.

Another form of public recording that has proved successful is a cumulative charting of progress toward some distant goal. For example, Henning (1987) described a "Miles Club" in which walkers and runners recorded their weekly mileage. As they reached certain designated intervals, they were rewarded with engraved paperweights and gift certificates. Another such program recognized employees who walked, biked, ran, or aerobic danced the equivalent distance from New York to Los Angeles (Legwold, 1987). Records of individual progress were logged on a hallway banner. There is no end of the possible variations of this idea.

The public recording of fitness data may raise concerns and questions of confidentiality. No one who objects to this procedure should be required to participate. For those who choose not to record their data publicly, an alternative record system that is accessible only to the client and the exercise leader should be implemented. This record should provide the same performance data, appropriately charted, as for other class members.

Recognition of Accomplishment

Although vehicles of communication such as newsletters and bulletin boards are primarily informational and educational, they can also serve a motivational function. Recognition for achieving certain goals tends to stimulate people to put forth even greater efforts. Listing names and accomplishments in a company newsletter or posting milestones that have been reached on a bulletin board are useful motivational techniques (Franklin, 1978). People like to see their names in print, especially if they are being honored for attaining some worthwhile goal. A key point in using this technique well is to mention many names rather than just a few. This is possible if there are many categories and milestones to make recognition accessible to all participants. The creative use of recognition can be a valuable tool for the exercise practitioner.

Another approach to recognizing achievements is to hold periodic award ceremonies. Certificates, plaques, T-shirts, or other inexpensive items can reward outstanding accomplishments such as best attendance record, most improved fitness, and greatest weight loss (Franklin, 1984). An awards luncheon or dinner lends additional significance to the achievements being recognized.

Family Involvement

As we have seen, family involvement can improve exercise adherence. The support of one's spouse and other family members may also increase motivation. They can show continued interest and enthusiasm for the involved family member's exercise program and accommodate that involvement within the dynamics of family life. Involvement of spouses in special events or parallel programs have proved to be particularly sound motivational techniques. An example of a parallel program might be to have special speakers for family members who address related topics of interest (Erling & Oldridge, 1985; Franklin, 1978; Oldridge, 1984b; Whitehouse, 1977).

Interpersonal Relationships

Few motivational techniques are as potentially powerful as the social support that occurs within a fitness class. By establishing a warm and nonthreatening relationship with the client, the exercise leader may influence the client's level of motivation. One way to help establish this relationship is to communicate an expectancy for the client's performance that is challenging yet attainable. The importance of a teacher's expectations on subsequent student performance has been established in education and, to some extent, in sport (Carron, 1984; Horn, 1984). Although we have not found studies of the relationship between expectations of exercise leaders and performance levels of clients, it is likely that leader expectations play an important role in exercise and fitness programs as well. Another way the exercise leader is likely to affect client motivation is through social reinforcement. Social reinforcement is one of the most effective methods of influencing behaviors available to the exercise practitioner.

The relationships among program members is another source of motivation. As relationships are formed within the exercise group, members begin to feel a greater sense of commitment and personal involvement, and a greater reluctance to let the other members down through poor attendance or lack of effort. Friendly rivalry and good-natured competition often encourage members to work harder than they otherwise might. Establishing a "buddy system" has been found to be effective in overcoming the initial anxiety of beginning a program. It can also be effective in encouraging continued participation (Hobson, Hoffman, Corso, & Freismuth, 1987). Based on the promising results of Wankel's (1984) research, class members should be encouraged to provide each other with social reinforcement. A program T-shirt, emblem, or some other item that everyone wears serves as a symbol of participation and helps to promote the feeling of belonging to a worthwhile group (Collis, 1977).

Competition

As we established in our discussion of intrinsic motivation, competition is usually not a recommended motivational technique in exercise and fitness programs. It may, however, have a role to play in some instances. Younger program participants and those who are already in good condition may not be sufficiently challenged by activities appropriate for older, more sedentary participants. In such cases, parallel program activities that include competition may help motivate these clients. Certainly, no one should ever be forced to compete unless they are so inclined. However, few situations are as likely to motivate maximum performance as competition with an opponent of similar skill.

One form of competition that is motivational but nonthreatening is to engage in friendly contests with similar fitness groups. Competition in attendance, total weight loss, or miles run can be fun and contribute to an "esprit de corps" (Collis, 1977). Henning (1987) described a voluntary competition of this type. Volunteers were randomly assigned to teams of five to six people, and the team that used the facility most during a particular month won a free lunch. A team challenge board posted in a prominent location generated interest and enthusiasm for the contest. As a result of the competition, overall participation and group morale increased. A similar program dubbed the "Battle of the Department Stars" featured competition among the various departments. Teams were comprised of at least one person over 45, one upper management person, and one woman (Legwold, 1987).

Music

One of the more popular motivational techniques in recent years has been the use of music in exercise and fitness programs. Although energy expenditure is only slightly higher with music, participants perceive exercise to be easier (Franklin, 1978). Listening to music while exercising can probably be considered a disassociation method, which as we have seen is a recommended procedure for beginning exercise participants. The distraction of attention from unpleasant physical sensations to more pleasant auditory sensations seems to make the entire experience more palatable for some participants. Indeed, the proliferation of portable radios and tape players worn by walkers, bikers, and joggers seems to validate this observation.

In some fitness programs, music plays an integral part. The Canada Life fitness program, which included music as a central focus, found that participants overwhelmingly preferred to work out with music (Employee Fitness and Lifestyle Project, 1978). Music for exercise must have an appropriate tempo for the activity. The correct tempo and mood of the music are so important that if an instructor cannot provide suitable music, it is better to leave it off altogether (Employee Fitness and Lifestyle Project, 1978). Some fitness instructors encourage students to bring their own music. In such cases, the instructor should screen the music for appropriateness. By teaching clients to count beats and use other specific criteria in choosing music for class, the instructor can reduce time spent screening the music. Music prepared especially for use in exercise classes is available commercially, and although it tends to be expensive, the time saved in searching for good music may justify the cost.

We should caution that the legal implications of using recorded music for classes or for background purposes are considerable. If music is for other than personal use, individuals and organizations are required under copyright law to pay royalties to one of two music licensing organizations—the American Society of Composers, Authors, and Publishers (ASCAP) or the Broadcast Music Incorporated (BMI). Payment of a fee provides a blanket license to use all music controlled by the licensing body.

Program Variety

To maintain client interest, the exercise professional must continually seek ways to infuse variety into the program. To insist on a rigid program of calisthenics or running for all clients is sure to prompt many to drop out. More attractive forms of exercise that offer comparable physiological outcomes should be encouraged (Franklin, 1984). Introducing new exercises, developing different routines, staging unique events, honoring birthdays, and adopting themes are a few ways of providing novelty (Collis, 1977). One source of innovation is the class itself. Soliciting volunteers as "leaders for the day" can introduce some interesting program permutations. Recreational games can also provide variety. To minimize the competitive nature or the level of skill required for successful participation, rules may need to be modified. In volleyball, for example, a reduction of court size, allowing one bounce of the ball, and forbidding spiking can prolong rallies, increase fitness outcomes, and provide more fun for participants (Franklin, 1984).

Bells and Whistles

Some clients will be motivated by what we call the "bells and whistles." Program accouterments, such as programmable electronic exercycles, isokinetic muscle-testing equipment, and other sophisticated exercise equipment, although expensive and unnecessary as far as fitness development is concerned, will attract people who like gadgets and technical devices. The added complexity that these items provide may be sufficient to motivate continuing participation. Although certainly not scientific, our observations have shown that when given the choice between a regular exercycle and a more advanced programmable exercycle, more people

choose the programmable one. Of course, economics is an important consideration, and we are not suggesting that large sums of money be spent on these items. We would, however, recommend that after acquiring the basic equipment, some representative items of this sort be purchased as it becomes financially feasible.

Emphasis on Fun

Many fitness programs are very businesslike and serious. Overemphasizing the serious nature of exercise may alienate some clients. People generally know the benefits of good health habits. Messages of gloom and doom may be just aversive enough to make people look for other, more enjoyable ways to spend their discretionary time. As Snyder and Spreitzer (1984) have concluded, most people do not exercise because it is good for them, but because it feels good.

A fun approach to fitness has proved to be more successful in promoting long-term participation and enjoyment (Franklin, 1984). One technique that has been effective, particularly with obese clients, is to emphasize pleasure and success through games and recreational activities (Franklin, 1984). Activities that stress successful participation and enjoyment draw on the reinforcing properties inherent in the activity, which motivates future participation.

Special Programs and Events

Special events can provide a motivational jolt to a stagnating program. Fun runs, charity runs, walkathons, or swimathons are examples of such events. Staging a comprehensive "fit fair" can be educational as well as motivating. Inviting a variety of "experts" to participate in such an event can rejuvenate flagging interest. Clinics, workshops, or lectures provided by local medical personnel or a fitness specialist with good credentials not only help renew interest but also reinforce what the regular staff has been communicating. Hearing similar information from another credible source seems to increase retention. Holding special events in conjunction with officially designated focus periods, such as heart month, or planning them to coincide with certain holidays can result in some interesting programs. A reunion of program graduates can also be an incentive for program maintenance (Martin & Dubbert, 1987). Not all special events need be fitness related. Purely social activities can have positive effects on morale and motivation. A picnic, a hike in the woods, a trip to the beach, a ball game, or a fishing trip are all examples of fun events that help to solidify group commitment. Including spouses and other family members in special programs helps to elicit their continuing interest and support.

Financial Rebate Systems

Most researchers agree that if people are to benefit from a fitness program, they should have some financial investment in it. Individuals with no financial interest in a program tend to sign up, but they also tend to drop out ("Motivation a key," 1981). An approach that has proved successful in corporate programs is for the company to pay most (but not all) of the program cost. Pollock and associates (1982) compared four methods of payment and found that program attendance was better when participants were either reimbursed based on attendance or split the fee with their employer. In this study, the lowest record of attendance was associated with programs in which the company paid the entire fee. The next lowest attendance was recorded for participants who paid the whole fee themselves. The Campbell Soup Company's program requires employees to pay $50 the first year. If they exercise 3 times a week or more during the second year, they pay only $25. If the employees continue to exercise at this rate, they pay nothing the third year (Legwold, 1987). A system that ties a financial rebate to improvement in fitness parameters rather than attendance is a motivational technique that also deserves consideration.

Active Participation of Top Managers

Corporate programs that not only have the moral support of management but also have the top managers actively involved tend to be very successful. Participation at this level is an excellent way to communicate the importance of fitness to the work force (Hobson et al., 1987). When employees see the company president running around the gym, they may see that individual in a new light and may be challenged to match the commitment ("Motivation a key," 1981). Moreover, observing one's supervisor struggling like everyone else conveys the message that exercise and fitness are important. Another message is that if managers can find time for fitness, employees can too. The participation of managers and employees together can also improve morale. The informal give and take of the exercise setting tends to promote "team spirit." It should be recognized, however, that some managers are uncomfortable exercising with employees and may prefer to work out alone or with other managers.

Leadership

Some believe that leadership is the single most important factor in client motivation to exercise (Oldridge, 1977). Chapter 9 is devoted to the skills and characteristics of effective exercise leadership. For now, we shall simply state that a knowledgeable, concerned, and enthusiastic professional is the point of departure when considering motivation for exercise and fitness.

SUMMARY

Client motivation, one of the most important tasks of the exercise professional, has been discussed from theoretical as well as practical perspectives. Incentives, both tangible and intangible, can be effective motivators of exercise behaviors if used judiciously. Incentives should be used primarily in the early stages of a program to stimulate client interest. Their use should be gradually reduced as exercise behaviors become established. To promote long-term involvement in exercise and fitness, one of the most promising strategies is to foster intrinsic motivation. Opportunities that enable clients to demonstrate competence and self-determination are most likely to develop intrinsic motivation. Clients need to have a major voice in planning their own programs. Rewards, if used, should have informational rather than controlling properties. Programs that emphasize enjoyment and client satisfaction are most likely to elicit intrinsic motivation. It is also highly desirable to emphasize positive feedback while minimizing pressure for ever-higher levels of performance.

Goal setting is another promising motivational technique available to the exercise practitioner. Goals focus client attention, mobilize energy expenditure, and prolong effort over time. Goals should be collaboratively set, important, specific, and challenging. Short-range, intermediate, and long-term goals should be set, and feedback on progress provided frequently.

Other "tried and true" methods of developing or increasing program interest and enthusiasm include public recording of attendance and performance, recognition of accomplishment, family involvement, fostering the development of interpersonal relationships, "friendly" competition, using music during workouts, offering program variety, providing technical equipment features, emphasizing fun and enjoyment, holding special events, assuring that individuals have a financial stake in the program, and securing the active participation of management.

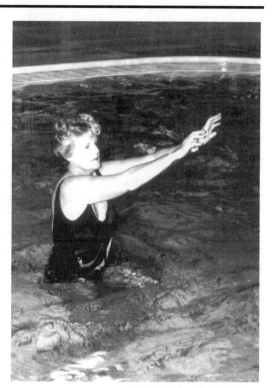

Chapter 7
The Principles of Cognitive and Behavioral Change Strategies

The evolution of learning theories of behavioral change have yielded a rich diversity of approaches and continually refined theoretical models. The study of behavioral change is a core area of psychological research. In this chapter we will address how an understanding of behavioral change can be of use to the exercise practitioner.

Engaging in exercise is itself an initiation of behavioral change. Both process (e.g., the participation in exercise for simple enjoyment) and outcome goals (e.g., participation in exercise to reduce weight and improve cardiovascular functioning) of a physical and therapeutic nature are formulas

for behavioral change. The exercise practitioner and client can factor the desired change into the exercise experience. If the exercise practitioner does not develop goals for desired change and monitor the client's progress, an undesired behavioral change may occur.

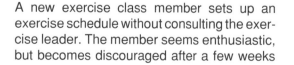

A new exercise class member sets up an exercise schedule without consulting the exercise leader. The member seems enthusiastic, but becomes discouraged after a few weeks

111

and drops out. It turns out that the participant has set up a grueling schedule way beyond the person's capability. The individual has not built in any reinforcers, social support, or sources of encouragement, and has decided that exercise is too punishing. The resulting cognitive-behavioral change is that the individual develops negative feelings about exercise (cognitive change) and discontinues exercise (behavioral change).

A key principle for success in exercise is the understanding of and ability to utilize cognitive-behavioral strategies. This chapter provides a comprehensive review of behavioral change approaches. Some of the approaches represent the foundation principles of learning and change, while others have more recently emerged as interdisciplinary forms of behavioral interventions. The major areas described are

- classical conditioning,
- operant conditioning,
- cognitive-behavioral approaches, and
- social cognitive theory.

The last section addresses the application of behavior change strategies to specific health concerns, including smoking, obesity, stress, alcohol abuse, and coronary heart disease.

CLASSICAL CONDITIONING

Behavioral change strategies that exemplify classical conditioning approaches focus on helping individuals to stop undesirable or maladaptive behaviors. The therapeutic intervention includes a component intended to decrease a maladaptive behavior as well as one that encourages a more desirable adaptive response. For the intervention to be effective, the desired behavior must be incompatible with the undesirable behavior.

Pavlov, a Russian physiologist, first demonstrated classical conditioning in the 1920s. This demonstration was based on his work with conditioned reflexes. A *reflex* is a specific, unlearned reaction mediated by the autonomic nervous system and elicited by a specific stimulus (e.g., pain elicits a physical withdrawal reaction). The response to the stimuli is automatic. No decision to respond is made. Because of the role classical

conditioning plays in the development of conditioned emotional response, such as fear and anxiety, it can affect participation in exercise. For example, if at some time in a person's past a traumatic experience paired exercise with a fear-provoking stimuli (e.g., being bitten by a dog while running), the anticipation of exercise may elicit a response of anxiety or fear from that individual. In such a case, controlled and moderated exercise can reduce the anxiety by (1) allowing the exercise behavior to occur without the feared consequence (being bitten) and (2) using exercise to reduce anxiety and tension as a result of increased levels of endorphins and norepinephrine (Dishman, 1982).

It is important to note that classical conditioning, unlike operant conditioning, always involves an unlearned innate reflex (e.g., fear). Classical conditioning never involves learning new behaviors, only conditioning existing responses to new stimuli. The most frequently used example of classical conditioning today is *systematic desensitization*, which includes *progressive relaxation*.

Systematic Desensitization

In the early 1950s, Joseph Wolpe developed the technique of systematic desensitization that uses relaxation to suppress anxiety. Systematic desensitization is based on the principle of counterconditioning. A response of anxiety is learned or conditioned and can, therefore, be eliminated or unlearned by substituting relaxation as an adaptive behavior. Because relaxation is incompatible with the anxiety response, an individual cannot be anxious and relaxed at the same time. If the relaxation technique is learned well, the individual can induce relaxation and inhibit anxiety. There are three basic steps in the systematic desensitization procedure:

1. Relaxation training
2. Creation of an anxiety hierarchy
3. Actual desensitization

An illustration of how desensitization can be applied in the exercise setting follows.

Relaxation Training

Jacobson (1938) developed the therapeutic technique of progressive muscle relaxation. Since that time, many modified versions of the relaxation technique have been used with systematic desensitization. Muscle relaxation involves the systematic tightening and relaxing of the major muscle groups. The effectiveness of the relaxation technique has been well documented for tension-related problems (Bernstein & Borkovec, 1973) and anxiety (Kazdin & Wilcoxon, 1976).

---■---

Anna is a 57-year-old who has had a mild heart attack, and part of her recommended cardiac rehabilitation is hydrotherapy. However, Anna is afraid of water. Although she wants to cooperate and contribute to her rehabilitation, she is reluctant to do the exercise activities.

The first stage of the relaxation procedure involves a thorough assessment of Anna's fear (or other aversive response, such as panic or anger), the circumstances surrounding the fear, and the intensity of the feelings associated with the fear (Morris, 1986). The assessment also helps Anna realize that the fear of water is being maintained by anxiety, not by aversive experience with water. Anna has been afraid of water for as long as she can remember, but does not recall any frightening experience associated with water. The practitioner questions Anna about what negative feelings she has, the intensity of the feelings, and the circumstances that typically evoke these feelings. The practitioner then leads Anna through relaxation training.

The progressive muscle relaxation training follows a standard procedure in which approximately 14 muscle groups are trained. This procedure can be done in five to six sessions and usually involves homework assignments of practicing the steps in Table 7.1. Exercise practitioners may note that relaxation techniques, besides being part of the desensitization process, can be used independently simply to relieve stress and tension. This technique can be conducted with an individual or in small or large groups, and is sometimes paired with visual imagery relaxation.

Creating an Anxiety Hierarchy

Midway through relaxation training, the practitioner asks the client to construct an anxiety hierarchy based on data from the initial interview. Wolpe developed a system called SUDS (subjective units of distress scale) in which each anxiety level is assigned a score. The hierarchy includes approximately 20 to 25 items, each of which is equally spaced in terms of eliciting anxiety. If the items are too closely related, the process will be too time-consuming, and if they are too far apart, the client may relapse and lose the level of desensitization already achieved. To accomplish this stage, the practitioner must consult with the client to develop a clear understanding of the nature of the problem and to establish a workable hierarchy. The entire range of anxiety-based items must be identified or the higher level anxiety may be missed. The practitioner should ensure that a 0-level control scene (one considered totally relaxing) is identified.

---■---

An abbreviated anxiety hierarchy for Anna looks like this:

Fear of Water

  10—Entering the pool area

  20—Walking toward the pool

  30—Sitting on the edge of the pool

  40—Dangling her feet and legs in the pool

  50—Standing in the shallow end

  60—Walking into waist high water

  70—Putting her head under water

  80—Walking toward the deep end

  90—Using an inner tube to paddle in water over her head

100—Being in water over her head and having to swim

Desensitization Proper

After relaxation training and the creation of an anxiety hierarchy, the client is ready to be desensitized.

---■---

The practitioner instructs Anna to establish a relaxed state by undergoing the relaxation procedure. When Anna is relaxed, the practitioner presents the least anxiety-producing item on the hierarchy and asks Anna to imagine the situation. If she feels any anxiety, she signals the practitioner, who then helps her reestablish relaxation.

The process is repeated with anxiety items being reintroduced until detectable anxiety is noted and relaxation is again reinstituted. The process

Table 7.1   An Introduction to the Relaxation Training Steps of Systematic Desensitization

1. Take a deep breath and hold it (for about 10 seconds). Hold it. Okay, let it out.
2. Raise both of your hands about half way above the couch (or, arms of the chair), and breathe normally. Now, drop your hands to the couch (or, down).
3. Now hold your arms out and make a tight fist. Really tight. Feel the tension in your hands. I am going to count to three and when I say "three," I want you to drop your hands. One . . . Two . . . Three.
4. Raise your arms again, and bend your fingers back the other way (toward your body). Now drop your hands and relax.
5. Raise your arms. Now drop them and relax.
6. Now raise your arms again, but this time "flap" your hands around. Okay, relax again.
7. Raise your arms again. Now, relax.
8. Raise your arms above the couch (chair) again and tense your biceps until they shake. Breathe normally, and keep your hands loose. Relax your hands. (Notice how you have a warm feeling of relaxation.)
9. Now hold your arms out to your side and tense your biceps. Make sure that you breathe normally. Relax your arms.
10. Now arch your shoulders back. Hold it. Make sure that your arms are relaxed. Now relax.
11. Hunch your shoulders forward. Hold it, and make sure that you breathe normally and keep your arms relaxed. Okay, relax. (Notice the feeling of relief from tensing and relaxing your muscles.)
12. Now turn you head to the right and tense your neck. Relax and bring your head back again to its natural position.
13. Turn your head to the left and tense your neck. Relax and bring your head back again to its natural position.
14. Now bend your head back slightly toward the chair. Hold it. Okay, now bring your head back slowly to its natural position.[a]
15. This time bring your head down almost to your chest. Hold it. Now relax and let your head come back to its natural resting position.[a]
16. Now open your mouth as much as possible. A little wider, okay, relax. (Mouth must be partly open at end.)
17. Now tense your lips by closing your mouth. Okay, relax. (Notice the feeling of relaxation.)
18. Put your tongue at the roof of your mouth. Press hard. (Pause) Relax and allow your tongue to come to a comfortable position in your mouth.
19. Now put your tongue at the bottom of your mouth. Press down hard. Relax and let your tongue come to a comfortable position in your mouth.
20. Now just lie (sit) there and relax. Try not to think of anything.
21. To control self-verbalization, I want you to go through the motions of singing a high note—not aloud! Okay, start singing to yourself. Hold that note, and now relax.
22. Now sing a medium note and make your vocal cords tense again. Relax.
23. Now sing a low note and make your vocal cords tense again. Relax. (Your vocal apparatus should be relaxed now. Relax your mouth.)
24. Now, close your eyes. Squeeze them tight and breathe naturally. Notice the tension. Now relax. (Notice how the pain goes away when you relax.)
25. Now let your eyes relax and keep your mouth open slightly.
26. Open your eyes as much as possible. Hold it. Now, relax your eyes.
27. Now wrinkle your forehead as much as possible. Hold it. Okay, relax.
28. Now take a deep breath and hold it. Relax.
29. Now exhale. Breathe all the air out . . . all of it out. Relax. (Notice the wondrous feeling of breathing again.)
30. Imagine that there are weights pulling on all your muscles making them flaccid and relaxed . . . pulling your arms and body into the couch.

[a]The client should not be encouraged to bend his or her neck either all the way back or forward.

From "Fear Reduction Methods" by R.J. Morris. In *Helping People Change: A Textbook of Methods* (pp. 159-160) by F.H. Kanfer and A.P. Goldstein (Eds.), 1986, New York: Pergamon Press. Copyright 1986 by Pergamon Press. Reprinted by permission.

continues until the highest item on the hierarchy elicits no anxiety. Each hierarchy scene is presented 3 or 4 times for 5 to 10 seconds each. The relaxation periods last from 10 to 15 seconds. Three or four different scenes may be presented per session and a single session lasts from 30 minutes to 1 hour.

During the last phase of treatment, it is often helpful to put the client in an *in vivo* situation, which entails causing the client to experience the actual anxiety-producing situation under controlled conditions. The practitioner must be certain that the client is ready for the experience. The practitioner should also ensure that the last part of every treatment session ends on a positive note and that enough time is allowed to debrief.

Systematic desensitization may not be recommended in the following circumstances (Carnwath & Miller, 1986).

■ Relaxation may be cathartic in that suppressed emotions or tension may become unleashed unexpectedly in an uncontrolled environment.

■ Muscle relaxation could cause pain in strained muscles or could affect recent surgical procedures.

■ If a personality disorder or psychological dysfunction exists, the condition could be exacerbated. Also, if severe disorders exist, relaxation does not help.

■ Medical conditions such as epilepsy may be adversely affected.

For those readers interested in relaxation training, Morris (1986) has written an extensive and detailed instructional description that we highly recommend.

OPERANT CONDITIONING

Operant conditioning focuses on the relationship between a behavior and its consequences. Operant approaches assume that the consequences of behavior affect the likelihood that the behavior will be repeated. To change certain behaviors, it may be necessary to modify their consequences. Our behaviors are not primarily maintained by overt and immediate reinforcement, but rather by secondary reinforcers that function subtly. Secondary reinforcers are associated with primary reinforcers. Money, a secondary reinforcer, has value only because it can acquire primary reinforcers, such as food and shelter. Exercise professionals must have a clear understanding of operant conditioning and other cognitive-behavioral methods to effectively design and implement exercise programs.

Operant principles provide a systematic approach to changing a behavior and verifying that the change has in fact occurred. Figure 7.1 is a schematic representation of the basic principles and components of behavior change. The nature of the consequence (positive/negative reinforcement

or punishment) determines whether the behavior will increase, decrease, or maintain the present rate. Figure 7.1 may be used as a reference throughout this section.

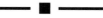

A 42-year-old man named Bill has begun an exercise regimen to lose weight. Bill is considerably overweight and has high cholesterol and high blood pressure. The exercise practitioner works with Bill to set up an exercise program appropriate for his goals and his baseline level of fitness. The instructor also explores the environmental, social, and personal aspects of Bill's lifestyle that might contribute to his overeating and helps him identify the reinforcing consequences of eating. They discover that Bill eats primarily when he is home alone. He dislikes being alone and realizes that eating is a way of comforting himself when he feels isolated and lonely. Had the instructor not pursued this information, the exercise program would probably have failed because the reinforcement for overeating would have been overlooked.

Antecedent Conditions

Habitual behaviors are the result of responsiveness to environmental cues or discriminative stimuli. These cues or stimuli affect behavior because of what people anticipate the consequences will be if they do not respond to the cue. Antecedent cues that signal that potential for reinforcement or punishment are called *discriminative stimuli* or *prompts*.

If someone is driving late at night on a deserted road, that person will probably stop at a red light and continue to drive on the right side of the center line. The stoplight and center line have no reinforcement properties. The power of antecedent cues lies in their ability to warn that a consequence (reinforcement or punishment) of the behavior is potentially imminent. An unseen police car could result in a ticket and if the center line is crossed, the probability of meeting an oncoming car has sharply increased.

Although antecedent conditions are not themselves reinforcers, their importance in behavioral change cannot be underestimated. Examples of antecedent cues that occur naturally in exercise settings are physical facilities and equipment, dressing for exercise, making plans with a friend to attend class, and interacting with other class members. An objective of exercise participation is

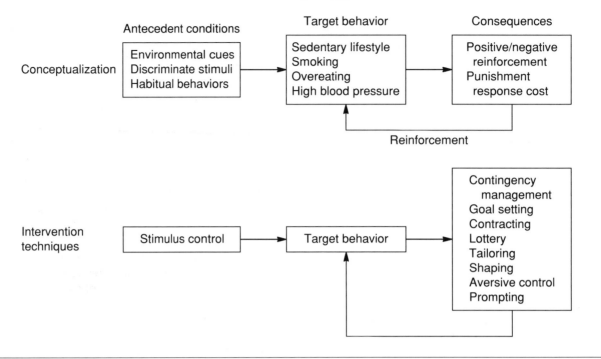

Figure 7.1 Schematic representation for operant behavior change.

to increase the frequency of a desirable activity (e.g., running or swimming).

The antecedent cues mentioned facilitate the occurrence of exercise. The exercise leader must also be aware of antecedent cues that support behaviors that compete with exercise participation. A more enjoyable activity scheduled at the same time as the exercise class, inconvenient exercise location, unpleasant facilities, driving by a favorite hangout on the way to exercise, or negative self-talk before exercise all discourage continued participation. A primary reason why exercise dropout rates increase after a program has ended is that supporting antecedent cues and reinforcements built into the class were not transferred to independent exercise. The exercise practitioner should help class members design an exercise plan that builds in reinforcements and antecedent cues for operating in a different exercise environment.

Stimulus Control

The process of manipulating antecedent conditions can be important in the exercise setting. It is often easier or more realistic to manipulate antecedent stimuli than to modify consequences of behavior (Karoly & Harris, 1986). Because a desirable behavior may not spontaneously or independently occur, stimulus control, such as instructions or encouragement, may initiate the behavior (Snyder, 1989).

Stimulus control can also reduce undesirable behavior. For example, an exercise class member often misses the noon class because she prefers to eat lunch and socialize. Her exercise instructor helps her design a stimulus control procedure in which she can skip exercise for lunch, but can only eat alone. The next week, the client can skip exercise and eat lunch, but only in her office. The following week, all of these conditions apply plus doing paperwork while eating. At this point, most reinforcers for missing exercise have been eliminated and there are more reinforcers for going to exercise class than for not going. Karoly and Harris (1986) identified a procedure for implementing a stimulus control program. We will apply this procedure to our earlier example of Bill and his problem of overeating:

1. Identify by individualized observation, not deduction, the anticipatory links between the antecedent cues and the desirable behavior. The desirable behavior for Bill is controlled eating and a change to healthier foods. The instructor and Bill structure some antecedent cues for healthier eating such as buying only healthy, low-calorie foods, making more social plans to avoid being home alone, and developing enjoyable activities he can do at home so that being alone is not so aversive.

2. Identify antecedent cues for the undesirable behavior. For Bill, cues for undesirable behavior are feeling sorry for himself for living alone, buying

favorite high-calorie foods, and spending long periods at home. The desirable antecedent cues are often the flip side of the undesirable antecedent cues.

3. Remove, through fading, or negative reinforcement, the cues for the inappropriate behaviors.

4. Strengthen the cues for appropriate behaviors. Make them more conspicuous and frequent.

5. Help clients develop the ability to control cues for their behaviors. The instructor helps Bill begin monitoring cues that have strong associations with eating.

An unusual application of stimulus control was implemented by Brownell, Stunkard, and Albaum (1980). They posted signs by elevators in public places that read, "Here's your chance to exercise your heart. It needs exercise." The frequency of individuals choosing the stairs rose from 5.3% to 13.7%.

Behavioral Consequences

Antecedent conditions create anticipation of behavior, but consequences determine the occurrence of behavior. Behavioral consequences may be categorized as reinforcement or punishment. Any event that increases the frequency of the behavior it follows is a *reinforcement*. The presentation of an aversive event or the removal of a positive event that decreases the frequency of a behavior is called *punishment*. Figure 7.2 may help clarify the different functions and effects of reinforcement and punishment.

Following are explanations of each of the four quadrants in Figure 7.2:

Positive Reinforcement

■ Praise and encouragement from the exercise leader

■ Documentation of physical improvement in heart rate, body fat, and weight after 6 weeks of exercise

■ Observation by the client and leader that endurance and length of time running has increased

The exercise practitioner must provide the appropriate reinforcement for the target behavior. Praise, special attention, rewards, and privileges are examples of effective reinforcers.

The exercise practitioner should note that identifying effective reinforcers is an individualized process. What works as a reinforcer for one person will not always work for another. There are, of course, commonly shared reinforcers. However, when working with an individual on specific target behaviors, individualized reinforcers are most important. The best way to determine appropriate reinforcers is to consult with the client. Ask specifically about consumable reinforcers, such as favorite foods; activity reinforcers, such as sport and leisure pursuits; social reinforcers, such as group activities; and acquisition of possessions, such as gadgets, games, or toys.

Negative Reinforcement

■ Elimination of tired, sluggish feeling as a result of jogging

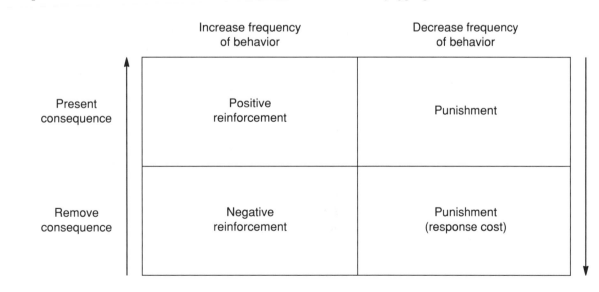

	Increase frequency of behavior	Decrease frequency of behavior
Present consequence	Positive reinforcement	Punishment
Remove consequence	Negative reinforcement	Punishment (response cost)

Figure 7.2 Principles of reinforcement.

■ Relief from tension and stress

■ Reduction in self-consciousness of body size as a result of weight loss from exercise

Negative reinforcement is often misunderstood. Punishment is frequently confused with negative reinforcement because both involve the presence of noxious or aversive stimuli. The difference is that punishment decreases a behavior and negative reinforcement increases a behavior.

Although response cost is sometimes used in self-management programs, punishment and response cost (a type of punishment) are not preferred modes of behavior change. If implemented, however, they would be better applied to noncompliance rather than to compliance, or as a consequence of an undesirable response incompatible with exercise.

Punishment

■ Bodily stress and tension are retained as a result of noncompliance

■ Weight gain

■ Difficulty in exercising at maintenance pace during the next exercise period

There are probably very few practical uses for direct forms of punishment in exercise and fitness programs. One of the disadvantages of punishment are the negative feelings that are invariably evoked. Hard feelings, ill will, and inhibited communication between the parties involved are common by-products of punishment (Presbie & Brown, 1977). Despite these disadvantages, some people do respond to punishment, and it can be effective, especially if it is necessary to stop behaviors quickly.

Response Cost

■ Loss of social contact and support of exercise class when absent

■ Loss of rating in goal-setting charts

Response cost is the removal of consequences, which reduces the frequency of the behavior. Presbie and Brown (1977) cited a study in which response cost was used to reduce undesirable behaviors of college students. When free weights were not returned to their racks when students were finished, a response cost procedure was successfully implemented in which students were told that the weight room would be closed unless the weights were returned to their proper places after use. In behavior modification terms, the continued use of the weight room was made contingent on the return of weights to their storage racks. The threat of the loss of access to the weight facility resulted in a decrease in this behavior.

Social Reinforcement

Social reinforcement is any social consequence, either verbal or nonverbal, that increases future behaviors (Presbie & Brown, 1977). Positive emotive behaviors by an instructor in the form of praise, reassurance, approval, encouragement, and support have consistently been proved to facilitate the learning of new behaviors or maintaining existing behaviors. On the other hand, negative emotive behaviors by the instructor such as disapproval, criticism, sarcasm, threats, or reprisals have not been as effective. The general rule for the effective use of social reinforcement is to minimize criticism and maximize praise and other forms of social reinforcement (Presbie & Brown, 1977).

Rushall (1980) developed a helpful reference guide to several forms of social reinforcement. The guide includes examples of key words, voice modulation, gesticulation, and instructor proximity as social reinforcements. Examples are given in Table 7.2. To be most effective, the exercise practitioner should develop a unique repertoire of social reinforcers comprised of key words, gestures, and expressions. There should be enough variety to avoid repetition. A periodic check on the use of social reinforcement, both in terms of amount and type, can be very informative to a fitness instructor as well as to his or her supervisor.

Verbal praise may be the single most important reinforcer for an exercise practitioner to learn from the behavior modification approach. Properly used, praise can have a powerful impact on client behaviors. Presbie and Brown (1977) identified some helpful principles for making verbal praise more effective:

■ Keep a daily count of verbal praises given to each individual. Try to praise each student 15 times in a 30-minute class period. When instructors cannot collect their own data, an assistant should record instances of praise.

■ Praise students equally. In a group situation, all clients should receive approximately the same amount of the instructor's attention.

■ Praise the students' behaviors as well as the students. Praise should be specific and descriptive. For example, instead of saying, ''Nice going over

Table 7.2   Reinforcement Synthesizer

Key words		Voice modulation	Gesticulation	Proximity	Subject
Top notch	A1	Pitch up	Wave arms	Touch	Individual
Capital	Grand	Pitch down	Punch air	Close	Subgroup
First class	Beautiful	Volume up	OK sign	Medium	Group
First rate	Incredible	Volume down	Clap	Distant	
Magnifique	Unbelievable	Pitch high	Smile		
Stupendous	Fantastic	Pitch low	Nod		
Superlative	Proud	Volume high	Pat on back		
Good	Superb	Volume low	Squeeze		
Super	Splendid	Pronunciation slow	Thumbs up		
Fabulous	Magnificent	Emphasis	Point		
Amazing	Terrific		Arm around shoulders		
Far out	Great				
Dynamite	Marvellous				
Phenomenal	Wonderful				
Tremendous	Gorgeous				
Out of this world					

Reprinted with permission of Macmillan Publishing Company, a Division of Macmillan, Inc. from *Psychology in Sport: Methods and Application* by Richard Suinn. Copyright © 1980 Macmillan Publishing Company.

there," say, "That is an excellent knee lift, Sue. That's the way to really get them up there!"

■ Ignore inappropriate behavior unless it disrupts others. Commenting on good behavior rather than dwelling on shortcomings is more likely to encourage good morale and enthusiasm. It will also communicate to other class members what is important, and what will be rewarded.

■ To maintain a positive class atmosphere, deliver at least five praise statements for each critical statement. Presbie and Brown (1977) have suggested that an instructor do "penance" for each critical statement.

To many, exercise is an unpleasant and even painful experience. Virtually all people who experience exercise in this way are dropout candidates. To try to minimize the perception of exercise as an aversive experience, the exercise professional should get background information on clients. A person with a minimal exercise history is not as likely to understand the sensations that accompany exercise nor be able to tolerate as much discomfort as a person with considerable former experience. In the early stages, intensity should be minimized and emphasis be placed on the enjoyable or reinforcing aspects of exercise. The practitioner should make the point that exercise makes you "feel good." By drawing attention to the pleasant sensations associated with exercise, the instructor can help clients learn to reinforce their own exercise behaviors. The eventual goal is for the exercise experience to become naturally reinforcing for the exerciser.

Operant Techniques Applied to Exercise Settings

Several operant approaches have been applied successfully in a variety of exercise settings.

Contingency Management

The process of changing the frequency of a behavior by controlling the consequences is called *contingency management* (Gatchel & Baum, 1983). Research has shown that contingency management increases the frequency of desirable target behaviors (Allen & Iwata, 1980; Allison & Ayllon, 1980; Perkins, Rapp, Carlson, & Wallace, 1986). Parents frequently use contingency management when they require children to rake the leaves, take out the garbage, or clean their rooms before using the family car. People set contingencies for themselves by requiring that they finish certain tasks before going to the movies, buying something frivolous, or going out to eat. Contingency management is a form of reinforcement. While reinforcement encourages the presence of a behavior, contingency management influences the frequency of a behavior.

Contracting

Written statements that outline specific behaviors and establish consequences for fulfillment are known as *contracts* (Kanfer & Gaelick, 1986). The contingency contract between the exercise practitioner and the client specifies expectations, responsibilities, and contingencies for behavioral change (Kirschenbaum & Flanery, 1983). The purpose of contingency contracts is to maintain clients' motivation to exercise. An effective contingency contract should include realistic goals, dates by which the goal must be reached, and consequences of meeting or not meeting the goal. The contingencies must be personalized to ensure the effectiveness of the consequence.

Kanfer and Gaelick (1986) identified the purposes of contracts or helping the client take action, establishing criteria for meeting goals, and providing a means for clarifying consequences. Contracts should have readily achievable short-range goals. The elements of a contract as outlined by Kanfer and Gaelick follow. The earlier example of Bill, the class member with a weight problem, will be applied here.

─────────── ■ ───────────

1. A clear description of the target behavior is stated. Bill and his instructor agree on a target loss of 10 pounds. Although multiple goals may apply (e.g., lowered blood pressure, lowered cholesterol, better cardiovascular functioning), for the purpose of clearly understood objectives, each target behavior should be considered separately.

2. Criterion for the time or frequency limitations of the stated goals is clear. The exercise class is extended to 10 weeks, which is the time frame for achieving the goal.

3. Specific positive reinforcements for goal achievement and aversive consequences for nonfulfillment are identified. Bill and his instructor identify effective reinforcements (e.g., a weekend vacation, an expensive purchase, or a party) as well as aversive consequences (e.g., being denied something he has wanted to buy or doing housework or home repairs).

4. A bonus clause for exceeding the goal is developed. Bill will allow himself to buy something extravagant.

5. A means of measuring progress during the program is established. Bill will keep a weekly chart of exercise and diet and the instructor will review the chart weekly.

6. The delivery of reinforcement contingencies is timely. The instructor ensures that the reinforcements are applied within 24 hours after a success.

─────────────────────────

Dunbar, Marshall, and Hovell (1979) cited several advantages of contracts:

■ Contracting involves the client in the behavioral change strategy. Often, the client's commitment is higher in a collaborative approach and the ability to individualize treatment is greater.

■ The written contract enables verification, while the verbal contract is sometimes unclear.

■ A public rather than private commitment may foster self-control over the behavior (Kanfer, Cox, Gruner, & Karoly, 1974).

■ Incentive value may be established through rewards for goal attainment.

If the client monitors the contract, the likelihood of treatment adherence increases. The role of the client in obtaining information, demonstrating intentions, and developing commitment are invaluable in fostering adherence (Kirschenbaum & Flanery, 1983).

Lottery

A technique frequently applied in conjunction with contracting is the lottery. All participants contribute an amount of money, and based on agreed upon criteria, the winner receives the money. Epstein, Wing, Thompson, and Griffin (1980) implemented a lottery in which subjects contributed $3 each and were required to attend exercise four out of five sessions per week to qualify for the lottery. At the end of the study, a winner was chosen randomly from among the qualifiers. Subjects in the lottery group had higher attendance in exercise sessions than did the control group.

However, in another study that included an attendance lottery component in addition to personal feedback and fixed versus flexible goal-setting, no significant difference was found between the lottery and the no-lottery groups. The presence of material and social reinforcers may well diminish the effectiveness of one or the other. In this study, the lottery was ineffective compared to the value of personal feedback (Martin et al., 1984). The consistent effectiveness of the lottery as a contingency technique without pairing it with other reinforcers is not yet known.

Several research findings seem to give direction to exercise practitioners who incorporate principles of motivation into behavioral treatment plans (Karoly & Harris, 1986). During the behavior acquisition phase, several rules may be followed:

■ Consequences should closely follow a behavior.

■ Tangible reinforcements are useful during behavior acquisition and the initial maintenance phase, but should be gradually reduced and eventually removed. It is critical to build in natural reinforcers and to identify intrinsic rewards as tangibles are removed, or the individual will be left with no reinforcement.

■ Increases in frequency and duration of exercise should be moderated to ensure success.

■ Contracts should be written, not verbal.

■ Public posting of goals with acknowledgment of meeting goals is effective for many people in increasing adherence. Public posting should be continued as tangible reinforcers are reduced.

■ Incentives should be associated with outcomes of exercise behavior, not attendance. The size of the incentive is not a determining factor in adherence.

■ Group contracts, at least in weight-loss programs, are more effective than individual contracts. The individuals feel a commitment to the group that may be stronger than the commitment to self.

■ Personal feedback is probably more effective than group feedback. The two could certainly be combined as an effective reinforcement.

Developing and Implementing an Operant Program

Operant principles are sometimes more easily understood than implemented. A set of procedural guidelines shows how to apply these principles to a target behavior in the exercise setting (Snyder, 1989):

Assessment

1. Describe the problem.

2. Identify and specifically define the target behavior.

3. Identify antecedent cues that promote or inhibit the behavior.

4. Identify and describe environmental cues (discriminative stimuli that promote or inhibit the behavior).

5. Identify and describe consequences that promote or inhibit the behavior.

When the problem is fully understood, a behavioral intervention program can be developed.

Program Development and Implementation

6. Identify desirable antecedent cues and environmental stimuli that are incompatible with the undesirable antecedent and environmental cues.

7. Carefully construct a set of consequences that includes positive reinforcement, contingency management, and negative reinforcement.

8. Monitor the target behavior. If the desired behavioral change does not occur, re-examine the antecedent cues, environmental stimuli, and consequences.

9. Help the client identify other contingencies, such as natural, social, and intrinsic reinforcers, that can operate after the formal program has ended.

10. Evaluate the effectiveness of the program by comparison with baseline data.

11. Conduct a 3-month, 6-month, and 1-year follow-up to give information on adherence and relapse possibilities.

COGNITIVE-BEHAVIORAL APPROACHES

Cognitive-behavioral approaches emerged out of traditional behavioral therapy in the early 1960s, and took form through the therapeutic intervention models of Bandura (1969), Ellis (1962), and Beck (1967). These models will be discussed later in the chapter. Since then, numerous therapeutic forms and approaches to cognitive behavioralism have evolved. Although these approaches differ in various ways, they all assume that private or internal representations, or thinking, may mediate behavioral change. This concept contradicts the traditional behavioral belief that only observable and measurable reinforcers affect behavioral change. The assumptions of the cognitive model are the following:

■ Cognitive activity can affect behavior.

■ Cognitive activity can be altered.

■ Cognitive change can facilitate desired behavioral change (Dobson & Block, 1988).

Carnwath and Miller (1986) identified some additional assumptions that further clarify and distinguish cognitive-behavioral models:

■ All behavior is mediated by cognition.

■ Cognitive processes affect the way in which people perceive the world and themselves in the world.

■ Therapeutic interventions will not be effective unless cognitive processes are addressed and appropriately altered.

Behavioral change, always a goal in the exercise setting, is not as simple as identifying effective reinforcers and contingencies. People are complex with individual differences and therefore respond to different reinforcers. They differ in perceptions of self and the environment, belief systems, values, assumptions about other people, and the meaning of others' behavior and their own behavior. Observable behavior is only half the story.

The exercise practitioner must know how to understand and interpret the clients' behavior, thoughts, and feelings. For example, two female exercise clients in a fitness class both want to lose 10 pounds. They are about the same height, weight, and age, and share a similar level of fitness. The exercise practitioner develops very similar programs for them, and they seem to have equal chances of reaching their goals. However, upon beginning the exercise program, participant A feels very unsure of herself. She sees herself as a failure, believes that others will immediately notice how inept she is, and feels very self-conscious about exercising. Furthermore, she continually berates and criticizes herself for being foolish enough to think she can change and succeed in a fitness program.

Participant B, on the other hand, feels very enthusiastic and confident about the program. She believes she won't do as well as some others, but feels okay abut that. She wants to be a part of a group and to challenge herself. She does not think

about how others see her and what they think about her. Instead, she focuses on her goal for the day, how she can improve her chances of meeting her goal, and how she will reward herself for a job well done.

All of these thoughts and feelings lie within the cognitive range, yet these thought processes will probably affect the behaviors, and therefore the exercise outcomes, of the two participants. The cognitive section of this chapter will help the exercise professional understand how to use cognitive processes to help reach exercise objectives.

Several cognitive-behavioral models have gained prominence as a result of their proven effectiveness in comparative studies. Those models that have been successfully applied to the exercise setting or that hold promise are Meichenbaum's cognitive-behavioral modification, Ellis's rational-emotive therapy, Beck's cognitive therapy, and self-management/self-control.

Cognitive-Behavioral Modification

Donald Meichenbaum's early research with severely disturbed patients and with hyperactive children led to the development of his cognitive-behavioral modification model (CBM). The core concept of CBM is the importance of covert speech and internal dialogue. Meichenbaum (1974, 1986) found that covert speech influences behavior just as overt speech does. The purpose of CBM, therefore, is to teach people to modify self-statements and replace dysfunctional or self-defeating dialogue.

CBM includes three concepts that guide the intervention strategy for conceptualizing and modifying behavior:

■ *Cognitive events* are conscious thoughts, attributions, and expectancies that are habitual and automatic. Cognitive events tend to occur most frequently when one makes a decision, anticipates an emotional experience, or learns a new skill.

■ *Cognitive process* is the means by which people select and process information. Cognitive processing, like the occurrence of cognitive events (internal dialogue), is automatic. Each person has a unique selection and interpretation process that is determined by how one assigns meaning to events and to what one attributes the cause.

■ *Cognitive structures* are the beliefs and assumptions that determine how a person perceives the world. Because these personal schemas influence how information is processed, they also influence behavior.

Meichenbaum emphasizes the assessment of present internal dialogue patterns and the replacement of dysfunctional patterns with healthy and useful patterns. His three-phase treatment strategy is designed to incorporate the core concepts in achieving this goal.

Phase I. Conceptualization of the Problem

People rarely realize that their thought process might contribute to their problems. Many people externalize their problems and see them as events in their lives over which they have no control. There are several steps to helping the client conceptualize the problem:

1. The practitioner encourages the client to explore and define all aspects of the problem.

2. The practitioner helps the client reconceptualize the problem through situational analysis. The practitioner helps the client identify events that precede the problem, the typical problem situation (environment), the people involved, the stressors, the reinforcements, general consequences of the events, and any other factors relevant to the problem.

3. The client reviews the problem situation by recalling all thoughts, feelings, anxieties, and self-statements made during the event. The client may need to keep a journal to gather data on these cognitive events. Meichenbaum suggests a self-monitoring procedure in which people record (a) the undesirable event or problem, (b) how they felt about it, (c) the automatic thoughts they had, and (d) other helpful thoughts they could have had.

———— ■ ————

Shawna is a 45-year-old woman who after years of a sedentary lifestyle decides to improve her physical health. She enrolls in a fitness class that involves an aerobic workout, flexibility exercises, and supplemental weight work. The exercise instructor's assessment indicates that Shawna is slightly overweight, has low muscle strength and flexibility, normal blood pressure, and slightly high cholesterol. After several weeks she has made little progress. She stops exercising and seems generally demoralized. The instructor meets with Shawna to discuss concerns about her progress. Through situational analysis, the instructor discovers that Shawna feels foolish working out. She fears that she looks silly, that people are laughing at "a woman her age trying to look younger," and that she is kidding

herself by thinking she can accomplish this goal. The exercise instructor asks Shawna to keep a record of the self-talk she has when thinking about going to exercise and when thinking about exercise after class.

Phase II. "Trying On" the Conceptualization

1. After the client has consistently recorded internal dialogue, the practitioner and client identify the relationship between the self-talk and the problem. The practitioner explains the effect negative self-talk can have and how the client is contributing to the problem by maintaining negative internal dialogues.

2. The practitioner helps the client reconceptualize the situation. It can be difficult to accept that one has a part in maintaining a problem. However, once that possibility is accepted, the person also has a sense of control over the problem.

———— ■ ————

The exercise instructor consults with Shawna and reviews the data from homework assignments, journals, and Shawna's recall about the nature of the internal dialogue. Once the instructor and Shawna clearly understand the dialogue, the instructor helps Shawna identify relationships between the internal dialogue and the problem events and points out occurrences of negative self-talk followed by a disappointing workout. They discover that before going to exercise class, Shawna tells herself, "I feel fat today and don't want anyone to see me; I don't feel like exercising; it's no use, I must be crazy. I should be home working." The days when she did not complete the exercise class or did not go at all were the days the internal dialogue was strongest.

Phase III. Modifying Cognitions and Producing New Behaviors

Once the practitioner and client share a common conceptualization of the problem, a treatment can be undertaken. Several methods for cognitive change may be chosen depending on the skills and specialty areas of the practitioner and preferences of the client. Examples are cognitive restructuring, coping-skills training, problem-solving training, and self-regulation or self-monitoring (Mahoney, 1974; Meichenbaum, 1977). The major component will probably be the collaboration between practitioner and client in developing constructive and useful cognitions that enable the client to affect behavior. These reinforcing events will lead the client to further reevaluate cognitions and continue to engage in new behaviors.

——————— ■ ———————

Shawna now collaborates with the exercise instructor to develop some realistic and helpful replacements for her internal dialogues. Some possibilities are: "Even though I'm tired, I really want to stick with my exercise routine, and I may be less tired if I exercise; several people in class are in about the same physical shape I'm in and are very supportive of me; I am pleased that I have been able to take on this project and stick with it; everyone here talks about some area of their lives they are trying to improve, so I'm not such an oddball after all."

There are two points to keep in mind when implementing this program. First of all, it is critically important that the modified or corrected cognitions be realistic and relatively easy to achieve (not grandiose or wishful thinking). It is better to modify a cognition only slightly than to adopt an ideal that the student cannot reach. Secondly, these interventions may be made at the cognitive events, cognitive process, or cognitive structure level. For example, the exercise instructor could encourage the student to examine either the event, or the literal, initial self-statement (e.g., "I'll never be able to do this"); the process, or how meaning is assigned to an event (e.g., "If I can't do this, its further proof that I am a klutz"); or the structure, or the beliefs the student has about herself, exercise, and the importance of fitness (e.g., "I am a person who is not capable of doing any physical activity right").

Rational-Emotive Therapy

Rational-emotive therapy (RET) is based on the assumption that psychological problems arise from irrational thinking (Ellis, 1962). Ellis developed the A-B-C-D-E paradigm to express his perception of how problems develop. Events (A) do not cause emotional disturbance. A person's belief (B) about the meaning of the event causes emotional or behavioral consequences (C). The task of the practitioner is to determine what event triggered a reaction, what the individual's belief

about that event is and dispute (D) the irrational beliefs. The successful refuting of these irrational beliefs then leads to a positive effect (E) or result.

Ellis (1977) identified typical or frequently occurring irrational beliefs, which fall into four categories described by Haaga and Davison (1986).

■ *Awfulizing* is the implication that a situation is catastrophic. For example, "Making a 'B' in this class is the worst thing that has ever happened to me."

■ *Shoulds, oughts, and musts* is the belief that only desirable events are meant to happen by a grand design. For example, "My friend Mary has a new car and lots of clothes. I should be able to have the same things she has."

■ *Comparative evaluation* is the act of measuring one's worth according to how one performed in a particular situation. For example, "I failed the exam, therefore, I am a worthless human being."

■ *Need statements* are really wishes that are perceived as needs. For example, "I need a good job and a beautiful home to be happy."

Let us continue with our earlier illustration of the 45-year-old woman. The instructor will apply RET instead of CBM, and implement the following procedure:

1. The instructor asks what the student tells herself about the class and her performance in it. The student's response is that she tells herself "I look fat and everyone will laugh at me; I should be home working." The student might express feelings of low self-worth because she is not as fit as others (comparative evaluation), or because if she does not lose weight people will not like her as much (shoulds, oughts, and musts).

2. The instructor asks the student what negative thoughts and expectations she has before class. The student reports that she thinks, "Here I go again, making a fool of myself. When am I going to stop doing this and wise up?"

3. The student is then asked to describe the feelings and emotions she has before and during class. She says she tells herself that the embarrassment of fat legs being seen by others is a terrible experience (awfulizing).

4. The instructor helps the student identify the irrational beliefs that are causing the negative feelings. Given the statements expressed by the student, the instructor identifies irrational beliefs such as (a) "If I am not as fit as other people then I have less worth as a person than they do," (b) "I need

for everyone to like me and if I don't lose weight they won't," and (c) "It is an awful thing that people will see my fat legs."

The instructor then helps the student dispute the irrational beliefs by pointing out advantages of giving them up and adopting rational beliefs. To show that the beliefs are irrational, the instructor asks questions such as, "What is the worst thing that can happen?" and "How awful can it get?" At this point, the student may begin to see her situation in a new light and be more willing to give up old belief systems.

RET emphasizes that if a person believes thinking and feeling are related, he or she can learn to modify thought patterns to alter emotional reactions and replace irrational patterns with realistic beliefs.

Beck's Cognitive Therapy

Beck's (1976) cognitive approach shares several assumptions with Meichenbaum's model. Both identify maladaptive cognitions, automatic thoughts (internal dialogue), distortions in information processing, and dysfunctional schemata (cognitive structures) as central factors in maintaining problem situations.

Beck has categorized seven types of cognitive distortions:

■ *Personalization.* Blaming oneself for external events ("If I weren't such a klutz, my exercise instructor wouldn't have to put so much effort into the class").

■ *Polarized thinking.* Thinking in absolutes ("I'm miserable because it's so much harder for me to lose weight than it is for anyone else in my class").

■ *Selective abstraction.* Focusing on one negative instance among positive ones ("The instructor doesn't like me because he corrected the way I was lifting the weights").

■ *Arbitrary inference.* Drawing a negative inference in the absence of negative feedback ("I must not be very important to the exercise class because I missed yesterday, and the instructor didn't even mention it").

■ *Overgeneralization.* Arriving at a sweeping conclusion as a result of minimum data ("I get winded so quickly that I must not have the capacity others do, so why try").

■ *Magnification.* Perceiving a minor negative event to be very important ("The fact that my fitness improvement rate was lowest in the class is a pretty clear sign to quit before it gets worse").

■ *Minimizing.* Discounting or disattributing positive accomplishments ("The instructor said I am improving only because he is supposed to give positive feedback to everybody").

Although Beck's therapeutic procedure is similar to Meichenbaum's, it has several distinctions.

The identification of automatic thoughts is similar to Meichenbaum's conceptualization phase. In this phase Beck also suggests rating the automatic thoughts for likelihood of being factual, and encouraging reality testing by setting up an experience that will verify or negate the automatic thought.

The generation of alternative ideas corresponds to trying on the conceptualization and modifying cognitions. Once the practitioner and client understand the meaning and perceptual pattern of automatic thinking, alternatives can be generated.

The uncovering and modification of dysfunctional schemata does not have an exact parallel in Meichenbaum's model. Beck perhaps places more emphasis on discovering the underlying beliefs that maintain automatic thoughts. Once these beliefs are identified, constructive beliefs can be introduced and tested. Beck emphasizes purposefully acting counter to the underlying beliefs. The individual would then record the thoughts, feelings, and consequences of the new behavior.

The exercise student in our illustration may well be operating under distorted automatic thoughts. "I wasn't able to make my goal today, so I'll probably never make it" shows selective abstraction and magnification. "Since I'm not improving as quickly as some others, the instructor probably wishes I would quit and put us all out of our misery" is an example of arbitrary inference. "After dropping that weight so hard, they probably will ban me from the weight room" is magnification.

Exercise instructors should be familiar with these distortions so they can recognize students who use distorted automatic thinking. The exercise leader who notices such thinking should talk informally with the student regarding his or her perceptions and thoughts about exercising. The instructor should always ask students if they would like to explore how their thinking affects emotions and behavioral outcomes before beginning the procedures. To proceed without total concurrence from the client would be self-defeating.

The instructor should assist the student in modifying automatic thoughts by developing constructive statements the student can incorporate into her thought patterns. It is critically important for the exercise instructor to monitor the modification of automatic thoughts to insure that (a) the change is not too ambitious, (b) the modified statements do, in fact, reconstruct the thoughts rather than subtly distort them in a different way, and (c) willingness to experiment rather than the success of testing out change is emphasized. For a more in-depth description of cognitive therapy, refer to Haaga and Davison (1986), Beck (1976), and Beck, Rush, Shaw, and Emery (1979).

Self-Management

In most of the cognitive change models discussed so far, the practitioner administers the treatment. Even though collaboration with the client is basic to the cognitive models, the practitioner is responsible for the therapeutic intervention. In self-management, the client is primarily responsible for the change process. Although self-management approaches vary depending on the orientation of the practitioner (Kanfer & Gaelick, 1986), they share several characteristics. To effect a behavior change, the client must have a strong motivation to change. The practitioner plays the role of motivator, negotiating and consulting with the client on his or her goal for change.

Kanfer (1970) describes the self-management process in three stages.

Stage 1. Self-Monitoring

In Stage 1, individuals carefully focus on their behavior. Kanfer (1970) found that people judge their behavior against performance criteria or standards. These criteria are determined by the person's past experience, perception of self and others, values, and social environment.

———— ■ ————

A middle-aged, heavy-set man named John wants to lose weight. His wife and children are worried about his health and have asked him to lose weight. John becomes very aware of his calorie intake and weight fluctuation. He keeps baseline records to track himself on these criteria for several weeks. The results of his monitoring and assessment will not be comprised solely of objective information on his caloric intake versus expenditure, but also on his observations of his environment, social comparison with others, and emotional and physiological reactions.

Stage 2. Self-Evaluation

At this stage, individuals make a comparative evaluation of what their actual behavior is and what they think it should be. If the self-monitoring phase was reasonably thorough, a person should be able to identify behaviors that need to change.

———— ■ ————

John realizes that his caloric intake far exceeds his caloric expenditure. He also notes that he eats more often and in greater quantities than others, and that the nutritional value of his diet is not as good as he thought.

Stage 3. Self-Reinforcement

After self-evaluation, people feel either satisfied with themselves or realize the incongruence between their desired and actual conditions. If they have identified discrepancies, people will then develop strategies to form new behaviors or to eliminate old behaviors. The client needs motivational support from the practitioner at this pivotal stage. The act of taking on a behavioral change may motivate an individual, but it could discourage and punish the person if the goals are unrealistic.

———— ■ ————

At this point, John has identified his discrepancies. He is slightly disappointed, but pleased to know where he stands and is enthusiastic about setting up his plan. His practitioner continues to support and encourage him, and give additional information as needed.

Self-management is a general therapeutic approach in which a person directs his or her own behavior and behavioral change. When the behavior to be learned or changed is conflictual, that is, the behavior results in equal positive and negative consequences, then a specific form of self-management, called self-control, may be implemented (Kanfer & Gaelick, 1986).

Self-Control

Individuals who practice self-control are regulating a response that has conflicting short- and long-term consequences. Usually, self-control means forgoing a short-term reinforcement to avoid long-term aversive consequences (Snyder, 1989).

Examples of this type of self-control include avoiding high-cholesterol foods and dieting. Self-control can also mean undergoing short-term aversive experience to achieve positive long-term consequences. All self-control behaviors involve choosing long-term positive consequence over the short-term positive consequence (Snyder, 1989).

Several techniques have been applied in self-control treatment programs (Mahoney & Arnkoff, 1978; Williams & Long, 1975). Two of these, stimulus control and relapse prevention are discussed in other sections of this chapter. Here, we will describe the therapeutic procedure for implementing self-control as illustrated by the technique of self-reinforcement.

As mentioned earlier, the success of a self-control program depends more on the motivation and commitment of the client than in other approaches, such as operant conditioning or social learning.

Self-Observation

An initial step in any self-control program is for the client to observe the target behavior as he or she enacts it. According to Snyder (1989), this step allows the client to become active in the change process immediately and provides a more accurate picture of the target behavior.

Asking people to observe themselves forces them to pay attention to the frequency, intensity, and duration of behaviors. Schacter (1971) conducted an unusual study in which overweight people were asked to report how much they had eaten during a specific period of time. They were then hospitalized and fed that exact amount of food at the reported rate. Every subject lost weight. Habitual behaviors are easily under or overestimated. Self-observation allows for a clear comparison of present and desired behavior and facilitates the identification of short- and long-term goals. Clients are asked to keep records of antecedent, concurrent, and consequential factors. This information is instrumental in the design of self-control strategies. Figure 7.3 illustrates one method of charting behavior. The specific system is not important, only that a written record of identifiable and measurable data be kept.

Snyder (1989) identified several steps that facilitate self-observation:

1. Discuss with the client the importance of the self-observation and self-recording stages.

2. Be specific about the behavior to be observed and give the client examples of the behavior.

It is important that the client understand the assignment.

3. Help the client identify manageable ways to record the behavior. If the client has logistical or technical difficulty with the assignment, the likelihood of failure increases.

4. Role playing and rehearsing the target behavior observation helps the client prepare for unpredictable obstacles during the actual observation.

5. Initially, assign only simple behaviors. As the client becomes more proficient, the observed target behaviors may become more complex.

6. Help the client determine the time and setting in which the behavior will be recorded. Other parameters may also be helpful depending on the client and the target behavior.

7. Check with the client during the initial weeks in case difficulties have arisen.

8. Consult with the client as data is collected to help the client correctly identify antecedent and discriminative stimuli, and consequences that evoke and maintain the target behavior.

After the self-observation data has been collected and the practitioner and client are confident that the record accurately reflects the target behavior, the client and practitioner can design a treatment program. The program should identify short- and long-term goals and implement some combination of technical approaches, such as stimulus control or self-reinforcement.

In exercise programs, self-observation typically records type of activity and measures duration and intensity, such as time, distance, or heart rate. The process of recording should not be so cumbersome that the client will fail to continue; however, if the client is committed to the task, the more detail, the better (Martin & Dubbert, 1984).

Studies in the area of self-monitoring have identified several factors that have implications for the effective functioning of self-regulation. Positive self-monitoring (recording successful performance) as compared to negative self-monitoring (recording unsuccessful performance) led to less accurate problem-solving, less time spent in self-monitoring, and lower rates of program attendance (Tomarken & Kirschenbaum, 1982). These findings corroborate earlier results that indicated that positive self-monitoring leads to these same problems when the task is well mastered or learned. In contrast, however, when the task has not been mastered, positive self-monitoring is at least as effective as negative self-monitoring in bringing about behavior change (Kirschenbaum & Karoly, 1977).

Day: _____ Thursday _____   Date: ____ 7/16 ____

Weight: _____ 183 _____   Calories eaten: ___ 3828 ___

                                     Calories exercise: ___ 100 ___

                                     Total "meals": ____ 7 ____

Time	Place	Activity	People	Mood	Amt. food		Calories
7:30	Dorm	Breakfast	?	Bitchy	1 o.j. 1 HB egg 2 toast, butter 1 coffee, cream & sugar	120 48 210 40	418
10:30	College Inn	Class break	Debbie, Alice, Tom	Bored	1 danish 1 coffee, cream & sugar	125 40	165
12:00	Dorm	Lunch	Barb, John	OK	1 milk 1 spaghetti 2 p. cake	160 not eat 500	660
4:30	Snack bar	After bio lab	Tom, Denise	Hungry	1 cheeseburger 1 fries	470 250	720
6:30	Dorm	Dinner	Barb, Alice, Jean	Good	1 meat (lamb) 1 peas 2 sm potato 1 choc. ice cream	470 115 120 100	805
10:30	Snack bar	Break from study	Tom, Jean	Tired	2 beers 1 potato chips	300 230	530
11:00– 12:00	Room	Studying	No one	Tired	10 chocolate chip cookies	500?	500

Exercise: ____ Moderate ____	____ Vigorous ____	____ Strenuous ____
Walk: ____ 15 min. ____	Walk fast: ____ 10 min. ____	Sports: _____
Bicycle: _____	Horse ride: _____	Dance: _____
Housework: _____	Swim: _____	Jog: _____
Total time: ____ 15 ____	____ 10 ____	_____
Calories: ____ 50 ____	____ 50 ____	_____

Figure 7.3 Self-observed behavior for weight control.

From *Health Psychology and Behavioral Medicine* (p. 241) by James J. Snyder, 1989. Copyright © 1989. Reprinted by permission of Prentice Hall, Inc. Englewood Cliffs, NJ 07632.

Self-Reinforcement

Self-reinforcement, the procedure by which individuals are responsible for their own reinforcement, corresponds operationally to operant reinforcers. Although positive reinforcement is the most frequently used method, a person could also employ negative reinforcement, punishment, or response cost. Self-administered aversive and punishing behaviors have different consequences than when they are imposed by others.

Kanfer (1975) has suggested several steps for designing a self-reinforcement program. In the following description of these steps, these principles are applied to a specific exercise setting:

1. As in operant conditioning, one of the most important initial steps is to accurately identify positive reinforcers. In the case of an exercise student, the instructor, after careful inquiry with the client, may identify several reinforcers to be administered daily. Preferably, the reinforc-

ers would already be part of the client's behavioral repertoire (e.g., watching a certain TV show or going to the movies with friends) and may already be self-administered, although noncontingently.

2. The practitioner and client define the specific target behavior and the reinforcement contingencies. They also discuss how the self-reinforcement should be implemented. The instructor and student may identify a target behavior of 1 hour of aerobic exercise 3 times a week. The student will monitor his or her own behavior and, if the exercise goals are met, he or she will go to the movies with friends on the weekend and go out to dinner twice during the week. It is very important that these reinforcers not be available to the student unless the goal is met. Therefore, behaviors that were formerly noncontingent reinforcement become contingent.

3. The practitioner rehearses the self-reinforcement procedure with the client so that the client has no confusion about the target behavior or the reinforcers. Rehearsal involves discussing each step of the procedure, possible obstacles, and methods for the student to manage the situation. This procedure should include rehearsal for both success and failure.

4. As the client progresses, the reinforcement schedule or particular reinforcers may need to be modified. The exercise client may tire of going to the movies or out to dinner. At this point, the instructor and student would simply identify new reinforcers.

The effectiveness of self-management depends on the motivation of the client, a shared conceptualization of the target behavior and treatment, and willingness to self-reinforce. The involvement of the instructor, however, must taper off during the maintenance period. Follow-up studies show successful behavioral change after at least 1 year for people who implemented self-control training. Those who dropped out of the training tended to relapse to former behavior (Brownell, 1982). A final recommendation, then, is to develop strategies to increase adherence and prevent relapse. Adherence is discussed in chapter 2 and relapse prevention is addressed in the social learning section of this chapter.

Attribution Theory

Individuals formulate explanations for the cause of events and behaviors (Heider, 1958). People engage in causal attribution to create a sense of control over their lives. Understanding attributions can be a valuable tool in interpreting behavior and in helping individuals to change behavior.

The research findings of Ross (1977) indicate that people attribute the same event differently because of individual distortions of inferences. A consistent distortion, which Ross (1977) called a fundamental attribution error, is the tendency to believe that the behavior of others is driven by internal or intrapersonal factors, known as *dispositional factors*. People view their own behavior as driven by environmental or external factors, known as *situational factors*. In judging another person, for example, one might say, "She behaved that way because of her personality, character, values, or beliefs," while one might say about oneself "I behaved that way because the situation I was in left me no choice." Weiner (1979, 1986) developed a three-dimensional attributional schema to describe the process people use to determine the cause of events, behaviors, or performance. Refer to Figure 7.4 during the following discussion for a clear understanding of this attributional process.

1. *Internality versus Externality.* Internal conditions are due to personal factors, such as physical ability or strength. External conditions are due to environmental factors, such as the exercise setting or the condition of exercise equipment.

2. *Stability versus Instability.* Stability refers to those factors that remain relatively constant, such as aptitude and personality. Instability refers to factors that may change, such as fatigue and mood.

3. *Controllability versus Uncontrollability.* In applying this third dimension, it was recognized that attributes such as mood, fatigue, and effort are all internal and unstable, yet they differ significantly from each other. Effort is typically considered controllable, whereas fatigue is viewed as a physical condition that cannot be controlled. Factors that are viewed as internal and stable also vary with regard to control. Aptitude is typically seen as uncontrollable, whereas commitment is considered controllable.

How can the exercise practitioner make use of this schema of perceived causes of behavior? First of all, the practitioner must listen for the attributions the participant makes. For example, a participant who says, "I fell short of my goal today because I really didn't put forth my best effort" is attributing performance to effort, an internal, unstable, and controllable condition. On the other

	Internal			External	
	Stable	Unstable		Stable	Unstable
Controllable	Industriousness Tolerance Laziness Long-term effort	Exertion Persistence Determination Commitment to exercise	Controllable	Teacher industrious- ness Teacher tolerance	Teacher effort
Uncontrollable	Aptitude Ability General body type Physical coordination	Mood Fatigue	Uncontrollable	Ability of the opponent Task difficulty Objective task characteristics	Luck Chance

Figure 7.4 Structure of causal perceptions.

Note. Adapted from *An Attributional Theory of Motivation and Emotion* (pp. 49-50) by Bernard Weiner, 1986, New York: Springer-Verlag. Copyright 1986 by Springer-Verlag. Adapted by permission.

hand, a participant who says, "I'll never be able to do this, the exercise is too hard. It's just not in the cards for me" is attributing performance to task difficulty and luck, which are external and uncontrollable factors. The exercise practitioner would respond to these participants differently when trying to motivate and encourage them.

The exercise practitioner must consider the individual's current attribution pattern before encouraging a shift in attribution. Forsterling (1980) has recommended several potential shifts with which practitioners could assist clients. All of these shifts assume the perception of some controllability:

■ An exercise student makes very little progress toward her weight-loss goal and attributes the problem to her lack of physical ability. The instructor might suggest that the difficulty is due to insufficient effort (movement from internal-stable to internal-unstable).

■ A person is afraid to join an exercise class and expects to fail because he remembers how incompetent he felt in an earlier exercise program. The instructor might encourage the student to think of the earlier class as an exceptional situation that would not happen again (movement from internal-stable to external-stable).

■ An exercise class member feels compelled to push herself beyond her exercise goals. She fears that if she lets up, she will eventually stop exercising and fail to become fit. The instructor might help the student look more objectively at her actual accomplishments, history of perseverance, and commitment to tasks. This approach may help the

student to see her exercise challenge differently (movement from internal-unstable to internal-stable).

■ An exercise student believes he can control the amount of weight he loses by regulating the amount of exercise and degree of dieting. The instructor might point out the likelihood that he will not be able to control everything and that rate of weight loss is going to be somewhat unpredictable (movement from internal-unstable to external-unstable).

SOCIAL COGNITIVE THEORY

In the early 1960s, Bandura and Walters (1963) introduced the principles of social learning. These principles were to become the cornerstone of a major movement from operant-behavioral theory to the emergence of cognitive-behavioral theory. Two organizing themes of social-cognitive theory are (1) the importance of acknowledging that personal, environmental, and behavioral factors all affect one another and (2) the importance of learning through observation of a model. Most behavior is learned through observing another person's behavior rather than through reinforcement of one's own behavior (Bandura, 1977b). If people had to directly experience every event in order to learn, their level of knowledge, information, and psychosocial development would be greatly constricted. Bandura (1986) noted that by observing others, people can form rules of behavior and increase their knowledge and skills by encoding information based on the behavior of others and the resulting consequences. As a result, people are able to learn new behaviors and modify acquired behaviors without the actual experience of reinforcement, punishment, or extinction of the behavior.

The principle of observational learning is a powerful teaching tool in the exercise setting and is an integral part of the practitioner's strategy. The practitioner does not wait for the participants to initiate exercise behavior on their own and then reinforce them with hopes that the participants will repeat the desired behaviors. Instead, the exercise practitioner models the desirable exercise behaviors for the participants. The participants initially engage in the behaviors not because there is an intrinsic or extrinsic reward linked to the exercise, but because they see that the practitioner is fit and healthy. The observation that fitness can be achieved through the behaviors modeled by the practitioner motivates the participants to adopt the exercise behaviors. Exercise participants also learn by observing classmates. Initially, the instructor may be the sole focus of observational learning, but gradually the instructor will share this role with class members who have achieved exercise goals still aspired to by other participants.

The instructor, therefore, must understand the principles of observational learning to use them effectively. Individuals do not always discriminate well when selecting behaviors to emulate. The exercise practitioner must be aware of how modeling affects the participants' patterns of behavior so that modifications can be made as needed.

Basic Processes of Observational Learning

Learning is the process that converts incoming information into symbolic representations, which then guide the selection and processing of certain information over other information (Bandura, 1977b). After all, we do not encode and retain all the information we observe. Instead a very sophisticated selection process enables us to manage the quantity and frequency of incoming information.

Bandura (1986) identified four basic processes involved in observational learning:

- ■ Attention
- ■ Retention
- ■ Production
- ■ Motivation (Figure 7.5)

Attentional Processes

To learn, the observer must accurately perceive, encode, and store in memory the relevant aspects of the modeled behavior. Selective attention is a critical aspect of observational learning. Several factors influence the selection process including cognitive skills and other characteristics of the observer; characteristics of the modeled behavior; and structural arrangements of the interaction, such as perceived value of the behavior, comparative attractiveness of modeled behaviors, and model availability.

A new member of a cardiac rehabilitation program may be cautious and fearful, uncertain that the program will help, and even concerned that exercise will trigger another heart attack. If the class is composed of members at varying stages of therapy, there will be modeling opportunities for the majority of members. As the new member acclimates to the class, the instructor can draw attention to several members who entered the program at a similar diagnostic level and treatment prescription. The instructor can encourage the new member to observe the level of functioning of the model members.

Retention Processes

To retain and replicate the modeled behavior when the model is no longer present, the information must be stored in memory in symbolic form. Human beings have the capacity for symbolization through representational systems. This ability enables people to vastly expand their observational learning potential. In the cardiac rehabilitation illustration, the new member may observe the model members and notice many behaviors, some of which are relevant to treatment and some of which are not. The model members will demonstrate characteristics such as a particular stride, arm movements, gestures, expressions, certain types of clothing, or a brand-name shoe. These characteristics simply describe the model's personal preferences. They have nothing to do with ability to accomplish the exercise goals. The new member must select behaviors related to treatment, and process the information so that the model behavior can be retained after exposure to the models has ended.

Production Processes

The observer must be able to produce the modeled behavior from the stored symbolic representation. Modeled activities are believed to be abstractly

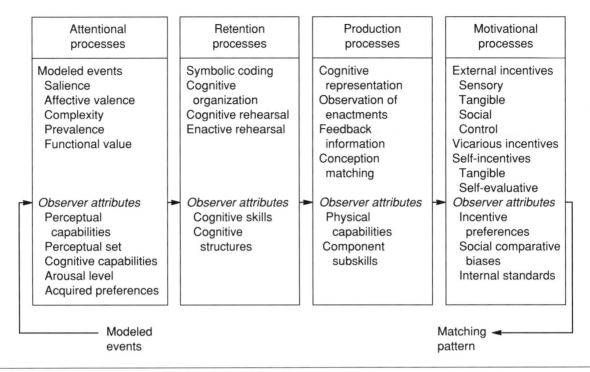

Figure 7.5 Subprocesses governing observational learning.

From *Social Foundations of Thought and Action: A Social Cognitive Theory* (p.52) by Albert Bandura, 1986. Copyright © 1986. Reprinted by permission of Prentice Hall, Inc., Englewood Cliffs, NJ 07632.

represented as conceptions and rules that give direction.

Practice of the modeled behavior is critical to production. Both intrinsic and extrinsic feedback are important to help the observer modify the modeled behavior and more accurately reproduce the behavior. In physical skill development and social skill development, performers cannot observe their own behaviors and so rely on feedback from others.

The new cardiac rehabilitation member will begin to produce exercise behaviors that are believed to match those of the model. As the instructor watches the member during stretching and floor exercises, it may become apparent that the member has retained the modeled behavior incorrectly, exaggerating exercise movements, which could cause muscular pain later, and the pace at which the member is exercising far exceeds the recommended rate. The instructor would observe the faulty behavioral response long enough to be able to describe the difference between the member's produced exercise behavior and the desired behavior. The instructor could also model both behaviors to help contrast the differences for the class member.

Motivational Processes

The difference between acquisition and performance is important. Many behaviors that are learned through acquisition are never performed. How the observer views the consequence of the modeled behavior will influence whether the behavior will be produced. If the model is rewarded for the behavior, the observer is more likely to attend to and model the behavior.

In the cardiac rehabilitation illustration, the observer may note that the models for the treatment program (1) are becoming stronger and more fit, and have improved ECG readings, (2) are in good spirits and report feeling better, and (3) receive praise and positive feedback from others. The new member is more likely to attend to, retain, and perform the model behaviors if the member believes that he or she will also receive positive reinforcement.

Enhancement of Acquisition of New Behaviors and Performance

Perry and Furukawa (1986) identified and summarized factors that enhance the acquisition and performance of new behaviors. Because these factors have generally been implemented together in behavioral treatment packages, the individual effect of each has not been clarified. These outlines are meant simply to provide guidelines for using observational learning for program enhancement.

Factors that reinforce acquisition can be categorized as characteristics of the model, the observer, and the model presentation. Research on differential effects of models has found that not all models are equally effective with different observers and in varying types of presentations.

Characteristics of the Model

■ A model who is similar to the observer in sex, age, race, and attitudes is more likely to be effective than one who is dissimilar. The observer must be able to identify with the model.

■ A model who has somewhat higher prestige than the observer, but not markedly higher, is more effective than low-prestige models, especially when the observer is anxious about performance.

■ A model who is slightly more competent than the observer is more effective than a highly competent model who is viewed as far superior to the observer.

■ Warmth and nurturance foster modeling. When given a choice, children identify with the warm, nurturing model over the cold, unfeeling model.

■ People the observer associates with reward are good choices for models.

■ Characteristics such as dependency, self-esteem, socioeconomic status, and gender of model may play a part in the effectiveness of the modeling presentation. There are no specific guidelines on these factors, only that practitioners should be aware of any interaction effect.

Characteristics of the Observer

■ The observer's ability to process and retain information is crucial to successful modeling. The exercise instructor should be aware of the strengths and weaknesses of the observer and make every attempt to adjust the modeling environment to increase the likelihood of success.

■ The observer who is unsure about his or her behavior and who needs information from the model to continue acquisition will be more attentive than more confident observers. An exercise practitioner who raises questions and issues that are not well known or understood by class members can increase the attention level of the observers.

■ High anxiety impairs learning while moderate anxiety increases motivation and selective attention. If class members suffer from high anxiety, relaxation exercises should be done before presenting the model.

Characteristics of the Modeling Presentation

■ Live models are usually more effective than symbolic models. Live models tend to be more interesting and hold attention better. A live model can also alter the presentation to suit the needs of the observer. However, the outcome cannot be controlled with a live modeling, and the potential for detrimental effects is higher.

■ Symbolic models, although not as interesting as live models, can be highly successful (Bandura, 1969). Symbolic models include presentations of behavior with tape, film, audio, and scripts. The presentation can be controlled, edited, and used again.

■ Multiple models can enhance the presentation by demonstrating variability. Multiple model use increases the probability that at least one model will be effective for an observer.

■ Research on the coping and mastery skills exhibited by the model has implications for the modeling presentation (Meichenbaum, 1972). A model who exhibits proficiency at the level of the observer and progresses to a higher competence level is demonstrating coping skills. Initially, the model may show uncertainty and anxiety. Then the model may increasingly improve coping ability to reach a level of desired competence. A mastery model exhibits a high level of proficiency at the outset. Studies, although not conclusive, have shown an increased incidence of success with the coping model.

■ Graduated modeling involves breaking the model behavior into component parts. This procedure is helpful when learning motor skills and complex behaviors such as swimming, tennis, and driving a car.

Factors That Enhance Performance

In an applied/clinical setting, the practitioner must understand the factors that enhance performance, and modify the learning environment and modeling program accordingly.

Incentives are factors that motivate the performance of modeled behaviors. Several types of incentives are discussed in the cognitive-behavioral section of this chapter and in chapter 6. Two incentives that are particularly relevant to observational learning are *vicarious reinforcement* and *direct reinforcement*.

Vicarious reinforcement occurs when the observer sees the model receiving reinforcement for a behavior that the observer has not performed. Vicarious reinforcement informs the observer about the model's performance and provides an incentive to perform the model's behavior. *Direct reinforcement*, on the other hand, is experienced by the observer after reproducing the model's behavior. Direct reinforcement is probably more effective than vicarious reinforcement.

The observer will often be able to reproduce the model's behavior, but not as well as desired. The practitioner can use several techniques to help the observer improve performance.

In *active rehearsal*, the observer rehearses a behavior following the model display to improve the approximation of the observer's performance to that of the model. A person attempting to improve diving techniques may watch films or live modeling interspersed with rehearsal. *Feedback* is recommended throughout the performance enactment to help the observer refine the component parts of his or her behavior. As the diving student rehearses, the model or coach may give feedback about various aspects of performance. *Participant modeling* involves direct interaction between the model and observer. The model may offer feedback to the observer to increase accuracy of performance.

The successful acquisition and performance of behavior must be transferable and generalizable. How can practitioners structure the learning experience and environment to increase transferability and generalizability? The training should occur in situations that simulate the natural environment for the behavior as much as possible. Repeated rehearsal increases the strength of the response and incorporates the response into the behavioral repertoire more efficiently. Incentives and reinforcements must be built into the natural setting as well as the training setting. Generalization is fostered by encouraging the performance of the desired behaviors in a variety of settings, not just the training setting.

Self-Efficacy

The concept of self-efficacy is central to Bandura's view of observational learning. Self-efficacy is the belief that one is capable of performing behaviors that produce a certain outcome. Bandura (1977a) asserted that self-efficacy expectations determine a person's choice to participate in events, the amount of effort the person expends, and the person's persistence.

Bandura sees behavioral change partially as a function of self-efficacy expectations (a belief that one has the ability to engage in the behavior) and outcome expectations (the belief that anyone engaging in the behavior can affect the outcome). This model focuses on an assessment of an individual's belief that he or she is capable, not on a measurement of actual capabilities.

Self-efficacy is influenced by four sources of information (Bandura, 1986):

■ *Enactive experience* refers to behaviors that have been successfully accomplished in the past. The exercise participant may have been successful in a walking program, but has not been able to transform that success to a jogging program.

■ *Vicarious experience* involves observing another person perform successfully. This observation can raise expectations that one will be able to perform as well as the model. If one views a classmate successfully making the transition from walking to jogging, the expectation for one's own success can be significantly raised.

■ *Verbal persuasion* is the attempt to talk an individual into believing that he or she can achieve the desired performance. This process is successful primarily when the observer perceives the desired performance to be realistically attainable. If the classmate exhibiting the modeled behavior and the instructor explain and describe the transition in terms of steps that the observer believes are doable, the observer is more likely to see the task as within his or her capability.

■ *Physiological states* that occur during a stressful situation are often interpreted as a sign of vulnerability. High arousal, therefore, can debilitate performance. Treatments that reduce arousal also heighten perceived self-efficacy and may improve performance (Bandura & Adams, 1977). The instructor should watch for physiological changes, describe the changes to the participant, and suggest ways for the participant to control the changes. Anxiety ratings, heart-rate measurement, breathing, and muscular responsiveness can be described to help participants monitor arousal in these dimensions and self-regulate the arousal response.

Performance attainment (successful production of desired behavior) is perhaps the most influential information source for self-efficacy interventions. When people actually see themselves successfully performing a new behavior or achieving a desired change in behavior, their belief in their capability for change increases.

Bandura (1977a) recommended a two-step process for appraising a class member's efficacy expectations: (1) Ask the individual whether he or she believes certain behaviors can be purposefully accomplished, and (2) ask if the individual believes he or she is capable of achieving the change and how the individual would rate the strength of his or her ability. For example, the practitioner might present the participant with a list of exercise activities with differing levels of difficulty and ask the participant to rate the activities based on his or her confidence level for achieving them.

The exercise practitioner should assess both self-efficacy and outcome expectancies when employing the self-efficacy model. If the participant believes he or she can accomplish the behavior but also that the behavior will not help bring about a desired change, then the focus must be directed to outcome beliefs instead of self-efficacy. Likewise, if the participant believes the behavior will lead to a positive outcome, but is uncertain of his or her ability to perform the behavior, then the focus must be directed to self-efficacy.

Most studies on the function of self-efficacy in health-related areas have found self-efficacy to be a consistent predictor of short- and long-term success in health behavior change (O'Leary, 1985; Strecher, DeVellis, Becker, & Rosenstock, 1986).

Kaplan et al. (1984) studied the application of self-efficacy in the exercise setting. They found that an actual increase in walking enabled the participants to feel greater competency and self-determined capability in walking. Self-efficacy expectations for other behaviors also increased as a function of their similarity to walking. Their results support the social-cognitive theory and confirm the influence of self-efficacy in behavioral and cognitive change.

Relapse Model

Traditionally, exercise professionals have focused on the acquisition of new exercise behaviors and the initial stages of maintenance measured by performance in a structured class. The majority of exercise participants experience lapses in their exercise regimen. How these lapses are perceived and dealt with determine whether or not the participant resumes exercise or drops out (Martin & Dubbert, 1984). Since researchers have begun to look at long-term outcomes of exercise maintenance, the need to understand and prevent relapse has increased.

The following section discusses Alan Marlatt's relapse prevention model and strategies for relapse prevention. The model has been applied mainly to addictive behaviors, such as alcoholism, drug abuse, and smoking. The model application attempts to reduce frequent undesirable behavior, whereas exercise adherence efforts attempt to increase an infrequent desirable behavior (Knapp, 1988). Nonetheless, the relapse prevention model has gained interest in the area of exercise behavior, and several studies have effectively applied the relapse model to the exercise setting.

Relapse in reference to health behaviors is the failure to abstain from an undesirable habitual behavior (Snyder, 1989). A lapse is a single event that may or may not lead to relapse. Marlatt and Gordon (1985) emphasize the distinction between a "slip" and total failure. Whether a lapse becomes a relapse depends on the individual's response to lapses and perceived loss of control (Brownell, Marlatt, Lichtenstein, & Wilson, 1986).

Marlatt and Gordon (1980, 1985) developed a cognitive-behavioral model of the relapse process. According to their model, a relapse begins with a high-risk situation (Figure 7.6). Without an effective coping strategy, self-efficacy is decreased and the undesirable behavior, often substance abuse, is initiated. This perceived loss of control results in the *abstinence violation effect*. The abstinence violation effect is the belief that once abstinence is broken, total relapse is certain. According to Knapp (1988), two potentially detrimental aspects of abstinence violation may develop: (1) The individual adopts the all-or-nothing perception that one cannot be a successful abstainer and slip at the same time. This dissonance cause the individual to feel out of control. The individual often attributes the lapse to personal weakness. (2) Self-attribution for the "failure" results in guilt, self-blame, and lowered self-esteem. The abstinence violation effect then increases the probability of relapse. If an effective coping strategy is available, the individual is likely to experience increased self-efficacy and perceive him or herself as in control, thereby decreasing the probability of relapse.

———— ■ ————

Two members of a cardiac rehabilitation program are faced with the high-risk situation of being apprehensive and uncertain about participating in the program. One member

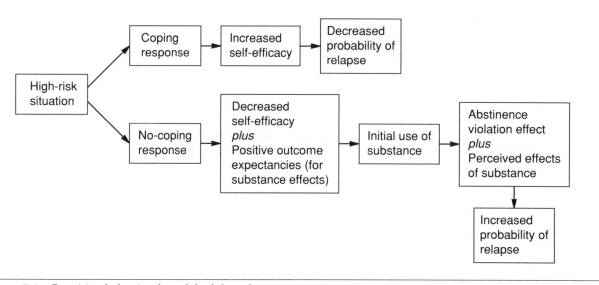

Figure 7.6 Cognitive-behavioral model of the relapse process.

From *Relapse Prevention: Maintenance Strategies in Addictive Behavior Change* (p.38) by G.A. Marlatt and J.R. Gordon, 1985, Elmsford, NY: Guilford Press. Copyright 1985 by Guilford Press. Reprinted by permission.

consults with the program director and seeks support from others to develop a self-management strategy. He identifies the negative factors of scheduling problems, fatigue, and anxiety about the physical activity, and then develops a variety of reinforcements and positive consequences for exercise compliance. The other member misses class occasionally. Each time he misses, he feels guilty, questions his ability to follow through, and feels like a failure. As a result, he drops out of class. He had no resources to help him develop a coping strategy.

Predictors of Lapse and Relapse

Several researchers have tried to classify relapse factors (Brownell, 1982; Cummings, Gordon, & Marlatt, 1980; Marlatt & Gordon, 1978). Three general categories have emerged from these attempts (Brownell et al., 1986).

Individual and Intrapersonal Factors. Negative emotional states, such as stress, depression, and anxiety, may account for as much as 30% of relapses (Cummings et al., 1980). Although inadequate motivation is a frequent obstacle, it is not always detectable. The practitioner should make every effort to detect high-risk subjects, screen for motivation, and explore methods for improving readiness for change. Initial responses to treatment may predict later success. Early compliance has been associated with success in weight loss (Graham, Taylor, Hovell, & Siegel, 1983) and smoking

cessation (Pomerleau, Adkins, & Pertschik, 1978). However, Brownell et al. (1986) observed that participants who have excellent adherence rates initially may have more difficulty after a slip than those who have had more difficulty throughout the process. Participants who have developed cognitive and/or behavioral coping responses are more successful. Self-talk was found to be a popular and effective cognitive response.

Social and Environmental Factors. Research studies continue to substantiate the association between social support and successful weight reduction (Brownell, 1982), smoking cessation (Lichtenstein, 1982), and alcoholism treatment (Moos & Finney, 1983). Social support is an important aspect of self-help groups, which grew in popularity in the late 1980s. Self-help groups such as Alcoholics Anonymous have been the outpatient treatment of choice for traditional, biomedical clinical settings. However, self-help groups are difficult to evaluate and very few empirical studies have been done on their effectiveness. Environmental stimuli are often involved in relapse. Social pressure, social cues formerly associated with undesirable behaviors, and other external contingencies can be problematic. Contingency management and self-management programs have been effective in diminishing environmental effects.

Physiological Factors. Physical dependency may influence both alcohol use and smoking. Food is not addictive in the same way alcohol and smoking are, yet physiological components and metabolic factors are likely to interact with the weight-loss process and create powerful physical pressure to maintain weight.

Relapse Prevention

Brownell and colleagues (1986) identified the important aspects of relapse prevention (Figure 7.7).

They also developed a three-stage approach to relapse prevention, which is applied here to a fitness class in which all the participants have had relapses while dieting. The class is for people who overeat.

Stage 1: Motivation and Commitment. The initial step involves screening to identify individuals who are likely to succeed and those who are likely to fail. Although consistently accurate and effective screening methods have not been well documented, several approaches have been successful. The exercise instructor might screen for motivation and commitment with a behavioral test. For example, a deposit-refund system would

presumably screen out those with a low commitment to the program. Another behavior test establishes criteria before the class starts, such as losing 1 pound per week for 2 weeks and completing self-monitoring diaries.

In the second step of stage 1, the exercise instructor works with each participant to develop methods to enhance motivation. They adopt contingency management procedures including (1) a contract with the instructor and the class to restrict types of foods eaten and calorie intake, (2) distal and flexible goals for maintenance of diet and time spent jogging, and (3) social reinforcers of planned leisure activities with friends when goals are met. The instructor then discusses how to prepare for relapse. The instructor explains that the participants should have a recovery plan if they binge over the weekend.

Stage 2: Initial Behavior Change. Specific treatment procedures are developed that focus on decision making, cognitive restructuring, and coping skills. A scheme for understanding the lapse and relapse process and using decision

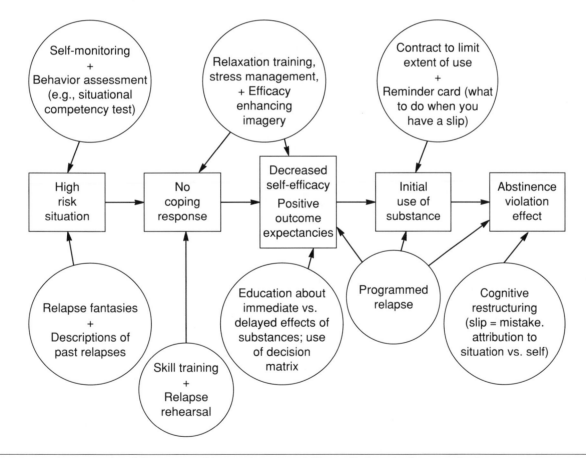

Figure 7.7 An example of decision-making and coping skills applied to the lapse and relapse process.

From *Relapse Prevention: Maintenance Strategies in Addictive Behavior Change* (p.54) by G.A. Marlatt and J.R. Gordon, 1985, Elmsford, NY: Guilford Press. Copyright 1985 by Guilford Press. Reprinted by permission.

making, coping skills, and cognitive restructuring is shown in Figure 7.6. The instructor and participants would use decision making to analyze the individual and environmental determinants of relapse. Then specific coping skills, such as self-talk and cognitive restructuring (reframing the lapse experience to a "slip" rather than loss of willpower) would allow the participant to reinterpret the situation.

Stage 3: Maintenance. Three areas of intervention are appropriate at this stage:

1. The instructor teaches the participants to monitor their behavioral change after leaving the exercise class and to self-administer an intervention when needed or to seek consultation at the time of a lapse or potential relapse.

2. The instructor encourages social support. An individualized identification of social support is important. For example, to enlist the support of family may be helpful for one participant, while it may be detrimental for another.

3. A change of lifestyle may help modify eating habits. Exercise is a highly recommended form of lifestyle change for everyone, not only for those with overeating difficulties.

Relapse Prevention Applied to Exercise Settings

Martin and Dubbert (1984) noted that several studies had yielded small but important findings that corroborate some of the relapse prevention hypotheses. They have incorporated some specific recommendations into their exercise programs based on these findings:

■ The probability of lapses is great. Exercisers should anticipate slips, be prepared, and view them as temporary and inevitable setbacks.

■ Exercise participants should be cautioned about the abstinence violation effect, which is quite potent especially for people with addictions. Exercise participants should be encouraged to view their exercise adherence on a continuum rather than as all or nothing.

■ Exercise participants should avoid high-risk situations that could unduly test their coping skills. High-risk situations are often incompatible with exercise, for example, watching T.V., double scheduling work time, and frequenting places with many antecedent cues, such as eating and drinking establishments.

■ Exercise participants should purposefully not exercise for 1 week and then resume the program. The purpose of this planned relapse is to experience the abstinence violation effect under controlled circumstances and with the practitioner's support. Also, if some participants have difficulty returning to exercise, the problem can be detected early and corrected.

APPLICATION OF BEHAVIORAL CHANGE STRATEGIES TO SPECIFIC HEALTH CONCERNS

Although little research has been done on behavioral change interventions with health-related behaviors, during the past 10 years there have been increasing numbers of studies in this area. These studies have investigated change strategies that have proven effective in nonhealth-related areas. We will review some promising studies that have been done in the health-related areas of smoking, obesity, stress, alcohol abuse, and coronary heart disease.

Smoking

Snyder (1989) noted that smoking is a major risk factor for cancer, heart disease, and other illnesses. About 54 million people in the United States smoke, and the costs, including medical expenses, are estimated at $27 billion. Most people in western cultures know about the risks of smoking. Even though many have stopped, young people continue to smoke, and many who wish to stop, cannot. Table 7.3 shows the various stages a smoker may experience.

It is believed that the persistence of the smoking habit can be explained primarily by psychological and physiological factors. Until recently, smoking was an integral part of social interaction. People who feel anxious, tense, or insecure in social situations often smoke to mask negative feelings as well as engage in a social ritual. Table 7.4 describes the various stimuli that initiate and maintain smoking. The habitual smoker is continually presented with a wide range of cues to smoke. Habitual smoking takes 2 to 3 years to develop (Snyder, 1989). Once the habit is established, the antecedent cues and short-term rewarding consequences create a powerful psychological need to maintain the habit.

Nicotine appears to produce no psychological damage, such as distorted perception, memory

Table 7.3 Developmental Stages of Smoking

Stage 1: Preparation (psychological factors before
            smoking)
            Modeling by significant others
            Attitudes concerning the function and
                desirability of smoking
Stage 2: Initiation (psychosocial factors leading to
            experimentation)
            Peer pressure and reinforcement
            Availability
            Curiosity, rebelliousness, and impulsivity
            Viewing smoking as a sign of adulthood and
                independence
Stage 3: Habitual (psychosocial and physiological
            factors leading to continued smoking)
            Nicotine regulation
            Emotional regulation
            Cues in the environment
            Peer pressure and reinforcement
            Urges to smoke
Stage 4: Stopping (psychosocial cues leading to
            attempts to stop)
            Health concerns
            Expense
            Aesthetic concerns
            Example to others (e.g., children)
            Availability of social support for stopping
            Notions of self-mastery
Stage 5: Resuming (psychosocial and physiological
            factors leading to recidivism)
            Withdrawal symptoms
            Increased stress and other negative effects
            Social pressure
            Abstinence violation effects

From *Health Psychology and Behavioral Medicine* (p. 43) by James
J. Snyder, 1989. Copyright © 1989. Reprinted by permission of
Prentice Hall, Inc., Englewood Cliffs, NJ 07632.

loss, or imparied functioning. It does, however,
cause physiological damage and is phyisologically
addictive. Carnwath and Miller (1986) note that
nicotine shares structural similarities with acetylcholine. Acetylcholine receptors respond to nicotine. Small amounts of nicotine create a stimulant
effect, and large amounts, a depressant effect. As
a result individuals can control their level of stimulation through nicotine regulation.

The withdrawal effects of nicotine also make
cessation difficult. Noradrenaline excretion is elevated for 2 weeks after a person stops smoking.
This physiological reaction causes restlessness,
anxiety, insomnia, and irritability (Carnwath &
Miller, 1986). Many people resume smoking because they are unwilling or unable to endure these
withdrawal symptoms.

Cognitive-Behavioral Treatment

Aversive strategies have been the most frequently
used treatments for smoking. The procedure entails pairing an aversive stimulus, such as electric
shock, noise, imagined vomiting, and smoke itself,
with the act of smoking. Although shock and imaginal techniques have not been successful, rapid
smoking (Lichtenstein, 1982), focused smoking,
and holding smoke (Snyder, 1989) show promise.
Rapid smoking is the inhalation of cigarettes at a
very rapid rate (6 to 8 seconds) until it can no
longer be tolerated. Sessions are repeated until the
desire to smoke ceases. Lichtenstein and Penner
(1977) found a little less than half of the clients
were still not smoking 2 to 6 years later. Lichtenstein (1982) cautions against use of this method
for people with heart problems and others who
may not be able to physically withstand the
treatment.

The focused smoking technique emphasizes concentration on negative sensory reactions while
smoking, and the holding technique entails holding smoke in the mouth for a given period of time.
Although few studies have used these methods,
they have been successful with some clients (Snyder, 1989).

Tension-reduction strategies include systematic
desensitization and relaxation training. This treatment is directed at alleviating the stress and tension
that lead to smoking (Gatchel & Baum, 1983).
Subjects are first asked to idenfity cues and consequences related to smoking; comply with a contingency factor, such as a monetary deposit; and
implement a self-monitoring procedure for track-
ing the frequency and circumstances of continued
use (Snyder, 1989).

Secondly, the subjects are asked to reduce antecedent stimuli and confine smoking to designated
locations and times (fading). A contingency contract may be developed that builds in a response
cost. Positive reinforcement should also be included in any contingency package, and, if possible, there should be a specific reinforcement for
behavior incompatible with smoking. For example,
people may reward themselves by going to places
such as theaters, galleries, and museums, where
smoking is not allowed.

Studies have found that people who have successfully stopped smoking used more stimulus
control techniques for a longer time and frequently
used self-reinforcement, problem-solving procedures, and cognitive restructuring (Perri, Richards, & Schultheis, 1977; Wax & Wax, 1978).
Relapsed smokers have reported a low sense of
self-efficacy related to failure (Blittner, Goldberg, &

Table 7.4　Antecedent Cues and Consequences of Smoking

Variable	Antecedent cues	Consequences
Physiological	Nicotine dependence Withdrawal symptoms	Stimulation, relaxation Nicotine regulation Decreased withdrawal symptoms
Psychological	Anxiety, tension Craving Excuses and rationalizations	Relaxation Pleasure Positive self-image
Social and cultural	Peer and adult models Invitations and peer pressure Norms and laws	Peer approval Group affiliation Stress reduction
Environmental	Commercials Situations that evoke smoking Situational stressors Automatic behavior	Oral, manual, and respiratory sensation
Behavioral	Multiple behavioral cues (e.g., with coffee, after meals)	

From *Health Psychology and Behavioral Medicine* (p. 44) by James J. Snyder, 1989. Copyright © 1989. Reprinted by permission of Prentice Hall, Inc., Englewood Cliffs, NJ 07632.

Merbaum, 1978), and cite stress as the main cause for relapse (Best, 1980). Therefore, cognitive-behavioral treatments should pay attention to internal dialogue and alternative coping skills (Turk, Meichenbaum, & Genest, 1983).

Although pharmacological interventions such as tranquilizers and stimulants are not recommended, nicotine chewing gum has shown some success in alleviating withdrawal symptoms. Nevertheless, it is not recommended as a primary treatment (Snyder, 1989).

Some research studies have recommended a multimodel approach to treat smoking. This approach has been successful in treating other health problems. The treatment plans described in Table 7.5 can be integrated in a way that recognizes and responds to individual differences and the many variables that affect addictive behavior.

Pechacek and Danaher (1979) also identified a multicomponent approach that includes the treatment strategies of self-monitoring, behavioral self-control, aversive smoking, skills training, and behavioral rehearsal of alternatives. The treatment plan must reflect the complexity of the smoking habit by addressing social aspects, beliefs, attitudes, and other cognitive processes.

Obesity

Each year over 400,000 people in the United States are involved in weight-reduction efforts in clinical settings (Stunkard, 1979). Most of the self-help groups and commercial programs include diet, exercise, and increasingly, cognitive-behavioral methods. Several studies have compared cognitive-behavioral treatments with other procedures or with combinations of approaches. Consistently, cognitive-behavioral techniques have been shown to be at least as effective, and often more effective, than other treatments (Barnstuble, Klesges, & Terbizan, 1986; Levitz & Stunkard, 1974; Polly, Turner, & Sherman, 1976).

Gatchel and Baum (1983) reported on several studies on the psychological and physiological differences between obese and nonobese individuals. These studies have suggested that obese people are not as sensitive to or accurate in interpreting internal cues of hunger as nonobese people, and that the obese individuals are much more responsive to environmental cues, such as the sight and smell of food (Schacter, Goldman, & Gordon, 1968). The amount of food eaten by obese individuals does not appear to be related to food deprivation or level of hunger. Other studies have shown that obese people are more sensitive to environmental stimuli, such as the presence of food (Nisbett, 1968) and react more than nonobese people to emotionally arousing events (Rodin, Elman, & Schacter, 1974). Apparently, obese individuals are strongly affected by external stimuli, whether the stimuli is food related or not.

Table 7.5 Options in Multicomponent Programs for Smoking Cessation

Preparation

Enhancement of client commitment and motivation
  Contingency deposits
  Review of risks of smoking and benefits of quitting
Assessment
  Self-monitoring to increase client awareness and
    identify situational cues and consequences for
    smoking
  Setting a target quitting date
Self-management to reduce smoking frequency
  Stimulus control
  Stress management, relaxation
  Use of substitutes for smoking

Quitting

Aversive strategies
  Imaginal sensitization
  Rapid smoking or satiation
  Focused smoking or smoke holding
Nonaversive strategies
  Nicotine fading
  Nicotine chewing gum
  Contracting

Maintenance

Booster sessions and extended contracts
Coping skills training
  Cognitive-behavioral coping skills for high-risk
    situations
  Avoiding abstinence violation effects
  Careful transfer of self-management skills to the
    client
Social support

From *Health Psychology and Behavioral Medicine* (p. 287) by James J. Snyder, 1989. Copyright © 1989. Reprinted by permission of Prentice Hall, Inc., Englewood Cliffs, NJ 07632.

The hypothalamus may function differently in obese and nonobese individuals (Schacter, 1971). This speculation is based on the finding that animals with a malfunctioning hypothalamus tend to become obese. The hypothalamus, as a satiation-regulation center, may lose the ability to regulate food intake. Animals with this malfunction and obese humans both demonstrate hyposensitivity to internal cues and hypersensitivity to external cues associated with food (Schacter & Rodin, 1974).

Cognitive-Behavioral Treatment

The most successful interventions cited by Snyder (1989) and Carnwath and Miller (1986) include a treatment package of

- self-control techniques (including contingency management),
- self-monitoring and goal setting,
- stimulus control,
- reinforcement, and
- coping skills.

Self-control techniques may include contingency factors such as depositing money or items with the practitioner or developing a set of rewards to be self-administered when increments of the target behavior are reached. Self-monitoring may include keeping records of daily caloric intake and observing the effects of antecedent cues and consequences. And, stimulus control may involve acting on the self-monitored data by altering one's environment, time expenditure, and other antecedent stimuli that affect eating. Reinforcement is important in eliminating the undesirable behavior and in maintaining and adhering to the new behavior. Reinforcement of behaviors incompatible with the undesirable behavior is also encouraged. Coping skills should be used to deal with urges to eat and with interpersonal experiences that include eating. It is often advisable to enlist the support of family and friends to achieve environmental control and minimize relapse potential. A comprehensive approach to weight loss should include the components of changed eating behavior, good nutrition, and exercise. The exercise professional should be prepared to incorporate all three components into a weight-loss program similar to the one described in Table 7.6.

Stress

Thoresen and Eagleston (1985) offered an integrated approach to stress control. Their stimulus model of stress describes external forces or pressures on a person. The reponse model describes how the organism responds to stress. They emphasize the physiological response measured by heart rate and blood pressure.

The transactional model of stress (Cox, 1978; Lazarus, 1976) takes into account the individual's perception of the demand and his or her appraisal of the resources available to meet the demand. That is, if people perceive themselves as resourceful and capable, they do not experience stress. If people do not perceive themselves as having the personal resources to cope, then stress levels will be high, even if they actually do have coping skills. The degree of stress, therefore, may be unrelated to the situational demand or the coping resources

Table 7.6 Options in a Multicomponent Program for Weight Control

Preparation

Enhance client commitment and motivation
    Contingency deposits
    Review risks of obesity and benefits of change

Alteration of eating behavior

Assessment
    Self-monitor eating to increase client awareness and
        to identify situation cues and consequences for
        eating
    Set short- and long-term goals for change in eating
        behavior
Self-management of eating behavior
    Stimulus control
    Incentive modification
    Coping skills training
Maintenance
    Relapse prevention training
    Enlisting natural social support systems

Alteration of exercise

Assessment
    Self-monitoring of current exercise to increase client
        awareness and to identify situations and times in
        routine available for exercise
    Medical examination to determine current fitness
        and potential risks of an exercise program
Increasing exercise
    Identify convenient and affordable programs
    Stimulus control
    Enlisting natural social supports
    Progressive shaping of exercise using the principle of
        overload
    Structuring and modeling exercise session: type,
        length, and phases
    Feedback about the benefits of exercise and other
        incentive modifications

Alteration of diet

Assessment
    Self-monitoring current food ingestion, amount, and
        type, using food chart
Dietary alteration
    Education to alter client's knowledge about
        "healthy" and "unhealthy" foods
    Dietary instruction and substitution to shape the
        amount and types of food eaten
    Stimulus control to develop "healthy" food shopping
        lists
    Incentive modification

From *Health Psychology and Behavioral Medicine* (pp. 296-297) by James J. Snyder, 1989. Copyright © 1989. Reprinted by permission of Prentice Hall, Inc., Englewood Cliffs, NJ 07632.

available. As a result, the appraisal of the situational demands and coping skills is critically important and should be assessed by both the practitioner and the client.

According to Snyder (1989), altering the environment or perceived demands involves

- providing information,
- creating social support systems, and
- planning the treatment environment.

Information may be both procedural (descriptive of what will happen, when and where it will occur, and how long it will last) and sensory (descriptive of bodily sensation and affect). People taking a gymnastics class for the first time may feel less stress if the instructor explains step-by-step what will happen during each activity and the bodily sensations they might expect.

Family and friends may be critical sources of support for clients. They may also influence the clients' motivation and perception of their coping skills. The practitioner should assess the clients' social support network and help them foster a positive support system. Additionally, support groups may be formed to specifically respond to the needs of class members. The practitioner can help facilitate the development of such groups.

Planning the treatment environment involves assessing the environment in which clients will be trying out their coping skills and identifying ways to make the environment more conducive to change, adaptation, and individual control. People who perceive that they have some control over their environment experience less stress than those who feel out of control. Exercise settings that accommodate individuals' needs to participate in decision making, establishing norms and regulations, increase clients' self-efficacy.

Coping-skills training must be based on an assessment of the clients' needs, strengths, and deficits in the areas relevant to the task at hand. Meichenbaum (1977) identified treatment components that underlie most coping-skills programs:

- Understanding the role of cognition in maintenance of the problem
- Accurately observing self-statements and monitoring maladaptive behavior
- Understanding the fundamentals of problem-solving
- Modeling self-statements associated with cognitive skills
- Modeling, rehearsing, and encouraging positive self-evaluation

■ Understanding and using procedures such as relaxation training and behavioral rehearsal

■ *In vivo* practicing of new skills

Alcohol Abuse

Several explanations for alcoholism have been considered in the attempt to understand and treat alcoholism. The two most prominent theoretical models of addiction have generated heated debate and have divided the professional community.

The biomedical or disease model espouses the importance of biological and genetic predisposition to addiction. According to this model, people are compelled and overpowered by biological forces and have no control over their drinking behavior. The treatment of choice is abstinence. The striving for successful abstinence is supported and enhanced by strong social support and self-help through active participation in Alcoholics Anonymous.

The second theory, based on a social cognitive model, maintains that addiction is a learned, acquired behavior. Addictive behavior stems from the development of maladaptive habits. Those who subscribe to this model are likely to look to operant, cognitive-behavioral, and social-learning techniques to treat alcoholism. They would also consider the determinants of drinking, such as environmental and situational antecedents, history with drinking, and the consequences of drinking.

A frequently used treatment combination involves stimulus control, self-reinforcement, coping skills training, and relapse management. Most of the research on relapse has been done with addictive behaviors, specifically alcoholism.

Marlatt and Gordon (1978) found that among subjects who had experienced some success in alcohol treatment, the most common reasons for relapse were negative emotional states, inability to resist social pressure, and interpersonal conflict. This and other studies indicate that treatments for alcoholism should include coping skills to deal with the high risk of relapse. Coping skills are built largely through mastery experiences. When individuals successfully recover from slips, perceived coping ability is strengthened. However, confidence in coping skills could create the belief that one can always recover. For the alcoholic, this confidence could reduce efforts in abstinence. Further study will try to determine whether strong resistive self-efficacy or recovery self-efficacy is better. Treatment approaches should allow the occurrence of lapse without the interpretation of failure and accept that lapses happen. Bandura (1986), however, does not propose planned lapse.

Perceived self-regulation efficacy has successfully predicted (Condiotte & Lichtenstein, 1981) which participants would relapse. Individuals with high self-efficacy tended to view a slip as a temporary setback, whereas people with lower self-efficacy tended to relapse completely after a slip (Bandura, 1986). Treatment strategies, therefore, should include measures of self-efficacy, provide individualized interventions, and enhance self-regulatory capabilities. For more information on this subject we recommend the work of Alan Marlatt & Gordon (1978, 1980, 1985), who developed the relapse prevention approach, and the work of Albert Bandura on the application of social cognitive theory in self-efficacy.

Coronary Heart Disease

Coronary heart disease is caused by a narrowing of coronary arteries when plaque accumulates on the arterial lining. The flow of oxygen to the heart is impeded, often causing angina pectoris or myocardial infarction. Snyder (1989) described a combination of factors responsible for coronary heart disease, most of which are psychological or psychosocial.

The psychobiological risk factors include high blood cholesterol, high blood pressure, smoking, a high-fat diet, and a sedentary lifestyle. Coronary heart disease is also influenced by genetic factors. People with a family history of heart disease have a higher risk of developing coronary heart disease. Although genetic risk may be mediated by health-promoting behaviors and lifestyle, behavioral and environmental influences cannot negate genetic predisposition.

Health-promoting behavior may also mediate psychobiological risk factors. However, only 50% of the cases of coronary heart disease are explained by these factors. Psychosocial factors and other stressors also contribute to the risk. Snyder (1989) reports that researchers who have focused on the psychosocial aspects of heart disease have identified several social and environmental factors. Social relationships and the presence of a social or familial network appear to be more important than once thought. A study of the social networks of 7,000 people found a significantly higher mortality among those who had less contact with others (Berkman & Syme, 1979). Other findings indicate that socioeconomic factors may also increase the risk of coronary heart disease. Jenkins (1976) identified higher mortality rates for individuals with little education, low occupational status, low income, and substandard housing.

Coping style is the most significant psychosocial factor for treatment. A coping style that appears to contribute specifically to the development of coronary heart disease is the Type A personality. The Type A behavioral pattern is characterized by time urgency, competitiveness, and hostility. The Type A coping style focuses on present or anticipated stress. Type A individuals may not discriminate between situations that are controllable and those that are not. The responses of working longer, denying fatigue, and reacting competitively influence physiological functioning and are thought to facilitate coronary heart disease (Snyder, 1989).

Behavioral Treatment

Attempts to decrease the risk of coronary heart disease for Type A people have focused on reducing physiological arousal by reevaluating the environment, reappraising resources, and restructuring perceptions.

Two studies by Roskies and colleagues (Roskies, Kearney, Spevack, & Surkis, 1979; Roskies et al., 1986) investigated the effects of different treatments on cardiac functioning. The first study compared male subjects across three treatment groups of psychoanalysis, behavioral therapy, and behavioral therapy with subjects who had preliminary indications of coronary heart disease (the other two groups had shown no such indications). At a 6-month follow-up, both behavioral therapy groups had lower serum cholesterol, lower blood pressure, less time pressure, and fewer psychological symptoms. In the follow-up study, Roskies and colleagues compared three treatments of aerobic exercise, cognitive-behavioral stress management, and weight training in modifying cardiovascular functioning and behavioral arousal in healthy Type A men. The stress-management strategies included self-monitoring, rehearsal, and coping strategies of relaxation, problem solving and cognitive relabeling, and stress inoculation. The results indicated a significantly greater change in behavioral reactivity in the stress-management group, but no differences in physiological measures between the groups.

In a study of 862 cardiac patients, participants were assigned either to a cardiac counseling group or to a behavioral counseling group that included cardiac counseling (Friedman & Rosenman, 1974). Those in the behavioral counseling group showed a 50% reduction in Type A behavior. The group

receiving cardiac and Type A counseling showed a 7.2% incidence of heart attacks compared to a 13% increase in the group receiving cardiac counseling only. These and other studies indicate that Type A behavior can be modified to reduce the arousal associated with heart attack (Snyder, 1989).

Several studies have supported the therapeutic and rehabilitative benefit of cognitive-behavioral interventions in the clinical treatment of heart disease. Coronary heart disease, unlike some other health-impairing conditions, affects one's physical efficacy and sense of control. Gruen (1975) found that after undergoing a treatment plan of coping-skills rehearsal, problem solving, and prompting of information seeking, cardiac patients spent less time in the hospital, were less anxious and depressed, and showed better follow-up rehabilitative progress than their counterparts who received normal cardiac care.

There is increasing evidence to indicate that perceived self-efficacy mediates health-promoting and health-impairing behavior (Bandura, 1986; Janz & Becker, 1984). If people do not believe they are capable of change or adherence to an exercise program, they will not put forth the effort necessary to test their physical efficacy and therefore will lose physical stamina. Paradoxically, individuals who are willing to test themselves increase their level of physical functioning, which in turn validates the initial perceived self-efficacy. Cognitive-behavioral treatment for coronary heart disease should, therefore, include self-efficacy training that emphasizes the individual's ability to alter health habits.

Treatment interventions for individuals with high coronary risk should be based on a thorough assessment of physiological, psychosocial, and environmental factors. Patient involvement in diagnosis, treatment, and development of psychosocial interventions increases a sense of control and self-efficacy. Cognitive-behavioral and social learning approaches continue to show promise in reducing high-risk, coronary-prone behaviors and inadequate coping styles.

SUMMARY

Exercise practitioners must understand how and why behavioral change occurs in order to help the exercise participant and contribute to the success of an exercise program. Behavioral change is a function of learning. The principles of the primary types of learning are classical and operant conditioning, cognitive-behavioral approaches, and social cognitive theory. Classical conditioning offers a means of modifying existing behaviors, rather than initiating new behaviors, through treatments such as systematic desensitization and relaxation. Operant conditioning enables the exercise practitioner to modify the consequences of behavior through control of reinforcements. The cognitive approaches focus away from control of the environment to understanding the role of cognitions and on internal, rather than external, events. The exercise practitioner must understand how the participants perceive themselves and the exercise setting if collaborative goal setting and treatment is to be successful. Social cognitive intervention focuses on the reciprocity of influence between environment, behavior, and internal mediating processes. Social cognitive theory allows the practitioner even greater flexibility in exercise treatment and intervention. Through observational learning, an organizing principle of social cognitive theory, participants can learn from another person's behavior and its consequence, rather than depending exclusively on their own experiences. The application of these learning principles to the exercise setting affords the exercise practitioner a clearer understanding of the transition from theory to practice.

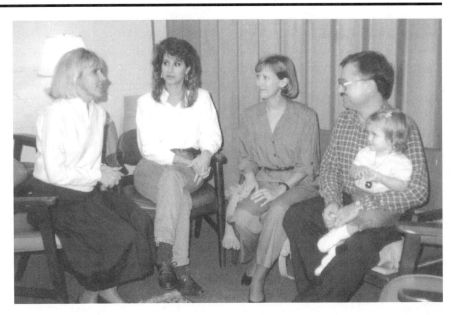

Chapter 8

Counseling in the Fitness Profession

In recent years, the holistic movement has significantly broadened the scope of traditional academic disciplines. Proponents of the holistic approach believe the physical, mental, and emotional processes of the individual to be inseparable (Gazda, 1989). As a result, many professions have reevaluated curricula, applied theory, and clinical treatments to respond to the needs of the total person. New integrated disciplines have emerged. Behavioral medicine, health psychology, neuropsychology, pschophysiology, and behavioral psychology are a few examples of the new interdisciplinary approach (Matarazzo, 1980; Schwartz & Weiss, 1977).

The fitness professional is being affected by the holistic movement in two ways: (1) The emphasis on physical fitness in the United States over the last 25 years has created a myriad of career options, ranging from sports psychology, exercise physiology, and aerobics to academic research and instruction. (2) Fitness professionals now value the total person in their work with students and clients, taking into account the psychological, emotional, and affective components as well as the physical aspects.

The counseling profession historically has supported the belief that people with certain characteristics or skills are capable of helping other people with life problems (Egan, 1986; Frank, 1973). One might think of psychologists, psychiatrists, mental-health counselors, and social workers as counseling professionals. There are many levels of counseling and many sources of help. Cowen (1982) identified important sources of psychological help in attorneys, doctors, ministers, teachers, and nurses. Frequently, psychological and socioemotional aspects of problems surface during professional interactions and need to be dealt with respectfully and responsively by the professional involved.

Fitness professionals are very much a part of the groups of professionals who increasingly play the role of counselor, and they are identifying the need to master basic interpersonal and communication skills. It is interesting to note that research has not always found counseling from mental-health professionals to be more effective than counseling from other sources (Lambert, Bergin, & Collins, 1977; Strupp, Hadley, & Gomes-Schwartz, 1977). Furthermore, a distinction is seldom made between competent and incompetent mental-health professionals (Ellis, 1984; Lebow, 1982).

These and other studies (Kagan, 1973) suggest that while many professionals are accredited, they may not have the interpersonal and therapeutic skills necessary to be effective counselors (Egan, 1986). Carkhuff (1969) emphasizes the importance of being effective. As Egan (1986) noted, the world is filled with informal counselors, and very little of the help provided comes from mental-health professionals.

Counseling is a very important function of exercise professionals. This role, however, has only recently been acknowledged, and formal integration of the role is still in process. How then can the exercise practitioner know when counseling is appropriate? How much counseling should be done and when should a client be referred to another professional? Is counseling formal or informal? These questions reflect the need to clarify and define the role of counseling for the exercise practitioner. Every exercise professional provides counseling on an ongoing basis. This chapter provides a framework from which practitioners may operate more effectively.

The importance of understanding the uniqueness of each exercise participant is primary. The exercise specialist needs counseling skills to develop a working relationship with a client and to understand how that person's individuality applies to exercise. Exercise participants all have their own perceptions of what fitness is all about. Unless there is a shared understanding of the goals of exercise, the practitioner and client may be working at odds.

The exercise specialist works not just with the goals identified by the participant, but with the total lifestyle of the individual. Failure to factor in variables in a person's life that affect adherence to

exercise objectives presents a major obstacle to success. A typical illustration is the case of the exercise participant whose spouse is already involved in exercise and has become impatient with the partner. The reverse scenario is equally common where the exercise participant's spouse is inactive and feels threatened by the partner's interest in fitness. The exercise specialist needs counseling and interpersonal communication skills to perceive these situations accurately and factor these variables into an exercise strategy.

In the exercise setting, counseling is both formal and informal. Typically, the exercise specialist will utilize some form of assessment to determine the baseline condition of the participants. At the beginning of an exercise program, clients often have questions and concerns. This is a time for formal counseling. In jointly identifying exercise goals, the practitioner and client consider variables affecting the accomplishment of the goals, such as lifestyle, behavioral patterns, habits, and other psychosocial factors (e.g., diet, sleep patterns, work habits, anxiety and tension, and smoking and alcohol consumption).

During class time, the practitioner is available for consultation. This is a time for informal counseling. The participants may seek help or the instructor may identify a potential problem for the participant. Some participants are very forthcoming with their feelings and thoughts, while others may need some prompting from the practitioner. Communication skills are most important. The practitioner needs to inquire appropriately, not simply question and probe.

The decision-making paradigm shown in Figure 8.1 may help the exercise professional determine counseling needs. The formal contact during the assessment and feedback session and the informal contact throughout the program can be used to clarify psychosocial variables that affect the exercise plan. When the practitioner believes he or she understands the participant's situation, the practitioner will decide how best to counsel the participant.

If the variables affecting the exercise program are integrally related to exercise (e.g., finding time to exercise), or the practitioner has knowledge in the area of the concern, the practitioner and client will plan a strategy for managing or resolving the problem. However, if the practitioner thinks that the variables are outside his or her area of expertise (e.g., chronic depression), the practitioner would refer the client to a mental-health specialist and continue to work with the client on the exercise program. The practitioner and mental-health

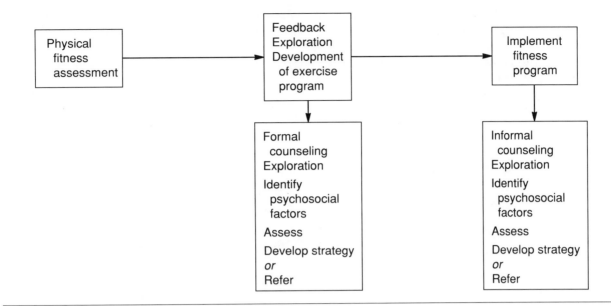

Figure 8.1 Decision-making paradigm.

specialist may also consult with each other to provide a comprehensive treatment.

This chapter will address the primary dimensions of counseling that are important to the fitness professional. These include (1) communication skills, (2) the core characteristics of the effective helper, (3) the helping models, and (4) ethical and professional issues.

COMMUNICATION SKILLS

There are three components of communication:

■ Attending
- Being aware of one's nonverbal behavior
- Observing nonverbal behaviors and characteristics of clients

■ Listening
- Understanding the feelings and content of verbal messages
- Identifying incongruities

■ Empathic responding
- Showing empathy
- Understanding core message

Think for a moment about a time when you brought up a concern in hopes of getting feedback or help from another person, and instead the person (1) used your statement to redirect the conversation to him or herself, (2) dismissed your concern by telling you that "everyone goes through the same thing," or (3) gave you advice without trying to understand your concern. Although it seems that communication skills should come naturally, training and practice are necessary to truly develop these abilities.

Through good communication, fitness professionals can enrich the quality of their interpersonal relationships, and manage and resolve problems. Good communicators can shift their focus of awareness from themselves to others. They understand what a person really means and accurately identify the feelings and thoughts the person is trying to express. This level of response shows clients that you are genuinely interested in helping them and that you have the capability to do so.

Attending

The ability to focus one's energy, attention, and thoughts on another person is the essence of *attending*. Egan (1986) defined attending as an intensity of presence, of "being with" the client. He further noted that attending demonstrates respect, which enhances the relationship, and helps the professional develop and maintain active listening. We will describe attending from two perspectives: (1) the nonverbal, physical, and psychological presence of an effective helper and (2) the nonverbal characteristics and behaviors of clients.

Counselor/Practitioner Attending Skills

Exercise instructors can improve their communication style by becoming familiar with their own nonverbal behavior. Ways to do this include requesting feedback from colleagues and students, and viewing themselves on videotape doing a consultation. The following attending skills have consistently been found to either enhance or hinder communication depending on how well the skills have been acquired.

Squaring.   Turning one's body to fully face another person emphasizes focused attention and interest. Standing with shoulders at a right angle or turned away communicates disinterest or rejection. Although in an exercise setting, the instructor and the clients are moving about, the fitness instructor needs to make every effort to physically attend to and be aware of the presence of the client.

Energy Level.   Truly focusing on another person requires mental and physical energy. Carkhuff, Pierce, and Cannon (1977) defined *energy level* as the amount of effort put into a purposeful task. The absence of energy is easily identified by clients and is frequently interpreted as lack of interest or preoccupation. The presence or absence of energy will affect the clients' willingness to make contact and be open to you.

Attending skills, in particular energy level, can affect how potential clients' view the instructor's approachability, even before the instructor has interacted with them. The influential "first impression" is especially important in exercise settings. If fitness professionals direct genuine interest by focusing energy on clients, they will have laid the groundwork for open communication and interaction.

What if the exercise leader experiences low energy? The most common causes of low energy include physical and mental stress, diet and exercise, and emotional concerns that cause worry, distress, anxiety, or depression. The energy deficit signals that corrective measures may need to be taken. If low energy persists, the practitioner may want to explore possible causes. Consulting a counselor or an exercise colleague could be helpful.

Posture.   Many interpretations are made about the meaning of folded arms, crossed legs, foot shaking, and other nonverbal behaviors. Fitness professionals should be aware of their body posturing as a sign of negative feelings or reactions to the client.

Eye Contact.   The most common and powerful nonverbal behavior is eye contact. Appropriate and natural eye contact varies somewhat across cultures. In our society, steady eye contact without staring indicates interest in an individual. Although occasional glances away are natural, following the activity, movement, or conversation of someone else is often construed as boredom and disinterest.

Cormier and Cormier (1990) have noted that more mutual eye contact occurs in counseling when:

■ physical distance is greater between the helper and client,

■ comfortable topics are discussed,

■ interpersonal involvement exists between the helper and client,

■ the person is listening rather than talking, and

■ the individuals are female.

Less eye contact is maintained when:

■ the helper and client are physically close,

■ difficult topics are discussed,

■ the person is talking rather that listening,

■ one of the individuals is disinterested in the reaction of the other, and

■ one of the individuals is embarrassed or hiding something.

Each of the nonverbal behaviors mentioned and other nonverbal behaviors, such as facial expressions, gestures, voice volume and rate, and mannerisms, convey a message. The counselor will probably be more effective if the nonverbal communication is congruent with verbal messages. The clients' trust and willingness to risk are contingent on the perception of helper congruence. Counselors should maintain a relaxed yet consistent focus on the client, even if the client is unable to make eye contact. The counselor's willingness and ability to look at the client sends a message of openness, acceptance, and availability.

Nonverbal Behavior of Clients

Knapp (1978) described nonverbal behavior as "all human communication events which transcend spoken or written words" (p. 38). The verbal and nonverbal components of communication are interdependent; however, the nonverbal component is often the most significant (Gazda, 1984). Birdwhistell (1970) believes that 65% of the meaning of any message is conveyed through nonverbal behavior. Many experts on communication style emphasize the importance of nonverbal cues in understanding of human behavior (Cormier & Cormier, 1990; Gazda, 1973; Mehrabian, 1971; Gazda, 1989).

One of the most effective ways to identify an unspoken problem is through the identification of incongruities. Incongruities can exist between (a) verbal and nonverbal messages, (b) two nonverbal responses, such as smiling and exhibiting a nervous gesture simultaneously, and (c) two different verbal statements.

In the following scenario, the instructor identifies a problem by accurately evaluating incongruent nonverbal behavior.

--- ■ ---

Jim signs up for a noontime fitness class at the university near his work. For the first 4 weeks Jim comes to class regularly and on time. He talks and jokes with the fitness instructor and his classmates. Then Jim begins to arrive late. He seems more nervous and serious. The instructor asks how he is doing. Jim claims to be just fine, but looks anxious when others ask about him. He stops his exercise early saying he is too fatigued to continue. The instructor tells Jim that he seems nervous, anxious, and frustrated, and expresses concern for Jim. Jim then confesses that his boss has reprimanded him for not being available to work through lunch and has challenged Jim's work commitment. Jim feels resentment toward his boss and frustration with himself for not being more assertive. The exercise instructor supports Jim in expressing his feelings, acknowledges Jim's predicament, and encourages him to pursue ways to improve his assertiveness skills and to evaluate his goals and priorities.

In this example, the instructor was aware of a cluster of erratic behaviors that were (a) incongruent with Jim's verbal response, (b) incongruent with Jim's earlier behavior, and (c) formed a pattern of being pressured, anxious, and frustrated. Had the instructor not noticed Jim's nonverbal behavior and accepted his cursory answer of "doing fine," the instructor would not have been able to help Jim with his problem.

Nonverbal communication is powerful partly because it is uncensored. As a result, nonverbal expression is a valuable tool for the practitioner in understanding clients. Incongruent nonverbal expression is particularly valuable because it signals that something important is going on that

cannot be expressed openly. The practitioner needs to both identify incongruence and interpret possible meanings of the nonverbal expression.

Table 8.1 shows an adaptation of Cormier and Cormier's (1990) categorization of nonverbal behaviors and probable meanings. Every person's verbal and nonverbal expression has special meaning for that particular person. Generalizations have been made after many observations of nonverbal behavior across cultures, gender, age, and other relevant variables. Interpretations of nonverbal behaviors must always be based on a cluster of observations that validate each other. Awareness and understanding of the context of expression is also most important in making accurate interpretations. Examples of contextual interaction are included in Table 8.1.

Listening

The purpose of listening is to understand what the other person is meaning. Effectively responding to a client requires active listening. The framework for listening, shown in Figure 8.2, includes several components that are interrelated but that contribute uniquely to understanding meaning.

People who listen actively can accurately identify congruities and incongruities in verbal and nonverbal communication. As the listener observes and understands the messages, themes and patterns begin to emerge that convey deeper meanings. The listener responds to the speaker by describing the meaning of the speaker's message as the listener heard it. Then the listener waits for further verbal and nonverbal responses from which to derive another meaning. This process is illustrated in the following exchange:

Exercise Participant (EP): I've been doing pretty well this week, nothing to complain about.

The exercise instructor (EI) notices the client has low energy, is not talking with other classmates as he usually does, and is reluctantly doing his exercise routine. This is an observation of an incongruence between the client's verbal statement and his nonverbal behavior.

EI: You know, even though you say you're doing okay, you don't seem yourself. (Stating the observed incongruence.)

EP: Well, I just had a hard time at work. The project I'm working on isn't going well.

Table 8.1   Inventory of Nonverbal Behavior

Nonverbal dimension	Observed behavior	Example of counselor/client interaction (context)	Possible effect or meaning
		I. Kinetics	
Eyes			
	Direct eye contact	Client has just shared concern with counselor. Counselor responds; client maintains eye contact.	Readiness or willingness for interpersonal communication or exchange; attentiveness
	Lack of sustained eye contact	Each time counselor brings up the topic of client's family, client looks away.	Withdrawal or avoidance of interpersonal exchange; or respect or deference
		Client demonstrates intermittent breaks in eye contact while conversing with counselor.	Respect or deference
		Client mentions sexual concerns, then abruptly looks away. When counselor initiates this topic, client looks away again.	Withdrawal from topic of conversation; discomfort or embarrassment; or preoccupation
	Lowering eyes—looking down or away	Client talks at some length about alternatives to present job situation; pauses briefly and looks down; then resumes speaking and eye contact with counselor.	Preoccupation
	Staring or fixation on person or object	Counselor has just asked client to consider consequences of a certain decision. Client is silent and gazes at a picture on the wall.	Preoccupation; possible rigidity or uptightness
	Darting eyes or blinking rapidly—rapid eye movements; twitching brow	Client indicates desire to discuss a topic yet is hesitant. As counselor probes, client's eyes move around the room rapidly.	Excitation or anxiety; or wearing contact lenses
	Squinting or furrow on brow	Client has just asked counselor for advice. Counselor explains role, and client squints and furrows appear in client's brow.	Thought or perplexity; or avoidance of person or topic
		Counselor suggests possible things for client to explore in difficulties with parents. Client doesn't respond verbally; furrow in brow appears.	Avoidance of person or topic
	Moisture or tears	Client has just reported recent death of father; tears well up in client's eyes.	Sadness; frustration; sensitive areas of concern
		Client reports real progress during past week in marital communication; eyes get moist.	Happiness
	Eye shifts	Counselor has just asked client to remember significant events in week; client pauses and looks away, then responds and looks back.	Processing or recalling material; or keen interest; satisfaction
	Pupil dilation	Client discusses spouse's sudden disinterest and pupils dilate.	Alarm; or keen interest
		Client leans forward while counselor talks and pupils dilate.	Keen interest; satisfaction

Nonverbal dimension	Observed behavior	Example of counselor/client interaction (context)	Possible effect or meaning
Total body			
	Facing other person squarely or leaning forward	Client shares a concern and faces counselor directly while talking; continues to face counselor while counselor responds.	Openness to interpersonal communication and exchange
	Turning of body orientation at an angle, not directly facing person, or slouching in seat	Client indicates some difficulty in "getting into" interview. Counselor probes for reasons; client turns body away.	Less openness to interpersonal exchange
	Rocking back and forth in chair or squirming in seat	Client indicates a lot of nervousness about an approaching conflict situation. Client rocks as this is discussed.	Concern; worry; anxiety
	Stiff—sitting erect and rigidly on edge of chair	Client indicates some uncertainty about direction of interview; sits very stiff and erect at this time.	Tension; anxiety; concern
	Repetitive twisting of hair, tapping of fingers	Client responds with short, minimal, non-self-revealing responses.	Feeling distracted, bored, or uncomfortable—or indication of some unexpressed emotion
	Breathing becomes slower and deeper	Client begins to settle back in chair and relate a positive event that occurred during the week.	Client is feeling more comfortable and relaxed; breathing changes reflect the decreased arousal
Shoulders			
	Shrugging	Client reports that spouse just walked out with no explanation. Client shrugs shoulders while describing this.	Uncertainty; or ambivalence
	Leaning forward	Client has been sitting back in the chair. Counselor discloses something about herself; client leans forward and asks counselor a question about the experience.	Eagerness; attentiveness, openness to communication
	Slouched, stooped, rounded, or turned away from person	Client reports feeling inadequate and defeated because of poor grades; slouches in chair after saying this.	Sadness or ambivalence; or lack of receptivity to interpersonal exchange
		Client reports difficulty in talking. As counselor pursues this, client slouches in chair and turns shoulders away from counselor.	Lack of receptivity to interpersonal exchange
Arms and hands			
	Arms folded across chest	Counselor has just initiated conversation. Client doesn't respond verbally; sits back in chair with arms crossed against chest.	Avoidance of interpersonal exchange or dislike
	Trembling and fidgety hands	Client expresses fear of suicide; hands tremble while talking about this.	Anxiety or anger

(Cont.)

Table 8.1 (Continued)

Nonverbal dimension	Observed behavior	Example of counselor/client interaction (context)	Possible effect or meaning
		In a loud voice, client expresses resentment; client's hands shake while talking.	Anger
	Fist clenching to objects or holding hands tightly	Client has just come in for initial interview. Says that he or she feels uncomfortable; hands are clasped together tightly.	Anxiety or anger
		Client expresses hostility toward boss; clenches fists while talking.	Anger
	Arms unfolded—arms and hands gesturing in conversation	Counselor has just asked a question; client replies and gestures during reply.	Accenting or emphasizing point in conversation; or openness to interpersonal exchange
		Counselor initiates new topic. Client readily responds; arms are unfolded at this time.	Openness to interpersonal exchange
	Rarely gesturing, hands and arms stiff	Client arrives for initial session. Responds to counselor's questions with short answers. Arms are kept down at side.	Tension or anger
		Client has been referred; sits with arms down at side while explaining reasons for referral and irritation at being here.	Anger

II. Paralinguistics

Voice level and pitch			
	Whispering or inaudibility	Client has been silent for a long time. Counselor probes; client responds, but in a barely audible voice.	Difficulty in disclosing
	Pitch changes	Client is speaking at a moderate voice level while discussing job. Then client begins to talk about boss, and voice pitch rises considerably.	Topics of conversation have different emotional meanings
Fluency in speech			
	Stuttering, hesitations, speech errors	Client is talking rapidly about feeling uptight in certain social situations; client stutters and makes some speech errors while doing so.	Sensitivity about topic in conversation; or anxiety and discomfort
	Whining or lisp	Client is complaining about having a hard time losing weight; voice goes up like a whine.	Dependency or emotional emphasis
	Rate of speech slow, rapid, or jerky	Client begins interview talking slowly about a bad weekend. As topic shifts to client's feelings about himself, client talks more rapidly.	Sensitivity to topics of conversation; or topics have different emotional meanings
	Silence	Client comes in and counselor invites client to talk; client remains silent.	Reluctance to talk; or preoccupation
		Counselor has just asked client a question.	Preoccupation; or desire to continue

Adapted from *Interviewing Strategies for Helpers: Fundamental Skills and Behavioral Interventions* (3rd Edition) (pp. 66-70), by W.H. Cormier and L.S. Cormier. Copyright © 1991, 1985, 1979 by Wadsworth, Inc. Used with the permission of Brooks/Cole Publishing Company, Pacific Grove, CA 93950.

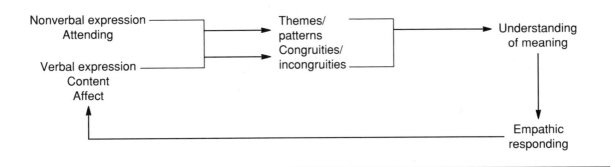

Figure 8.2 The listening paradigm.

EI: That must be discouraging. (Empathic response.)

EP: Yeah, it wouldn't bother me so much except that the car broke down this month and my daughter had to have her tonsils out. Now my knee is acting up again when I run.

The instructor realizes the theme of everything going wrong at once and that it is all beyond the participant's control. His verbal message implies that he has to keep up a good front and be strong.

EI: There sure are things going on in your life that are hard to handle all at once. I can see why you might feel discouraged and frustrated. It's hard to ask for help or to think anyone would be willing to listen, but others can't tell what you need if you don't ask. (Understanding meaning and empathic response to meaning.)

Content

The part of a message that conveys information about a situation or event is called *content*. The content becomes known through the "5WH" journalistic formula: Who, What, When, Where, Why, and How? An easy way to evaluate listening skills for content is to listen to a 3-minute verbal statement and try to repeat it. Most people are surprised at the selective forgetting that occurs. A common phenomenon is to forget statements that describe certain kinds of negative events such as sickness, misfortune, or unpleasant experiences, or to remember only negative events. Sometimes people recall details of events, but not names and places. Or they may recall a decision, but not the decision-making process or who made the decision. These are examples of faulty patterns of listening for content.

In the counseling role, the accurate understanding of content is important because the feelings

and meaning of the message are grounded in the content. The content is a frame of reference from which the individual develops a perspective. In the process of identifying themes and patterns, the counselor may want to note the content of the client's problem statements. Often, there is a common theme that contributes to understanding the meaning of an experience.

Affect

The feelings and emotions that accompany the content are known as *affect*. Often feelings are not expressed, especially negative ones, and these hidden feelings may be difficult to identify. Feelings control the energy and meaning behind the experience. The first step in understanding the meaning of an experience is to identify the cluster of feelings and the degree of intensity attached to the event (Table 8.2).

The chart in Table 8.2 gives an overview of categories and intensity levels of feelings. Happiness, sadness, fear, uncertainty, anger, strength, and weakness represent the range of feelings. These categories contain feeling words of strong, moderate, and weak intensity. It is important to be able to accurately identify the category and range of intensity. For example, if an exercise participant says, "I felt discouraged today," and the instructor responds, "Yes, I see your despair and feelings of hopelessness," the instructor would have greatly overstated the intensity. The helper must try to respond in the most accurate feeling category and then identify the appropriate intensity level within that category.

Correctly identifying feeling and content statements provides the foundation for the understanding of meaning. According to Carkhuff et al., (1977), content provides intellectual meaning and feeling provides emotional meaning.

The following dialogue between a fitness instructor and student illustrates the use of content and affect in effective responding:

Table 8.2   Commonly Used Affect Words

Level of intensity	Category of feeling						
	Happiness	Sadness	Fear	Uncertainty	Anger	Strength, potency	Weakness, inadequacy
Strong	Excited Thrilled Delighted Overjoyed Ecstatic Elated Jubilant	Despairing Hopeless Depressed Crushed Miserable Abandoned Defeated Desolate	Panicked Terrified Afraid Frightened Scared Overwhelmed	Bewildered Disoriented Mistrustful Confused	Outraged Hostile Furious Angry Harsh Hateful Mean Vindictive	Powerful Authoritative Forceful Potent	Ashamed Powerless Vulnerable Cowardly Exhausted Impotent
Moderate	"Up" Good Happy Optimistic Cheerful Enthusiastic Joyful "Turned on"	Dejected Dismayed Disillusioned Lonely Bad Unhappy Pessimistic Sad Hurt Lost	Worried Shaky Tense Anxious Threatened Agitated	Doubtful Mixed up Insecure Skeptical Puzzled	Aggravated Irritated Offended Mad Frustrated Resentful "Sore" Upset Impatient Obstinate	Tough Important Confident Fearless Energetic Brave Courageous Daring Assured Adequate Self-confident Skillful	Embarrassed Useless Demoralized Helpless Worn out Inept Incapable Incompetent Inadequate Shaken
Weak	Pleased Glad Content Relaxed Satisfied Calm	"Down" Discouraged Disappointed "Blue" Alone Left out	Jittery Jumpy Nervous Uncomfortable Uptight Uneasy Defensive Apprehensive Hesitant Edgy	Unsure Surprised Uncertain Undecided Bothered	Perturbed Annoyed Grouchy Hassled Bothered Disagreeable	Determined Firm Able Srong	Frail Meek Unable Weak

From *The Skills of Helping* (p. 77) by R.R. Carkhuff and W.A. Anthony, 1979. Copyright 1979 by Human Resource Development Press, Inc. Reprinted by permission of Human Resource Development Press, Inc., 22 Amherst Rd., Amherst, MA 01002, 1-800-822-2801 (U.S. and Canada) or (413) 253-3488.

Student: I am excited about getting back in shape, but I don't know how I'll do in a class with other people. (The student feels excitement, which was expressed, but also apprehension, which was not overtly expressed. The content statement about the exercise setting signals the presence of apprehension.)

Instructor: Even though you're excited about exercise, you also sound apprehensive about being in a class. (The instructor responds to feeling and content.)

Student: Yes, whenever I've been in groups doing physical activities, everybody else seems better than me. (The content statement is that the student has been in several situations where the student's performance was not as strong as others' performance. There is also an implied competitiveness in the content statement. The student does not give a feeling statement, so the instructor puts herself in the client's shoes. The feelings would be in the range of discouraged, uptight, uncomfortable, or defensive.)

Instructor: It sounds like you see the group activity as a competitive thing and then you end up feeling discouraged or uptight because somebody usually has a stronger performance than you. (The instructor takes the content statement and interprets probable feelings from it.)

The counselor must try to identify the feeling category as well as the appropriate intensity level. Becoming familiar with feeling categories enables the counselor to hit upon the correct feeling or group of feelings more frequently.

As identified in the Myers-Briggs Type Indicator (Myers, 1962), individuals have a patterned preference for operating in either a thinking or feeling mode. Those who prefer thinking will most likely speak exclusively in terms of content, often with great capacity for detail and description. For example, an exercise practitioner says to a student, "How are you feeling about your progress?" The student responds, "I have increased my distance by a mile a week and have leveled off at 5 miles a week. My pulse rate is down and I'm decreasing time per mile." Because counselors cannot depend on "thinkers" to provide feeling statements, they must be able to discern, through active listening and empathy skills, the underlying feelings and help the clients identify these feelings.

Conversely, people who prefer the feeling mode talk almost exclusively about their feelings without giving the counselor any content or descriptive events with which to connect their feelings. For example, the practitioner says to an exercise participant, "What are the objectives you would like to set for yourself in this class?" The participant responds, "I just can't tell you how exciting this is. I feel really good, like I'm already energized." These people often feel out of control of themselves and their life events, partially because they do not have a solid cognitive framework with which to understand their feelings.

Neither of these participants are purposely withholding information from the counselor. Part of empathic responding is to help the client identify the "missing part."

Empathic Responding

Empathy is the ability to understand the experience of another person from that person's frame of reference. Accurate understanding of content and awareness of nonverbal expression enables the counselor to "lock in" on the client's frame of reference through the following process:

1. Identify several nonverbal behaviors.

2. Note whether the nonverbal behaviors are congruent.

3. See if the behaviors cluster in a way that can support an underlying theme.

4. Be aware of your nonverbal reactions to the client and how you interpret your reactions.

5. Note any content information the client has provided.

6. Compare the experience (content) the client recounts to the client's previous experiences and/or patterns already identified.

7. Ask yourself how you would feel if this experience happened to you and you were exhibiting the same nonverbal behaviors as the client.

8. Test out your feeling statement through empathic response.

As Carl Rogers (1957) observed, research continues to support the conclusion that empathy may be the most potent factor in bringing about change and learning. A good rule of thumb for counselors is to ask, "How would I feel in this person's shoes?" Following are some examples of empathic exchanges:

---■---

Exercise Client: I just don't know if I want to continue in this class. Everyone else is in better shape than I am and it's a lot easier for them to meet their goals.

Instructor: (How would I feel if I had just said that?) It sounds like you might be discouraged and frustrated because exercise seems more difficult for you than for others.

---■---

A successful business executive accustomed to tight schedules, high pressure, and high expectations has joined a fitness class. He is middle-aged and considerably overweight.

Exercise Client: I'm used to getting things done in record time and never falling short of my goals. That's the way I'm going to handle this exercise class too. I'll have that weight off in a matter of weeks.

Instructor: (How would I feel if I were on that schedule?) I can see you're used to accomplishing what you set out to do and are probably really proud of that, but it sounds like that kind of schedule would require enormous energy and leave you exhausted.

The empathic response is formulated out of the counselor's identification of content, feeling, and nonverbal behavior. The effective empathic response is directed at a slightly higher level of awareness than the client has already achieved. The client may then immediately understand ("aha!") what has been said.

Empathy from the counselor enables clients to explore themes, emotions, and patterns of behavior they were previously unaware of (Patterson & Eisenberg, 1983). As clients tell stories and describe their circumstances, the professional should look for patterns and themes that run through the stories.

■

Susan is a 24-year-old graduate student in a fitness class. She is quite personable and talks easily about herself. She expresses to the instructor her discouragement about not keeping up with her friend, who had the highest mileage for running in the class. After several sessions, the instructor notices Susan talking about not being as productive as the top agent in her office at work, and not measuring up academically to her sister who always made "As." The instructor becomes aware not only that Susan continually measures herself against other people (theme), but that she also compares herself to the highest achieving people in any area (deeper theme). This pattern causes Susan to discount herself and feel inferior.

The ability of the instructor to perceive and understand such patterns is highly valuable for two reasons. First, accurate understanding enables the instructor to have a more accurate picture of the whole person, including what motivates and reinforces the person, as well as what must be addressed for the person to change. This information can help lay the groundwork for a behavioral change strategy. Secondly, conveying an accurate understanding tells the person that the instructor is really listening, which is vitally important in building trust. It also helps the person increase understanding of self.

CORE CHARACTERISTICS OF THE EFFECTIVE HELPER

Every fitness professional has a unique personality, skills, and interests. Holland (1977) noted that people of differing personality types are attracted to different work environments and that a good match is important for optimum work performance and job satisfaction.

Personal Characteristics

Research has indicated that factors such as sex, age, and level of education are not successful predictors of counselor effectiveness, but that the personality of the counselor is (Wiggins & Weslander, 1979). Many mental-health professionals have described several personality characteristics associated with being an effective counselor. Frequently mentioned characteristics include honesty, warmth, self-respect, patience, and sensitivity (Cavanaugh, 1982; Corey, 1985). Cormier and Cormier (1990) identified six qualities important in effective counseling. These qualities are equally important in the exercise setting.

Self-Awareness

Exercise professionals must be committed to their own growth and self-understanding. Being accessible requires being open to feedback from clients. Those who block out self-awareness, emotional reactions, and perceptions of self in the environment seriously hinder the ability to observe accurately and interact effectively. Exercise practitioners need to know at all times how they are affecting the interaction within the class.

Goodwill

Exercise practitioners need to work on behalf of the client in a positive and trustworthy way. Willingness to invest effort toward the welfare of a client without personal gain affects the degree of influence the client will accord the instructor.

Support

Therapeutic support takes the form of engendering hope and control by encouraging clients to make their own decisions and become self-reliant. Although support is sometimes construed as caretaking and rescuing, a caretaking response is detrimental because it enables the client to continue self-defeating behaviors. Exercise participants need to know they are supported. This awareness will enable them to believe they can be successful.

Flexibility

Exercise professionals must choose the therapeutic intervention most applicable to the client's problem and the practitioner's style. Effective counselors resist forcing a particular set of methods or favored treatment plan.

Energy

It is important to bring energy to the exercise setting and to interpersonal communication with the clients.

Intellectual Competence

Fitness professionals must have a working knowledge of both communications skills and the theoretical foundations of their particular discipline of exercise physiology.

Trustworthiness

Strong (1968) identified the importance of trustworthiness as a perceived trait of an effective counselor. There are several behaviors that clients tend to label as trustworthy:

■ Confidentiality. The client believes the counselor will not disclose information given in confidence.

■ Credibility. The client believes the counselor is dependable and reliable.

■ Consideration in the use of power. The client believes that the counselor will not use power or authority to control or manipulate.

■ Understanding. The client believes the counselor can accurately interpret the client's core message.

Professional Values

Core values (or dimensions) must be present for effective counseling to take place (Egan, 1986; Gazda, 1989; Rogers, 1957; Truax & Carkhuff, 1967). The core dimensions are the common threads running through many divergent theories and clinical approaches that are integral to all therapeutic models.

In 1967 Rogers began to refine his early work on identifying the necessary components of therapy. Carkhuff, Truax, and others joined the research effort and eventually isolated a group of core dimensions. With further study, they found that

when the counselor exhibited these core conditions, the client improved, and when these conditions were not present, the client showed no change (Gazda, Asbury, Balzer, Childers, & Walters, 1984).

Following the early studies, predictive studies measured the level of functioning of the counselor on interpersonal dimensions. It was consistently demonstrated that the behavior of clients changed according to the counselor's level of interpersonal functioning (Pagell, Carkhuff, & Berenson, 1967). Later studies corroborated the finding that a high-functioning person influences a low-functioning person, as exemplified in relationships such as parent-child, counselor-client, and teacher-student (Anthony & Vitalo, 1982). So far eight core dimensions have been identified. These dimensions are not simply skills to be learned, but qualities to have or be developed. Egan (1984) regards core conditions as values that are expressed behaviorally.

Empathy

Gladstein and Feldstein (1983) refined empathy as it applies to counseling and have identified two types. *Emotional empathy* refers to the capacity to be affected by another person's emotional experience. For example, one person may feel sad because another feels hopeless. The feelings are not the same; however, one feeling is a response to the other. *Role-taking empathy* is the ability to understand another person's emotional point of view. For example, one person may clearly understand why another feels angry, while not sharing the feeling. The counselor can help the client through the emotional experience simply by understanding the client and communicating that understanding.

Respect

Regard for another person that conveys that the person is valued is a demonstration of *respect*. However, respect for others because they are human beings does not convey an appreciation for the individuality of another person. The client needs to experience an appreciation of his or her uniqueness and a sense of "being deserving."

Individual differences in level of fitness and physical ability are apparent to the practitioner and class participants. It is important for the exercise professional to acknowledge these differences and make it clear that differences are natural. Many people suffer from some lack of self-respect. When the exercise participant receives respect from an instructor or role model, two phenomena tend to occur. First, through effective modeling, the participant learns to respect others and begins to develop self-respect as well. Learning from the instructor also develops and enhances personal qualities. Secondly, if the participants have high regard for the instructor and believe that the instructor values them, then the instructor has validated the class members. Just as children look to parents to validate their worth and value, clients, students, patients, and others look to the professional for approval and assurance.

Warmth

Gazda (1973) defines *warmth* as a physical expression of caring most often communicated through gestures, tone of voice, touch, and facial expression. Showing warmth conveys an appreciation for another person and a willingness to be open to that person. Just as being "cold" erects a barrier through which another person may not pass, warmth communicates the absence of barriers between the practitioner and client.

Genuineness

Rogers (1967) expressed *genuineness* as demonstrating congruence. Being the same person with different people and in different circumstances shows genuineness. If a client cannot be sure that the practitioner is being honest, the relationship and the therapeutic experience are undermined.

Egan (1984) identified several principles for counselors to follow in maintaining genuineness:

■ Refuse to overemphasize role. Helping should be role-free in that the "role of the helper" should not be put on and taken off in a way that manipulates or controls the client.

■ Be spontaneous. Tact is important, but it is also important not to filter needlessly.

■ Be assertive. The helper is ultimately responsible for the direction of the counseling.

■ Avoid defensiveness. If the practitioner becomes defensive, the client will fear the potential negative impact and will begin taking care of the practitioner.

■ Be consistent. Stability and the assurance that the client can rely on the practitioner is necessary for trust to develop.

Concreteness

Clients are frequently confused about how to deal with a problem and sometimes have trouble defining the problem. Clients will commonly express vague feelings, speak in generalities, or express only feelings unrelated to the problem. In these situations, the practioner must be concrete. Although the exploration and questioning may seem picky or trite, a confused client needs grounding and specificity to make sense of his or her experience.

Self-Disclosure

The practioner must be willing to share his or her experience to promote a foundation of trust. The key aspect of the professional's openness is appropriate self-disclosure. Self-disclosure is appropriate when the disclosure could be helpful to the client, the feeling or experience is relevant to the professional relationship itself, or the practitioner's unexpressed reaction is interfering with the ability to work with the client.

Inappropriate disclosure is exemplified by practitioners who refocus the session from the client's experience to their own situation as a self-indulgence. If the instructor keeps the focus on his or her personal experience and does not relate it to the participant, the disclosure is probably inappropriate and possibly self-serving.

Appropriate self-disclosure is especially important with clients who have difficulty opening up because they fear rejection or ridicule. The influence of the exercise professional as a role model applies in this situation. Self-disclosure allows the client to observe the practitioner as vulnerable, but also as coping successfully to resolve problems.

Immediacy

Making self-involving or self-observational statements about the present moment is *immediacy*. The counselor's willingness to identify feelings, reactions, themes, or personal dynamics going on during a transaction uses immediacy in a powerful way.

Confrontation

The concept of *confrontation* is frequently redefined as *challenge* in a counseling relationship. A challenge should be made only after a solid foundation of trust and mutual respect has been formed. Many professionals have more difficulty with challenge than with any other core condition, primarily because they fear a hostile confrontation, intrusion into the client's world, and mistrust or possible rejection from the client.

Challenge, done in a healthy and caring way, is the process of identifying incongruities in (a) what the client has said, felt, experienced, or expressed nonverbally, (b) what the helper observes versus what the client says, or (c) what the client did or said at an earlier time versus what he or she says or does now.

An example of healthy confrontation follows. A fitness instructor notices a self-defeating characteristic in Dion, one of the class participants.

———— ■ ————

Dion attends exercise class faithfully and tries very hard to put forth his best effort. The instructor notices that when a classmate compliments or supports Dion's performance, he discounts the compliment by saying, "There are lots of people here who are in much better shape than I will ever be." He often makes derogatory comments about his own ability in comparison to others. The instructor feels positive about the interpersonal relationship with Dion and decides to confront him on his attitude. The instructor tells Dion what he has observed and says, "I see you working very hard to do your best. Then when you put yourself down, it seems like a way to always end up feeling bad about yourself. I would like to see you change that and would be willing to help you figure out how to be more appreciative of yourself."

The practitioner makes these observations in a caring way that demonstrates (a) willingness to take a risk and be truly involved and (b) desire to help the client identify and overcome incongruities.

The personal and professional qualities mentioned in this section are often considered indicators of character and professional integrity. The presence of these characteristics is a function of personality, sociocultural influences, childhood and familial experiences, and other factors that shape behaviors and beliefs. The appropriate application of these qualities in an exercise setting requires skill in knowing when and how to influence the client.

HELPING MODELS

Several helping models are widely used in human services training and educational settings. Each of these models provides a framework from which exercise practitioners can systematically help their clients manage or resolve problems.

Exercise practitioners can adapt helping models to the variety of settings and problem circumstances they encounter by (a) first selecting a model that seems most applicable given the practitioners' needs or (b) combining aspects of more than one model to individualize the counseling approach. The practitioner should begin by developing a clear picture of the exercise setting, probable clientele, and typical problem scenarios. Then, the practitioner should visualize applying each model to his or her specific setting and professional needs. The practitioner can begin to experiment with approaches that seem to fit with the goal for creating an effective, individualized approach.

We will present three models that incorporate communication and training concepts applicable in the exercise setting. These models share underlying assumptions, principles of helping, and beliefs about health and well-being. These common characteristics enable exercise practitioners to adapt aspects of the models to their own exercise environments and still maintain continuity in their counseling styles.

Human Resource Development

Robert Carkhuff developed a step-by-step interpersonal-skills training model from Carl Rogers's client-centered therapeutic approach (Anthony & Vitalo, 1982). The Human Resource Development (HRD) model, as defined by Carkhuff (1969), consists of three helping phases (Figure 8.3). Each phase focuses on a goal for the client and a corresponding skill level appropriate for the trainer. The various client goals are (Anthony & Vitalo, 1982):

1. exploration—assessment of how well clients are functioning in their own environments,

2. understanding—identification of the gap between the clients' present level of functioning and their goals, and

3. action—development of strategies to achieve their goals.

An important part of the HRD model is an understanding of the skills required to be an effective helper and the developmental phases of helping.

Pre-Helping: Attending

During this preparatory phase, the trainer communicates genuine interest and concern for the client.

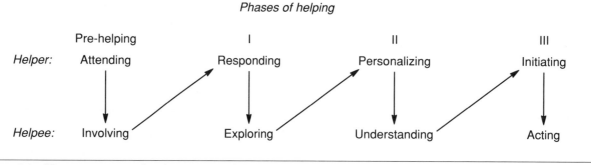

Figure 8.3   Human resource development model.

From "Human Resource Development Model" by W.A. Anthony and R.L. Vitalo. In *Interpersonal Helping Skills: A Guide to Training Methods, Programs, and Resources* (pp.70-71) by E.K. Marshall, P.D. Kurtz, and Associates, 1982, San Francisco: Jossey-Bass. Used with permission.

The groundwork for the helping relationship is laid with the development of trust and positive regard.

Phase I: Responding

The trainer strives to understand the client's concerns by clarifying their feelings and content statements. The trainer should understand the client's experiences at least as well as the client does. Effective responding encourages the client to further explore and understand the problem situation.

Phase II: Personalizing

Based on an understanding of the client's feelings and content gained through the responding phase, the trainer attempts to identify the personal meaning the client attributes to the problem. Because the same problem will be experienced at least slightly differently by every individual, the trainer must work with clients to understand their framework of personal meaning and how it affects their thoughts, feelings, and decision making. This process helps the client identify personal goals and desired outcomes.

Phase III: Initiating

Based on the goals identified in the personalization phase, the trainer and client develop an action plan for accomplishing the goals. Small steps can be built into the action plan to maximize the likelihood of success.

The following scenario illustrates movement through the helping phases and the development of trainer skill levels. Figure 8.3 further clarifies this process.

———— ■ ————

Helper Attending: A fitness instructor begins a new class in which a 35-year-old woman named Jane is enrolled. Through active listening and empathy, the instructor begins to understand the class members' problems that affect their exercise goals. The instructor notices that Jane seems particularly ambivalent and tentative about exercise. Although she says she wants to develop a healthier lifestyle, she does not convey that attitude nonverbally (incongruence between verbal and nonverbal message).

Client Involvement: Jane feels that the instructor listens to and understands her. She senses the instructor is trying to be helpful and wants her to be successful in the class.

Helper Responding: Through exploration and clarification, the instructor begins to understand that Jane has mixed feelings about exercise participation. She sincerely wants to improve her fitness and is very motivated, but also feels guilty because her husband does not exercise. She worries about spending time in an activity that does not include her husband and is afraid he will feel left out. She is also concerned that he might feel threatened or criticize her for inconveniencing the family schedule.

Client Exploration: Jane has not thought through her feelings about exercise before. She is surprised at the different issues and concerns she had without realizing it. This experience encourages her to explore her feelings more.

Helper Personalizing: The instructor helps Jane discover the personal meaning of what she is experiencing and to understand her part in the dilemma. Jane kept the problem going by not telling her husband about her concerns and making assumptions about what he would think, feel, and do.

Client Understanding: As the instructor and Jane explore further, they discover the actual problem is not Jane's guilt about exercising nor her concern for time conflicts with her husband, but rather her frustration with herself for not being straightforward with her husband about what was important to her.

Helper Initiating: The instructor helps Jane identify goals of improved communication with others and further personal clarification of values and important areas of her life.

Client Acting: Jane decides to join an interpersonal communications group to learn how to talk more freely with her husband. She also considers asking him to participate. Jane decides to further clarify her values by reading, talking with friends, and possibly talking with her interpersonal communications group.

Life Skills Training

Numerous theorists have developed models of the human development process (Dupont, 1978; Erickson, 1963; Piaget, 1954; Super, Starishevisky, Matlin, & Jordaan, 1963). The life skills model developed by George Gazda (1989) focuses on structured skills training for both remediation and prevention. The model assumes that people develop deficits in one or more areas of human development because they have not acquired the necessary coping skills to successfully accomplish the developmental tasks of a given stage.

As illustrated in Figure 8.4, Gazda, Childers, and Brooks (1987) drew from a pool of life skill descriptors frequently identified in human development research. They condensed seven areas of development into four general life skills areas: (1) interpersonal communication/human relations, (2) physical fitness and health maintenance, (3) identity development/purpose in life, and (4) problem solving/decision making. These skills apply to the four major living environments of home, school, work, and community.

In helping clients develop life skills, the practitioner may assume the roles of trainer, counselor, teacher, model, evaluator, motivator, and facilitator (Gazda, Childers, & Walters, 1982). Although

the life skills model is most easily applied to the exercise professional in the roles of teacher and counselor in the physical fitness/health maintenance generic skill area, the fitness professional may well be called on to help a client acquire other skills as well. Most clients will identify an area in which they want to improve, but as the practitioner and client begin exploring the chosen area, a related concern from a different area may surface. The fitness professional should be able to respond to client concerns in other areas as well.

The following scenario illustrates the use of the life skills model in an exercise setting.

—————■—————

Marcus, a 40-year-old businessman, joins an exercise class. As the class progresses, the practitioner learns that Marcus is somewhat depressed and anxious, and suffers from frequent insomnia. He seems nervous about fitting into the class. The practitioner notices that he is self-conscious in group situations, and later discovers that he is also concerned about his future at his company and "jokes" about being "over the hill."

Step 1

The practitioner classifies the symptoms and characteristics of the client into areas of development.

—————■—————

Marcus has shown mild to moderate concerns in the affective area (depression, anxiety), physical area (insomnia), psychosocial area (nervous about group interaction), vocational area (concern about job), and ego area (fear of being over the hill).

Step 2

The exercise professional responds primarily to the skill area of physical fitness and focuses on the client's physical deficit. The practitioner would identify the areas of concern that relate directly to physical fitness. Those concerns are then pursued with the client. Deficits are further clarified and assessed, and goals for overcoming those deficits are set.

—————■—————

Marcus's insomnia (physical area), nervousness about being in the group (psychosocial area), and fear of loss of physical

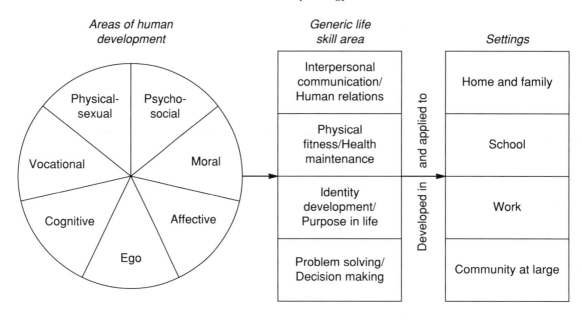

Figure 8.4   A model for the development and application of generic life skills.

From *Foundations of Counseling and Human Services* (p. 146) by G.M. Gazda, 1987, New York: McGraw-Hill Publishing Company. Copyright © 1987 by McGraw-Hill Publishing Company. Reprinted by permission.

stamina (ego area) are directly related to the physical fitness generic area. The practitioner works with Marcus to set goals to overcome these concerns.

Step 3

The instructor and the client discuss how these identified areas of concern affect the client in the home, school, work, and community settings.

——— ■ ———

Marcus is being affected at home by insomnia, at work and in the community by self-consciousness in a group situation, and at home and at work by fear of being over the hill. The instructor measures improvements or changes in these deficit areas by monitoring changes as they occur in these settings.

Because both affective (depression) and vocational (concern about job) areas are not directly related to physical fitness, the instructor refers Marcus to other professionals to deal with these concerns.

Integrative Problem-Solving

Gerald Egan (1986) developed a framework for problem solving that outlines the tasks of helping

and identifies the relationships between tasks. One of the strengths of this model is the collaboration between the counselor and client. Counselors act as consultants to the clients, who are primarily responsible for change through the therapeutic process (Figure 8.5).

Egan's model consists of three stages, with three steps within each stage.

Stage I: Present Scenario

Although clients usually know they have problems, they often cannot identify, clarify, and understand their problems without help. The counselor helps the client explore potential problem areas and identify and understand the problem situation. The most important helper skills at this stage are active listening and empathy.

Step I-A.   *Telling the story* is the process in which the client explains his or her problem to the counselor. Trust is enhanced and the professional relationship is developed.

Step I-B.   *Focusing* is the process of helping the client to accurately identify and clarify the problem. It is important to respect the client's perspective.

Step I-C.   *Identifying blind spots* is helping the client gain new interpretations and perspectives.

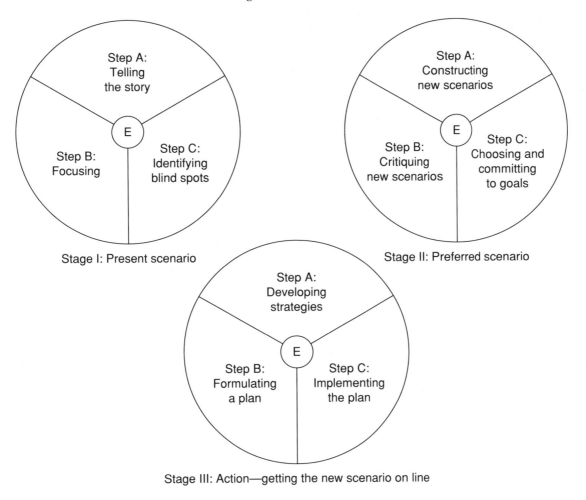

Figure 8.5 Integrative problem-solving model.

From *The Skilled Helper*, 3rd Edition, (p.332) by Gerard Egan. Copyright © 1986, 1982, 1975 by Wadsworth, Inc. Used with the permission of Brooks/Cole Publishing Company, Pacific Grove, CA 93950.

——————— ■ ———————

Tony, who has resisted joining an exercise class, confides his confusion about his resistance to his fitness instructor (Step I-A: Telling the story). Together they explore his reluctance and soon touch on childhood experiences in which he was labeled as nonathletic and "wimpy." He remembers that he did not feel as good as the other kids and he did not like himself very much. He is now afraid that others in the class will see him in the same way and reject him (Step I-B: Focusing). The instructor encourages him to relate this present feeling to earlier experiences and feelings related to his self-concept. Tony realizes that he has a poor self-concept, and that this could affect his relationships with others (Step I-C: Identifying blind spots).

Stage II: Preferred Scenario

Once clients understand their problem, they must do something about it. They frequently need help in setting goals. The helper skills most applicable to the stage are effective consulting, providing relevant information, inviting clients to challenge themselves to accomplish goals, and being empathetic.

Step II-A. *By constructing new scenarios*, a client can visualize how the situation would be different if changes were made.

Step II-B. *Critiquing new scenarios* involves determining whether newly conceived options move the client closer to the desired outcome. The second and equally important part of critiquing new options is the consideration of likely consequences of those choices. Understanding the connection between options and their consequences is crucial in sound decision making.

Step II-C. *Choosing goals* helps the client develop a sense of responsibility and initiates change. Helping the client maintain motivation for and commitment to the chosen goal is important at this phase.

The fitness instructor helps Tony realize that his feelings about himself are a greater obstacle than his fear of other people's opinions. The instructor consults with him to find ways to improve his self-concept (Step II-A). Tony decides to (a) seek out personal counseling, (b) confide his concerns to his wife and friends, and (c) join a personal growth group. The instructor and Tony assess the value of exploring his self-concept in addition to continuing the exercise program and consider the consequences of both (Step II-B). Tony decides to continue the fitness class as well as pursue means of self-exploration and personal growth (Step II-C).

Stage III: Action

The counselor and client translate goals into various action plans, then select and implement the preferred program. The skills and techniques applicable during this stage include reinforcement of creativity, helping the client be specific in selecting strategies, and monitoring strategies to ensure that they are realistic.

Step III-A. *Developing strategies* to implement goals helps to anticipate factors that might influence the outcome.

Step III-B. *In choosing a strategy and formulating a plan* to implement the strategy, it is important that the strategy fit the individual's needs, values, and resources.

Step III-C. *Implementing the plan* is the action phase. During this final step, the strategy is tested and, hopefully, the goals are accomplished.

The fitness instructor helps Tony explore appropriate services and resources. They determine that professional counseling, self-help books and materials, talking to others with similar problems, and an interpersonal communication group are all suitable options (Step III-A). The instructor and Tony decide that personal counseling and the communication group are the best strategies. The other options are unstructured, and Tony thinks he would be less likely to follow through (Step III-B). The instructor refers Tony to the appropriate professionals (Step III-C).

The integrative problem-solving model lends itself to a strategy that employs other techniques. The strength of the model lies in that tasks are specifically identified, yet it does not prescribe methods by which the tasks must be accomplished.

The human resource development model, life skills training, and the integrative problem-solving model have all been acknowledged as effective teaching models in counseling and related mental-health training programs. Each model has unique strengths and training components, yet they all share common philosophical foundations, a theoretical base, and beliefs about the therapeutic process. Each section of this chapter has incorporated integrated themes and drawn from common concepts. Because training in counseling is a developmental process, it must be based on various interpersonal and communication theories.

ETHICAL AND PROFESSIONAL ISSUES

Ethical standards are guidelines for professional conduct that direct decision making and provide a set of values for the members of a profession. According to Gladding (1988), ethics are normative principles that govern professional relations. Professionals are frequently confronted with circumstances that cannot be clearly understood in terms of societal, cultural, or familial values. However, Hayman and Covert (1986) found that less than one-third of all respondents in an ethics study relied on their professional ethical standards to make decisions. The reliance on personal views, tradition, or "common sense," although often practiced, is risky because of the nature and purpose of the professional relationship. Ethical codes ensure commonly held values and beliefs among a set of professionals and protect the quality of the professional interaction for the client.

In contrast to ethics, law is a set of governing standards developed to ensure legal and moral justice (Hummel, Talbutt, & Alexander, 1985). Although legal and ethical codes often agree, an action that is legal is not necessarily ethical and vice versa. For example, a counselor who refuses to reveal to the court information gained through confidential disclosure could be acting ethically but illegally, and could be cited for contempt of court. Conversely, a counselor who reveals to a 32-year-old client's mother that the client was contemplating suicide is acting legally but unethically, and could be cited for breach of confidentiality.

It is incumbent on professionals to seek out and understand the ethical guidelines of their profession and the state laws governing the area in which they practice.

Purpose of Ethical Standards

Ethical standards

■ enable a profession to regulate and monitor itself, which allows a degree of autonomy from legislative control;

■ promote consensual decision making and stability, and offer a framework for negotiation within the profession; and

■ protect members from liability if the professional has been compliant with the accepted standards (Van Hoose & Kottler, 1985).

Professional Codes of Ethics

Because specialty areas in the helping profession have different codes of ethics, a professional may need to abide by several different codes. The three most widely known codes are those of the American Psychological Association (1981), the American Association of Counseling and Development (1981), and the American Association of Marriage and Family Therapy (1981). The American Psychological Association (APA) addresses 10 principles of ethical consideration:

■ *Responsibility* in roles such as researcher, teacher, or practitioner refers to accountability for behavior and decisions that affect the public to ensure integrity of professional interactions.

■ *Competence* addresses the need to be aware of boundaries and limitations of professional abilities, skills, and use of techniques.

■ *Moral and legal standards* outlines areas of conduct in which awareness of community standards and deviation from or conformity to such standards influence professional effectiveness.

■ *Public statements* emphasize the importance of accurately representing credentials and professional qualifications and providing truthful information about products, publications, and services.

■ *Confidentiality* describes the obligation to respect and treat carefully information acquired through one's professional role.

■ *Welfare of the consumer* addresses the limitations and expectations of professional services rendered to a client. This principle covers conflict of interest between an institution and a client and business aspects of the profession.

■ *Professional relationships* describes acceptable and unacceptable interactions between people within the same profession and across professions.

■ *Assessment techniques* describes proper use of investigative instruments and the interpretation of results.

■ *Research with human subjects* protects the civil and human rights of clients, research subjects, and all who participate in a professionally conducted research investigation to prevent mistreatment and exploitation.

■ *Care and use of animals* addresses the welfare, respectful treatment, and quality of care of animals in experimental settings.

Although these APA guidelines apply specifically to psychologists, they are widely used in helping professions and related fields.

Although not practicing in a mental-health setting, the exercise practitioner who follows established ethical guidelines can feel confident of upholding a standard of care that is highly defensible. Exercise professionals will find many aspects of these 10 principles relevant to their work. These guidelines can be applied to a wide range of settings.

Following are recommendations for applying these principles to the exercise setting.

The exercise practitioner should become familiar with the APA's *Ethical Principles of Psychologists* (1981) and other professional guidelines that apply to the client population and work setting. For example, in a center that serves families or adolescents, the practitioner should be familiar with the American Association of Marriage and Family Therapy's ethical standards. A practitioner who leads groups should know the Association for Specialists in Group Work's guidelines for group leaders.

Exercise practitioners should also know the policies and procedures practiced in their institution or agency. If the agency's ethical policies conflict with a professional association's guidelines or with personal professional standards, the practitioner must clarify and resolve discrepancies before an issue arises.

During an initial session, exercise practitioners should disclose to their clients any professional requirements so that the clients can act accordingly. For example, a practitioner would explain on the first day the institution's policy of providing information from physical examinations to parties who prove a need to know, such as employers or insurance companies. The class members can then decide their course of action. If this information were withheld, a class member could charge the practitioner with wrongful disclosure of records.

If an ethical dilemma arises, the practitioner should consult with another professional, a supervisor, a professional association, or the state certification/licensure board. Although direct action may seem unwarranted, professional behavior is judged by compliance with ethical standards not the outcome of the incident. If a practitioner is judged as behaving responsibly and in accordance with professional standards, he or she would be in a strong legal and professional position even if the outcome of the situation were adverse.

Special Areas of Consideration

Confidentiality

Confidentiality is an agreement between the helper and the client to disclose no information about the client except under conditions agreed to by the client (Siegel, 1979). The prohibition applies only to the professional. The client may disclose what he or she wishes.

Legal issues, including imminent danger to others, inadequate care for potentially violent individuals, and child abuse, have redefined confidentiality so it is not so restrictive (Boylan, Malley, & Scott, 1988). The best policy on disclosure is to decide before beginning professional contact what one's privileges and limitations are and fully inform the clients of these decisions. Group leaders should inform their clients not only of the degree of confidentiality they can expect from the leader but also of the confidentiality all group members must respect.

Record Keeping

Administrative procedures of an institution or agency also affect confidentiality. Gazda (1989) identified the following guidelines:

■ When consulting with another professional, only personal information necessary for consultation purposes should be revealed.

■ Data gathered from clients for research purposes must be obtained only after written consent from the client.

■ Any identifying data used in publications or instruction must be disguised.

■ Practitioners should be familiar with the procedures and policies of their work site with regard to records, their storage, use, and access.

■ Practitioners must inform clients of the policy for clients accessing their own records.

■ The practitioner should not release confidential records without the informed consent of the client.

■ If records are stored on a computer, the practitioner should know the policy for confidentiality of records and make every effort to limit access.

■ The practitioner should provide only limited and necessary information for insurance reimbursement. The entire set of records should never be sent to insurance companies and clients should be informed of how much information is provided to the company.

Clients' Rights

As Gladding (1988) noted, provisions of the Buckley Amendment enable an individual to access his or her records and, in some circumstances, enable others with just cause to access information without the consent of the client. Standard practice, however, requires that all records be kept confidential. No information should be given over the phone. Information should be given in person only after the client has signed a release form. Professionals must make a practice of being familiar with legal codes, statutes, and case law in the state where they are practicing (Hummel et al., 1985).

Informed Consent

The formal follow-through on the previously described right to privacy and full disclosure of professional parameters is the informed consent agreement. The three most common circumstances that require informed consent are when (1) conducting a research project that requires human subjects, (2) testing physiological or psychological variables on subjects or clients, and (3) performing professional services that require knowledge of client behavior that would not be revealed under ordinary circumstances.

Some professionals believe that asking for fully informed consent focuses on extreme scenarios and scares clients away from the service. Others believe that this willingness to risk negative response builds confidence and encourages a trusting relationship. Malley (1988) has identified several issues that should be addressed during the initial interview with a client. The following issues have been adapted for the exercise setting:

■ The exercise and/or interpersonal or group techniques that will be used

■ The appropriateness of various techniques

■ How long the exercise course or treatment will take

■ The risks involved in the exercise treatment

■ The professional background and credentials of the instructors

■ The benefits of the exercise treatment

■ Whether questions can be asked after the exercise treatment has started

■ When and with whom the client can review his or her records

■ Whether the client can withdraw from the exercise treatment at any time

■ Whether the client is free to not participate

■ The electronic systems that will be used

■ Who will view any existing tapes and how long they will be kept

■ Who will have access to the client's exercise records and physical data

Exercise professionals should review this list, identify those issues that apply to their work settings and clientele, and brainstorm with colleagues about other issues not mentioned.

Leaders' Values and Qualifications

The exercise leader should possess the educational and professional credentials that are necessary to perform the professional service and that are presented to potential clients through advertisement, marketing, or personal description. If the exercise professional's personal, moral, social, or religious values might affect his or her interaction with clients, or if there is potential conflict of interest, the professional should address the issue with the clients.

Personal Relationships Between the Professional and Clients

The APA Ethical Standards prohibit sexual contact between the practitioner and client. An extension of this policy that applies to relationships with former clients is currently under consideration. Many professionals already abide by the extended interpretation because of the strong belief that a role change of that nature is harmful to the client.

Professional relationships that take on other roles such as a friendship are not prohibited. Nevertheless, the professional should consider postponing extended relationships with the client until the professional relationship has ended to prevent conflict of interest.

The Right of Members to Leave the Professional Relationship

The client should be allowed to terminate the professional commitment at any time without coercion, harassment, or negative reaction. The professional may want to do an exit interview to learn more about the client's experience for future referral.

The Right to Participate Without Coercion or Pressure

Some exercise professionals encourage competitiveness among group members. In a sports setting, choosing this approach is a judgement call for the leader. In exercise settings with nonathletes, competitiveness should be encouraged without pressure or implication of consequences. The leader also has the responsibility to intervene if a group member attacks, ridicules, or negatively challenges another person.

The Leader's Role in Making a Referral

It is incumbent on the exercise professional to determine whether a client needs further professional help.

Following are suggestions to help exercise practitioners identify participants who need to be referred to another counseling professional:

1. Individuals with physical, emotional, or interpersonal difficulties can be identified by observation, comments by classmates, or self-disclosures by the individual.

2. Take time to observe the individual before initiating contact to confirm that there is observable behavior or documentation that warrants concern and that the problem situation has continuing effects.

3. Describe the problem to a colleague and ask for the colleague's opinion. Occasionally, you may miss the possibility of different perceptions and interpretations.

4. If the colleague is not concerned, continue to observe the individual and reassess your perception. If you continue to be concerned, follow through with the next suggestion.

5. Talk with the individual in confidence and explain your concern. If the person acknowledges the problem, you would offer to refer the client to an appropriate professional. You should be prepared with specific referral recommendations at this point so the individual can seek help immediately if necessary.

6. If you are in a university setting, establish a relationship with the counseling center. Students qualify for services at the counseling center. If your client is not a student or if you are in a corporate, agency, or private setting, network with the city or county mental-health services. Nonprofit agencies often publish community mental-health services guides. Identify several services and develop a consulting contact in those agencies. You will feel much more confident if you have professional support and resources.

7. Most clients will relate problems to you or other classmates in a peripheral way or in a way that relates to their exercise goals. When personal difficulties continue to affect exercise progress, you should feel confident in continuing to monitor and work with the client in the exercise program. However, a client who continues to present problems that are unrelated to the exercise class and the member's exercise goals should be referred to another professional.

Following are three categories of high-risk clients. Such clients should be referred to a mental-health professional if exercise professionals observe or suspect these risk behaviors.

Potential for Suicide

Exercise professionals are not held responsible by law or by APA Ethical Standards for suicidal clients. However, knowing the risk factors for suicide and understanding procedures for referral can determine successful intervention with a client.

Fujimura, Weis, and Cochran (1985) and Patterson, Dohn, Bird, and Patterson (1983) have identified risk factors for potential suicide:

■ Age. There is a bimodal distribution with peaks in the teen years and elderly years.

■ Depression. Risk of suicide is 30 times greater if the client is depressed. Fifteen percent of chronically depressed people commit suicide.

■ Previous attempts. Twenty-five to fifty percent of all people who commit suicide have made previous attempts.

■ Alcohol abuse. Fifteen percent of all alcoholics commit suicide.

■ Lack of social support. Suicidal clients frequently have no friends, are single, and have no close family members.

■ Organized plan. The client who has a detailed, well-thought out plan for suicide is at much higher risk than those with less organization.

■ Sleep disruption. Insomnia may increase depression and, subsequently, the risk of suicide.

Substance Abuse

Although exercise professionals are not obligated to report illegal drug use, they are obligated to help clients deal with deficits and problems that he or she would like to change. The exercise professional should know the policy on drug and alcohol abuse and the roles, if any, played by the staff. The professional should also have an appropriate and effective system of referral.

Fertman, as cited by Boylan et al. (1988), identified symptoms of substance abuse:

Alcohol

■ Growing preoccupation with drinking at uncommon times

■ Growing need to drink during times of stress

■ Growing rigidity in lifestyle, particularly when drinking is involved

■ Growing tolerance to alcohol

■ Loss of self-control, deteriorating lifestyle and social network, physical repercussions, defensiveness, legal problems

Drug Dependency

■ Growing preoccupation with drug use and increased stress

■ Activities revolve around drugs

■ Increased dosage, ingenuity in taking drugs without others knowing, cheating on refills, jumping from doctor to doctor to keep prescriptions, using a variety of drugstores, combining several prescription drugs for the synergistic effect

■ Blackouts, taking larger dosages of medication than prescribed, physical incapacitation, dealing in illegal drugs, loss of social network, job absenteeism, increasing hospitalizations

Child Abuse and Neglect

Exercise professionals in teaching roles are obligated by law to report any knowledge of child abuse. There are mandatory reporting laws in all 50 states. Because these laws vary among states, exercise professionals should be familiar with the legislation in their state of residence and practice.

Child abuse is usually detected through reports from the child or from another person, or indirectly through the helping process. The professionals should not concern themselves with the legitimacy of the report, but report the incident directly to the county family and child services. Erickson, McEvoy, and Colucci (1984) identified general characteristics of abuse victims:

■ Directs inappropriate hostility toward authority figures

■ Displays disruptive and destructive behavior

■ Is passive and withdrawn and cries easily

■ Is sometimes fearful and does not want to go home

■ Is absent from school or tardy frequently

■ Is inappropriately dressed for the weather

■ Has bruises and burns

■ Has untreated medical needs

■ Is continually hungry

■ Makes sexually oriented remarks

■ Has high anxiety

SUMMARY

Professional counseling requires communication skills, certain professional and personal characteristics, and practice of ethical standards. The primary communication skills of attending, listening, responding, and showing empathy enable the exercise practitioner to accurately identify problem areas and concerns of clients and effectively respond to them. This ability greatly enhances the relationship between the professional and the client and lays the groundwork for successful intervention and collaboration.

The ability to practice communication skills depends on certain personal and professional characteristics of the helper. Research studies have consistently identified personal characteristics that enhance relationships and professional characteristics that contribute to therapeutic growth and development. Professional and personal qualities are not always distinct and are manifested by the helper in an integrated way.

The helping models provide a framework through which communication skills and helper characteristics are integrated and systematically channeled to maximize the effectiveness of the helper. Problem management, life skills training, and human resource development are three helping models that can guide the fitness professional in the role of the counselor.

The ethical guidelines described apply to all helping professions and set the professional helper apart from paraprofessionals and skilled lay helpers. Different professional disciplines have different codes of ethics.

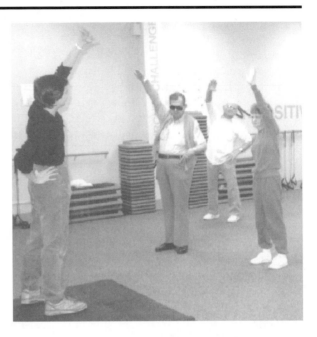

Chapter 9

Leadership and Group Dynamics

Imagine that you have just left your roommates to go to your aerobics class. You wait with a group of people at the bus stop. Because you arrive at the fitness class early, you go to the snack bar where there are people sitting around tables. You leave and go to class where you participate in the exercise program. Afterward, you and some people from class go out to dinner. Which of these collections of people could be defined as a group? What is a group? What characteristics and behaviors separate a group from a collection of people?

Group theorists have not been able to develop one definition of *group*. Some of the more accepted definitions include (a) a collection of individuals who are interdependent to some significant degree

(Cartwright & Zander, 1968); (b) individuals who see themselves as pursuing interdependent goals (Deutsch, 1973); (c) a dynamic whole determined by interdependence, not similarity (Lewin, 1948); and (d) shared norms and interlocking roles (Newcomb, 1943).

Winston, Bonney, Miller, and Dagley (1988) enumerated characteristics of a group as follows:

- Shared goals
- Perceived benefits from membership
- Anticipation of group continuance
- Willingness to cooperate in goal attainment
- Trust and acceptance of other members

- Shared perceptions of group structure
- Members identify themselves as members
- Shared network of informal interpersonal relationships
- Shared standards of behavior

The common denominator in all definitions of group is interdependence and reciprocal influence through interaction. Now review the collections of people previously mentioned and consider whether or not they meet these criteria.

With this frame of reference in mind, we will shift our focus to group dynamics. Kurt Lewin (1951) created and popularized the term *group dynamics*. Lewin made significant contributions to early research in group dynamics theory, and, in 1945, he established the first research institute for group dynamics at Massachusetts Institute of Technology. Lewin's field theory emphasized the interrelatedness of groups and proposed that behavior is determined by the individual's personal characteristics and the environment. Correspondingly, the behavior of group members is influenced not only by personal characteristics, but also by group functions, such as the characteristics of the members and the leader, and the roles and norms of the group.

Group dynamics, therefore, has come to be defined as the study of the behavior of groups. This chapter will address the more frequently studied aspects of group dynamics in the areas of

- leadership,
- the structure of groups,
- group communication, and
- group conflict and problem solving.

At the end of this chapter is a series of exercises. These exercises allow the reader to participate in an in-class experience that operationalizes the major concepts described in each section.

LEADERSHIP

The concept of leadership is easily comprehended, yet professional agreement on the function and process of leadership continues to elude researchers and educators. Who within a group emerges as the leader and why? Does the group, the situation, the environment, or the task influence choice of leader? Does the effectiveness of the leader lie in form or substance?

Lewis (1974) observed that there is no society in the recorded history of the human species that appears to have been absent of leadership. All dimensions of our lives—family, school, religion, workplace, social groups, and government—depend on formal or informal leadership to function successfully. It seems that when two or more people are present, one person will exercise more influence than the others.

Definition of Leadership

Definitions of *leadership* have varied with the changing criteria, such as personal traits, personal values, behavior, group needs, and group situation (Bass, 1981; Gibb, 1969). No single definition of leadership has become widely accepted. Nevertheless, there are generally acknowledged aspects of leadership that contribute to an evolving definition. Lassey and Sashkin (1983) describe leadership as a role that involves influence and interaction, leads toward goal achievement, and results in structural change within groups.

Stogdill (1974) developed a collection of perspectives on leadership. Depending on the leader's style, the situation, and the interaction, leadership may be defined as:

- a function of group process,
- personality,
- an inducement for compliance,
- the exercise of influence,
- a form of persuasion,
- a set of acts or behaviors,
- a power relationship,
- an instrument of goal achievement,
- an effect of interaction,
- a differentiated role, or
- the initiation of structure.

Theories of Leadership

Several leadership approaches have sustained continued investigation and empirical scrutiny. We have organized these approaches under six headings: (1) trait theory, (2) contingency model, (3) participation theory, (4) power, (5) multidimensional model, and (6) normative model.

Trait Theory

Trait theorists believe that leaders possess personality characteristics or clusters of attributes that ensure their success in leadership roles. Exhaustive studies conducted over the past 40 years have yielded mixed results.

Two early overview studies extensively reviewed traits that seemed to differentiate leaders. However, the first study found that only 5% of the traits appeared in four or more studies using trait theory (Bird, 1940) and the other found that only 5% of the participants were consistent across different situations requiring leadership (Borgatta, Couch, & Bales 1954). After conducting several comprehensive reviews from 1948 to 1974, Stogdill identified several traits that are more prominent in leaders than in nonleaders: achievement orientation, adaptability, alertness, ascendancy, energy, responsibility, self-confidence, and sociability. Although a clear relationship was demonstrated between these personality traits and leadership, no causal inference could be made. However, Stogdill suggested that leadership ability may be affected by the interaction of personality and situational factors (Forsyth, 1983).

During the investigation for notable personality traits, Stogdill (1948, 1974) and others found correlating personal characteristics. According to these findings, leaders tend to be taller and older than their subordinates, be slightly more intelligent, and have high task ability (i.e., they are highly capable and competent).

The leader's effectiveness may be diminished, however, if personality traits and style convey lack of enthusiasm, energy, self-confidence, or responsibility. These impressions can be quite subtle yet can negate the positive influence of skill and competency.

Contingency Model

Trait theory and other early theories supported a one-dimensional model that assumed the personality style of leaders was constant and that certain leader characteristics would be desirable across all situations. In studies of leadership styles, Fiedler (1978, 1981) postulated that a leader's style changes in different situations and that the same leadership style is not equally effective in all situations. This research gave rise to the contingency model.

The contingency model defines leader effectiveness in terms of the personality of the leader and the leader's control over a situation. Fiedler and other theorists believe that *personality or motivational style* is either relationship-oriented or task-oriented. Relationship-oriented leaders foster a cooperative and positive interpersonal relationship with coworkers. The maintenance of these relationships is more important than the tasks to be accomplished. Task-oriented leaders, on the other hand, see the work of the group as the primary goal. Task progress and completion are more important than maintaining relationships.

To assess dominant motivational style, Fiedler developed the Least Preferred Coworker Scale (LPC). Fiedler's instrument is unique in its method of indirect self-assessment by the leader rather than a group rating of the leader. People who score high on the LPC describe their least preferred coworker in positive terms that support the importance of relationship. These people are relationship-oriented. Even though the coworker is difficult to work with, the leader sees positive personal attributes. People who score low on the LPC are task-motivated. They value task completion enough so that difficult coworkers are viewed as having negative personality attributes.

Situational factors determine the effectiveness of a leader by the degree of control or influence the leader has over a situation. The factors most often considered in assessing control are (a) leader-members relations, or group cohesion and the degree to which the group accepts the leader; (b) task structure, or clarity of task and goal consensus; and (c) power, or the leader's ability to gain compliance through reward and punishment.

Fiedler determined that the interaction of motivational style and situational factors provide a measure of leader effectiveness. Several important concepts that emerged from these findings enabled Fiedler to develop a prediction model of leader effectiveness (see Figure 9.1).

The graph in Figure 9.1 describes situational factors on the horizontal axis from most to least favorable, and motivational style on the vertical axis. The model predicts that high-LPC leaders (relationship-motivated) will perform more effectively in situations of moderately favorable leader-member relations, task structure, and leader power. The low-LPC leaders (task-motivated) will be most effective in either highly favorable or highly unfavorable conditions. When conditions are favorable, a positive relationship is already established and the conditions are set for task accomplishment. When conditions are unfavorable, the instability, disorganization, and uncertainty require task orientation to regain direction. Nurturance of the relationship becomes important when the group is on task but at risk for losing cohesion, motivation, or morale.

The contingency model is particularly applicable to exercise leaders because it emphasizes task goals while attending to the reinforcement value

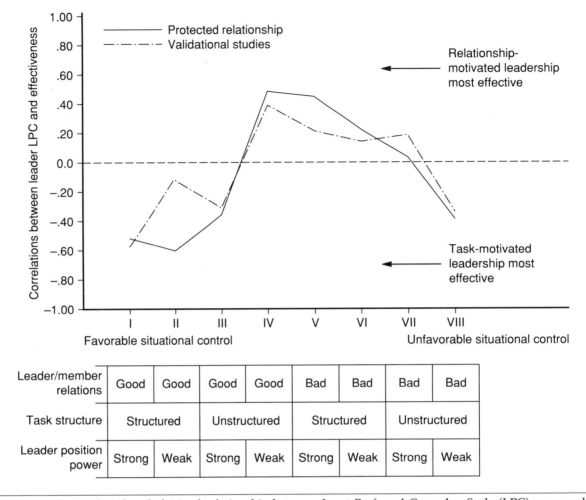

Figure 9.1 The predicted and obtained relationship between Least Preferred Coworker Scale (LPC) score and leadership effectiveness in eight group situations. The correlations from Octant I to Octant VIII, for the original studies, are −.52, −.58, −.33, .47, .42, xx (Octanct VI is missing), .05, −.43. The correlations, from Octant I to Octant VIII, for the validational studies are, −.59, −.10, −.29, .40, .19, .13, .17, −.35.

From "What Triggers the Person-Situation Interaction in Leadership?" by F.E. Fiedler. In *Personality at the Crossroads* (pp. 154-163) by D. Magnusson and N. Endler (Eds.), 1977, Hillsdale, NJ: Lawrence Erlbaum Associates. Copyright © 1977 by Lawrence Erlbaum Associates. Reprinted by permission.

of relationship nurturance. Task-oriented leaders risk member dropout if they do not realize the importance of verbal reinforcement and the need for a sense of belonging to a group. Relationship-oriented exercise leaders, on the other hand, may nurture and reinforce class members very effectively, but lose sight of how important it is for exercise members to see improvement in their level of physical fitness (by charting, for instance, distance run or length of time in anaerobic exercise).

The contingency model can also describe the task or relationship orientation of the class members. A task-driven leader may be very effective with task-driven class members because such members would have less need for social interaction and external reinforcement. Likewise, a relationship-motivated exercise leader may be more effective with relationship-oriented members who are more concerned with recognition and support than they are with task accomplishment.

Effective exercise leaders must assess both the class environment (situational controls) and the task/relationship orientation of class members. Some members may need task emphasis while others need support and reinforcement. The leader must be able to shift orientation to respond to circumstances and specific class members.

A final recommendation is to pair a task-oriented leader with a relationship-oriented leader to blend the strengths of these different leadership styles.

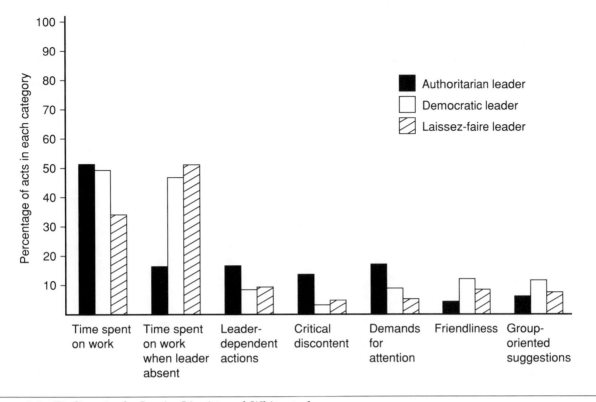

Figure 9.2 Findings in the Lewin, Lippitt, and White study.

From *Autocracy and Democracy* by Ralph K. White and Ronald Lippitt. Copyright © 1960 by Ralph K. White and Ronald Lippitt. Reprinted by permission of HarperCollins Publishers.

Participation Theory

An exercise instructor plans and publicizes a fitness class. When the class begins, the instructor realizes there are decisions to be made throughout the course regarding scheduling, prescribing exercises, class procedures, sequencing in class activity, and others. The instructor wonders whether to (a) make decisions as done in precourse planning, (b) include the class in decision making, or (c) allow the class to decide. How should the instructor make this decision and on what criteria should the decision be based?

Lewin, Lippitt, and White (1939) investigated group member participation in decision making. These efforts resulted in their classic study of authoritarian, laissez-faire, and democratic leadership. In the study, preadolescent boys were asked to participate in hobby activities after school and were assigned an adult leader for the activity. The leader practiced one of the three leadership styles. The autocratic leader made all decisions, capitalized on authority, determined the work environment, and gave instructions autonomously. The democratic leader discussed all decisions with the group and invited participation and feedback. The

democratic leader also encouraged decision making within the group and fostered shared responsibility. The laissez-faire leader functioned primarily as a consultant, allowing group members to make all decisions and determine work activity and pace.

A comparison across the three groups indicated differences in group atmosphere, coping skills, and relationship with the leader. As shown in Figure 9.2, the authoritarian-led group and the democratic-led group were both more productive than the laissez-faire group when the leader was present. However, the autocratic group dropped in productivity when the leader left the room, while the democratic group maintained the same pace. The productivity of the laissez-faire group increased when the leader left. Democratic group members were friendly, whereas the autocratic group members were more hostile and aggressive. The boys indicated that they preferred the democratic style.

Although group members reported greatest satisfaction with democratic leaders, studies of leadership style (Stogdill, 1974) continue to confirm that no one style is always preferable. Personality, situation, task objectives, and other factors influence whether a leadership style is effective.

Power

Power is an abstract concept that has many meanings given the context and the frame of reference of the observer. Common definitions of power range from manipulation, deception, and illegitimate control to benevolent influence exercised at the will of the group. Very few social concepts have such extremely positive and negative connotations as the term *power* does. These bipolar connotations contribute to confusion and tentativeness on the subject of power.

Power in the leadership role is viewed as a means of accomplishing group goals. The emphasis is not on group resistance, but on the leader's ability to motivate group members toward a goal that cannot be reached without the leader's direction. This is a form of power with which the leader can influence the actions of others. How and why does this dynamic occur? What is it about leaders that enables them to exercise power over others?

French and Raven (1959) developed a conceptual scheme of the origins of power by identifying five common power bases. This scheme has become the standard way to categorize power.

A person influenced by *referent power* identifies with the person in power and may model that person's attitudes, behaviors, or characteristics. People with referent power may be high in intellect, ability, or charisma and style. Certain leader attributes can influence change in members' behavior, often without the awareness or intent of the leader. Examples of the influence of referent power are young children emulating older siblings, students admiring a teacher and imitating the teacher's behavior, high school football players following the lead of a professional football idol, and adolescents identifying with movie stars. Advertisements for consumer goods, such as clothes, cars, and cigarettes, often show attractive people having fun and enjoying life. The intention is that the consumer will admire and identify with the actors and use the product to be more like the actors. As these examples illustrate, referent power can be either a positive or manipulative force.

How might referent power apply to exercise professionals? Referent power is more elusive than other power bases because the leader is often unaware of it. Exercise class members may admire and strive to develop attributes they identify in the leader. These attributes may range from personality style, interpersonal skills, and intellectual ability to physical appearance. If an exercise professional is in much better shape than the class members, the members will, often unconsciously, perceive the exercise leader as a role model and emulate the leader's behavior to become "more like" the leader. The exercise professional should try to be aware of the leadership image being conveyed and to assess the effects of the image through feedback from group members or through peer consultation.

Legitimate power emphasizes a leader's right to make decisions for the group based on position and official authority. A person elected or appointed to a position within a government, a company, or institution would have legitimate power. Legitimate power is one of the most effective and efficient power bases because the power structure has been agreed upon by the group. Congressional representatives, policemen, teachers, coaches, judges, and military officers have legitimate power by virtue of their official authority over constituencies and members.

The exercise professional has varying degrees of legitimate power depending on the professional setting. For example, a professor of exercise physiology has legitimate power by virtue of the fact that students sought membership in the class thereby accepting the norms, rules, and expectations of the professor and the group. Moreover, students who do not acknowledge the power of the professor may not be able to complete the course. An aerobics instructor has a similar degree of legitimate power over members who have joined the class and accepted the authority of the exercise leader. On the other hand, the voluntary nature of an aerobics class diminishes the legitimate power of the leader over class members who are not motivated, committed, or who simply reject authority because there is no response cost. Exercise professionals in settings where members must acknowledge legitimate power to pass a course will not need to spend as much time as the private-industry or noncredit-course instructors in fostering involvement, commitment, and motivation.

Expert power is often closely aligned with legitimate power. Expert power is based on specialized information, knowledge, or skill, which are often requirements for leaders in legitimate power positions. Examples of individuals with expert power include doctors, auto mechanics, teachers, and dentists.

Expert power transcends status, social norms, referents, and socioeconomic class. Professionals defer to working-class experts when the car, an appliance, or the plumbing is not working. An illustration of this is a story in which a high-powered lawyer suffered plumbing problems the morning of an important trial. The lawyer called a plumber who promptly arrived, fixed the plumbing in half an hour, and charged $150.00. The lawyer said, "This is outrageous. I don't make this much money per hour." The plumber responded, "Neither did I when I was a lawyer."

The exercise professional has a great deal of expert power over group members because of actual or perceived special knowledge. The extent of the leader's expert power often depends on the knowledge of the group members. For example, an exercise instructor leading an aerobics class of other exercise professionals will not receive the same recognition as an expert exercise instructor in a cardiac rehabilitation program with people whose lives depend on improved fitness. However, leaders may remain just as highly respected if they have other sources of power and acknowledgment.

Reward power is based on the leader's ability to dispense positive or negative reinforcement and punishment. The effectiveness of reward power depends on several basic behavioral principles.

■ The members will respond more to positive reinforcement than to negative reinforcement or punishment. An exercise class member will respond to reward power of an instructor who compliments improvements rather than one who looks for deficiencies.

■ If the reward is not as desirable as other reinforcements, it loses value. An exercise instructor may informally reinforce class members for progress made toward fitness goals, but if members are also reinforced by classmates, the behavioral effect on the members will be greater.

■ The leader will have more reward power if no one else is able to reinforce. Exercise students in individualized prescriptive exercise programs are more likely to depend on the instructor for reinforcement and feedback. Even if there are others in the class, the instructor is the only person with direct knowledge and ability to monitor progress. The instructor's power to reward will therefore be enhanced.

■ The reward must be truly desired by the members. A reward of chocolate only reinforces someone who likes chocolate. It is critically important for the leader to do an individualized assessment of each class member to determine appropriate rewards.

Coercive power is the use of threats, punishment, denigration, or physical violence to achieve compliance. Although coercive power can be effective, compliance does not entail acceptance or internalized belief or attitude change (French & Raven, 1959). Common forms of coercion are parents grounding adolescents, teachers requiring a student to stay after school, or a policeman giving a parking ticket.

Coercive power should be a last resort, particularly in educational and training settings. Motivation and internalized desire to succeed are critical factors in exercise adherence.

Multidimensional Model

The multidimensional model (Chelladurai, 1985) attempts to integrate major concepts of the primary theories to provide a more comprehensive understanding of leadership (Figure 9.3).

The model identifies three aspects of leader behavior: required, preferred, and actual. The antecedent variables that affect leader behavior are situational characteristics, leader characteristics, and member characteristics. The outcome or consequences of leader behavior is measured by group performance and member satisfaction.

Required leader behavior is determined by the organization or environment. For example, the norms, roles, codes of conduct, and behavioral interactions differ between a classroom and a coach's bench. These situational factors can control required leader behavior and are often task oriented.

Preferred leader behavior is determined both by situational and member characteristics. Members who need affiliation may prefer a socially oriented leader while members who need achievement may prefer a task-oriented leader. A person in a teaching role might be expected by class members to be democratic in style, but that same person in a coaching role may be expected to be authoritarian.

Actual leader behavior is the result of leader characteristics and the influences of required and preferred behavior. How well the leader integrates these influences will be determined by the leader's (a) knowledge of the group's goals and the procedures necessary to accomplish the goals, and (b) ability to analyze problems and to persuade members toward group tasks and goals.

Performance and satisfaction depend on congruence among the three categories of leader behavior. For example, if the fitness instructor adapts to required behaviors (e.g., high degree of structure, formality, and inflexibility) that are unpopular within the group, required and preferred behaviors will be incongruent and group satisfaction will be low.

The multidimensional model identifies the situation, leader, and members as influential factors over required, preferred, and actual leader behaviors. Group performance and member satisfaction

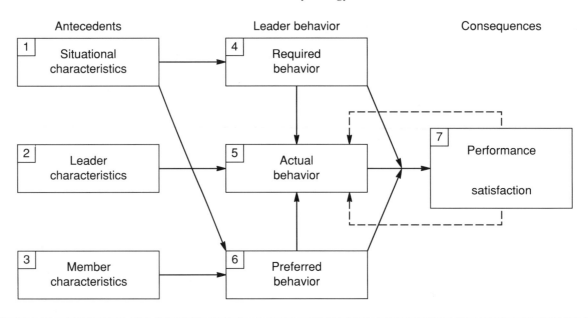

Figure 9.3 A multidimensional model of leadership.

From *Sport Management* (p.159) by P. Chelladurai, 1985, London, ON: Sports Dynamics Publishers. Reprinted by permission.

are related to the degree of congruence among these leader behavior categories.

Normative Model

Vroom (1973) addressed the question of member participation in leadership and decision making through the development of his normative model of leadership theory. According to Vroom, a leader can determine how much group involvement in decision making is desirable by using the decision tree (see Figure 9.4).

Vroom describes an autocratic-participative continuum that includes five types of leadership:

■ *Autocratic I:* The leader acquires necessary information and makes a decision.

■ *Autocratic II:* The leader depends on the group for information, but makes the decision independently.

■ *Consultative I:* The leader solicits information, opinions, and suggestions from key group members, then makes a decision.

■ *Consultative II:* The leader solicits ideas and suggestions from the entire group, then makes a decision.

■ *Group II:* The leader and group discuss the problem and agree on a solution (there is no *Group I*).

The problem attributes to be considered in the decision-making process are covered by the seven

questions in the decision tree. These questions focus on the integration of situational factors and leadership style. Each question is charted to help the leader arrive at the best choice given the descriptive profile of the group. Every instructor has a leadership style that emerges from the strongest and most stable aspects of his or her personality. Vroom's normative model enables the leader to integrate personality and leadership style with a method of leadership.

Leadership Roles

As a result of empirical studies on leadership and descriptions from leadership theorists (Fiedler, 1967; Hersey & Blanchard, 1977; Lewin et al., 1939; Vroom, 1973), a new perspective has emerged that emphasizes group characteristics and situational factors in determining leadership roles. The role of the leader includes helping the group achieve its goals and influencing the behavior of group members. Effective leaders must also set group goals, guide members toward goals, improve group interaction, build cohesiveness, and identify group resources (Cartwright & Zander, 1968). But although various roles of the leader can be identified, continually changing variables prohibit an exact definition of effective leadership. These variables include the uniqueness of the group and the traits of the leader and group members. Situational factors such as structure, goals, and attitudes and

A. Is there a quality requirement such that one solution is likely to be more rational than another?
B. Do I have sufficient information to make a high-quality decision?
C. Is the problem structured?
D. Is acceptance of decision by subordinates critical to effective implementation?
E. If I were to make the decision by myself, is it reasonably certain that it would be accepted by my subordinates?
F. Do subordinates share the organizational goals to be attained in solving this problem?
G. Is conflict among subordinates likely in preferred solutions?

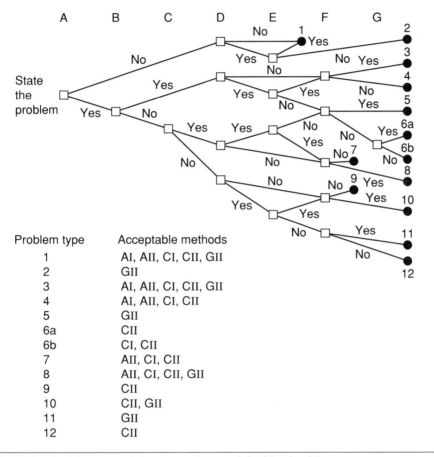

Problem type	Acceptable methods
1	AI, AII, CI, CII, GII
2	GII
3	AI, AII, CI, CII, GII
4	AI, AII, CI, CII
5	GII
6a	CII
6b	CI, CII
7	AII, CI, CII
8	AII, CI, CII, GII
9	CII
10	CII, GII
11	GII
12	CII

Figure 9.4 The decision tree of the normative model of leadership.

Adapted and reprinted from *Leadership and Decision–making*, by Victor H. Vroom and Philip W. Yetton, by permission of the University of Pittsburgh Press. © 1973 by University of Pittsburgh Press.

expectations of the group also vary. However, identification of these factors can help determine group objectives (Cattell, 1951; Stogdill, 1974). Bales (1950) and Benne and Sheats (1948) delineated group functions in terms of group objectives (Table 9.1). The group objectives, either task or maintenance/socioemotional, help determine appropriate leadership roles.

Task Roles

The task roles described in Table 9.1 correspond closely to the leadership roles of the exercise professionals. Following are examples of functions

appropriate to exercise professionals in the task role category:

■ The *initiator* suggests effective exercises for individual needs.

■ The *information seeker* gathers information about the students before prescribing a regimen.

■ The *opinion seeker* looks for feelings and reactions the students have to the exercise program schedule and their rate of fitness improvement.

■ The *information giver* educates students who are unfamiliar with fitness principles and terminology.

Table 9.1 Task Roles and Socioemotional Roles in Groups

Role	Function
Task roles	
Initiator contributor	Recommends novel ideas about the problem at hand, new ways to approach the problem, or possible solutions not yet considered.
Information seeker	Emphasizes "getting the facts" by calling for background information from others.
Opinion seeker	Asks for more qualitative types of data, such as attitudes, values, and feelings.
Information giver	Provides data for forming decisions, including facts that derive from expertise.
Opinion giver	Provides opinions, values, and feelings.
Elaborator	Gives additional information—examples, rephrasings, implications—about points made by others.
Coordinator	Shows the relevance of each idea and its relationship to the overall problem.
Orienter	Refocuses discussion on the topic whenever necessary.
Evaluator-critic	Appraises the quality of the group's efforts in terms of logic, practicality, or method.
Energizer	Stimulates the group to continue working when discussion flags.
Procedural technician	Cares for operational details, such as the materials, machinery, and so on.
Recorder	Provides a secretarial function.
Socioemotional roles	
Encourager	Rewards others through agreement, warmth, and praise.
Harmonizer	Mediates conflicts among group members.
Compromiser	Shifts his or her own position on an issue in order to reduce conflict in the group.
Gatekeeper and expediter	Smooths communication by setting up procedures and ensuring equal participation from members.
Standard setter	Expresses, or calls for discussion of, standards for evaluating the quality of the group process.
Group observer and commentator	Informally points out the positive and negative aspects of the group's dynamics and calls for change if necessary.
Follower	Accepts the ideas offered by others and serves as an audience for the group.

From "Functional Roles of Group Members" by K.D. Benne and P. Sheats, 1948, *Journal of Social Issues*, **4**, pp. 41-49. Copyright 1948 by the Society for the Psychology of Social Issues. Reprinted by permission.

■ The *opinion giver* helps students who seek advice on exercise pacing and scheduling.

■ The *elaborator* explains complex terms and ideas that are important to the success of the student's prescriptive program.

■ The *coordinator* explains the relationships between different exercises and the importance of integrating them into the exercise regimen.

■ The *orienter* guides students to the appropriate exercise tasks and helps them stay on track.

■ The *evaluator* assesses the progress of the group and the individual members toward their fitness goals.

■ The *energizer* motivates the class when morale is low.

■ The *procedural technician* monitors the condition and accuracy of the exercise equipment and explains how the equipment works.

■ The *recorder* keeps progress logs of the students to track performance, provide feedback, and evaluate progress.

Certainly, all of these roles will not be played out simultaneously. However, these examples illustrate the relevance of task roles in exercise leadership. It is also important that exercise professionals know when various leadership functions are needed.

Socioemotional Roles

Following are examples of socioemotional roles that apply to the exercise setting:

■ The *encourager* reinforces class members who have reached an exercise goal and those who are having difficulty reaching an exercise goal but continue to persevere.

■ The *harmonizer* resolves conflicts between competitive class members or between a class member and co-leader who do not get along.

■ The *compromiser* finds the middle ground when half of the class chooses one option and the other half chooses another. Even though the exercise leader has a degree of control over the group, the leader compromises to increase cohesion and reduce conflict.

■ The *expediter* ensures fair play within the class and increases effective communication by developing operational procedures for the group.

■ The *standard setter* asks for group input on the quality of class interactions and activities or receives feedback on the pace of the class and the effectiveness of the leader's approach to attaining goals.

■ The *group observer* identifies ways to help the exercise class proceed more effectively or identifies self-defeating behaviors that impede progress.

■ The *followers* enable the group movement and motivate or reinforce the leader. Exercise participants who are enthusiastic and motivated to carry out the leader's goals enhance the credibility of the leader with other members and nurture motivation in the group.

Task and maintenance/socioemotional roles are present in all groups and can be developed in many ways. These roles are frequently held by different people in the group and are determined partly by personality of the group member and partly by situational factors (see Figure 9.1). The very process of playing two quite distinct roles in the same group would require a highly skilled leader. For example, the leader who fulfills task roles identifies problems, occasionally confronts members, makes unpopular decisions, gives orders, and performs other behaviors that cause tension. Because reactions to conflict are directed to the task leader, the leader could probably not play an emotional or supportive role effectively. Conversely, if a leader is effective in the socioemotional role of promoting goodwill, harmony, and empathy, it would be difficult for that leader to confront members, set limits, or give negative feedback.

Group Cohesion

Task and socioemotional roles have long been acknowledged as integral concepts in group dynamics theory. In recent years, sport and exercise research has increasingly focused on these concepts largely due to the studies of the Waterloo group (Carron, Widmeyer, & Brawley, 1985, 1988). Group cohesion is recognized as a variable in sport team performance, adherence to physical activity, and level of group functioning. The Waterloo group identified the need to develop an instrument to assess group cohesion and to create a conceptual model to understand the dynamics of group cohesion. The instrument, called the Group Environment Questionnaire (GEQ), comprises four scales that reflect the constructs of the conceptual model:

■ *Group integration (task)* represents bonding and closeness within the group related to group goals and objectives.

■ *Group integration (social)* represents closeness and bonding within the group related to social aspects of the group.

■ *Individual attraction to group (task)* represents the individual's feelings about the group and his or her involvement with the group members on matters of group goals and objectives.

■ *Individual attraction to group (social)* represents the individual's involvement with other group members on aspects of social relationships.

Exercise practitioners value group cohesion because it can enhance the group and individual's experience of the fitness class. Weak cohesion can be detrimental to members' attitudes, cooperation, and adherence.

The exercise practitioner who wishes to use the Waterloo research might follow these general guidelines:

1. Become familiar with the group cohesion conceptual model.

2. Give the GEQ to class members at the beginning of a fitness program.

3. Look for distribution of scores across the four construct areas.

4. Members with high scores on any index are likely to have some investment in the class and may be less likely to drop out or become disengaged from the group.

5. Members with no high scores should be monitored to assess the probable reason for low involvement and to develop some interventions to increase cohesion.

6. If a member is strong in only one category, it does not necessarily indicate weakened cohesion. The instructor should monitor these individuals. If they continue to stay involved, it may be that they simply have concentrated either on task or on social roles. However, if an individual with only one strong category begins to falter, he or she should be treated in the same way as a person who scored low in all categories.

7. Administer the GEQ halfway through or at the end of the program to compare pre- and post-scores. This procedure could be helpful in shaping the exercise program.

THE STRUCTURE OF GROUPS

Let's say an adult fitness class is being held through the physical education department in a nearby university. The class instructors are advanced students in the department and the class members work for or near the university. If we visited this class to observe the group functioning, the most notable aspects of the group would be the roles played by the members. The members, both men and women, may range in age from 22 years to 60 or more. Some members are in excellent physical condition, while others are in moderate to poor condition because of obesity or physical limitations, such as arthritis, high blood pressure, ulcers, or back pain.

We might notice that even though there are strong individual differences among members, they all comply with the instructor's directions. Certain members might communicate more with the instructor than others, and some members might be sought more for conversation, while others may be sought more for advice.

We might describe the instructor's role as highly respected by the class because we observe that the advice and information given by the instructor are heeded by all. The instructor might be sought out before and after class for advice, casual conversation, and joking.

These observations identify some of the structural properties of a group. Structure is the unseen framework that maintains the group and accounts for regularities in group behavior (Forsyth, 1983). Group structure is both formal and informal and highly to marginally stable. All groups have informal structure and most have at least some degree of formal structure. A group that has acquired stability through relationships among members is considered structured (Cartwright & Zander, 1968). The formal structure is typically known to all participants, while the informal structure is usually not verbalized. In a fitness class, the instructor would expect the members to comply with the formal structure by arriving on time, staying for the entire class, complying with departmental policies and guidelines, and acknowledging the instructor as the primary information giver and the class members as primarily information receivers.

Let's imagine for a moment that an informal structure developed in which a group member perceived to be competent and skilled gained an informal leadership role in the class. Depending on the personality, leadership power, and situational control of the instructor, the group members might be influenced more by the informal leader than by the formal leader. If the instructor understands the principles of group structure, the situation could be dealt with knowledgeably. However, if the instructor perceives only the formal structure, he or she would miss much of what happens in the group.

We will identify several select properties of group structure. These structural properties are stages of group development and norms.

Stages of Group Development

Several group and counseling theorists have identified predictable stages through which a functioning group is likely to pass. Figure 9.5 compares three of the most representative models of group development. Each of these models identifies characteristics of group evolution with which the exercise leader should be familiar. These models have a shared foundation and common themes, although there are slight differentiations. The following illustration applies the stages of group development in a fitness class. As you read through each stage, imagine yourself as the exercise instructor in the class. Would you be aware of these developments in your own class experience? How might the awareness of these dynamics affect your teaching approach or your effectiveness?

The exercise leader may describe the first session or two as the *exploration, establishment, or forming stage.* The leader would discuss the formal ground rules, goals, and expectations:

———————— ■ ————————

1. The leader introduces the group goals with regard to exercise objectives and any interpersonal or socioemotional goals. The leader also encourages individual group members to express at least general individual exercise goals.

2. Certain group norms begin to form, such as acceptable attendance standards. The tone and atmosphere of the group settles into a norm of being lighthearted or serious, task- or relationship-oriented. The atmosphere is usually determined by the leader.

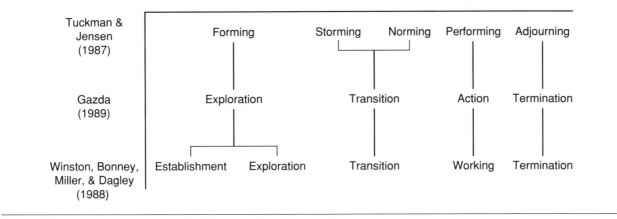

Figure 9.5 Comparisons of models of group development stages.

3. The group members informally evaluate the exercise leader based on knowledge of exercise physiology, ability to convey knowledge, interpersonal skills, and personality style.

4. Roles and status begin to form. Members who are physically fit assume higher status unless they lack interpersonal skills or compete with less fit members. Those who demonstrate strong group commitment and encouragement and help others become influential members. The leader identifies how roles and status are being assigned in order to understand the informal structure of the group.

The next phase could be referred to as the *transition or norming stage*:

■

1. A small percentage of members test the ground rules by frequently being absent, arriving late, or disrupting the class. Some avoid doing certain exercises.

2. Group commitment and cohesion are enhanced through self-disclosure and deeper levels of interpersonal communication between members. Individuals speak with the leader or other members about insecurities regarding appearance, fear of not meeting the exercise goals, or fear of looking foolish. The leader is sensitive and perceptive during this stage so that the individuals will not feel rejected or unheard. If the members do not feel accepted and fail to develop a sense of belonging at this stage, they will not be able to move forward.

The third phase, the *performing, working, or action stage*, is the beginning of actual exercise goal accomplishment:

■

1. Members seek feedback about their progress more readily.

2. A high degree of group cohesion and cooperation is evidenced by members remembering how many miles or how long classmates run each session and encouraging them in that goal for the day. Members recall difficulties or infirmities classmates have experienced and inquire about them. If a member returns after an absence, other members are genuinely interested in why the member has been gone.

3. Members meet for lunch, after class, and to run together on off days. They no longer communicate strictly through the leader.

4. The leader gently challenges members who are not progressing by exploring motivational or other causal factors.

The last phase, is the *termination or adjourning stage*:

■

1. The leader formally ends the class. The leader designs certificates or awards for class members to recognize some area of achievement. The leader also makes observations about progress by the group as a whole.

2. Members identify significant occurrences in the group and describe the impact of the events on them. Members also discuss

actual progress toward exercise goals and share feedback with each other.

3. Members speak about their exercise plans after the group experience has ended. The members make contracts with themselves on further exercise goals they wish to achieve.

Norms

Group *norms* are rules of behavior endorsed by the group and the standards against which the group and leader regulate the performance of the group members. Norms are usually informal and implicit. Following is an example of the elusiveness of norms.

———————— ■ ————————

An exercise leader had announced that the group exercise begins at noon. As people drift in late, the instructor shows no reaction until one or two people come in 20 minutes late. Then there is a noticeable negative nonverbal reaction from the instructor, who later speaks privately to the two latecomers.

The formal norm in this example is that members should be present at noon, but the informal norm is that members should be present by 12:15 p.m.

Development of Group Norms

The group leader must understand how norms work within the group to be able to control both the informal and formal functioning. In the previous example, the instructor had no understanding of informal norms and probably lost the role of the leader to a group member who possessed leadership qualities and understood the functions of the group.

Two popular explanations for the development and maintenance of norms are behavioral reinforcement and social influence.

The *behavioral reinforcement approach* explains the development of norms simply as individuals engaging in behavior that will be reinforced and avoiding behavior that will be punished. Social learning theorists maintain that social reinforcers may operate on such a subliminal level that the individual is unaware of being influenced.

The leader of a fitness class could unconsciously reinforce those who are punctual by making announcements at the beginning of class and not repeating them (punishment through covert conditioning); or the instructor may compliment and spend more time talking with those who are punctual than those who are not (reinforcement through covert conditioning). As a result, a strong norm of punctuality could develop without anyone being aware of the dynamics involved.

To illustrate social influence over individual perspective, let's say the group leader notices on the first day of class that group members are dressed in a variety of outfits. After three or four sessions, the instructor notes that the variety of dress has decreased, and that those members with less status (often those perceived as less fit) have begun to dress more like the members with higher status. The instructor also notices that even though etiquette had not formally been discussed, the class members are alert to behaviors and interactions of others who are using the same track and equipment. These are examples of compliance with social norms. The influence of social norms stems not from avoidance of punishment, but from desire to fit into the group.

GROUP COMMUNICATION

Studies of group communication have had a slightly different focus than research on leader-member or individual communication. Studies have suggested that successful groups are characterized by highly motivated leaders who encourage communication by focusing group attention on the tasks (Harper & Askling, 1980). Also, a high correlation between quality of communication among members and group problem-solving abilities has been shown (Katz & Tushman, 1979). These and other studies point to the importance of communication in group productivity and efficiency.

Influential Factors in Group Communication

Several aspects of group communication have been identified as factors that contribute to or hinder effectiveness (Napier & Gershenfeld, 1987).

Size

There is no optimum group size that ensures quality communication. However, studies have identified some directional trends.

■ As size increases, the group breaks into subgroups, which increases the complexity of communication.

■ Small groups encourage more participation than larger ones, and members of small groups report greater satisfaction.

■ Two-person groups usually cause tension because a dominant-submissive relationship develops.

■ Three-person groups are more successful than two-person groups because there is no possibility of an equal split.

■ A group with 10 members or more becomes too large and restricts participation.

The exercise practitioner should consider group size primarily in terms of types of exercise, special populations, and physical setting. A class that involves mainly floor exercises, running, or walking could accommodate more participants (providing adequate space allocation) than could a class that requires use of equipment (e.g., weight machines or stationary bicycles). Control of class size is even more important when using specialized equipment (e.g., heart monitoring or treadmill). Members of special populations, such as a cardiac rehabilitation group or people with physical disabilities, would need more individual attention from the instructor than other groups. The instructor must also consider the amount of space in relation to the number of participants and type of activity.

Time

As the size of the group increases, the time available for interaction decreases, which in turn diminishes participation (M. Shaw, 1981). If an activity requires individual time or special instruction, the practitioner should control the size of the class, the duration of the class, or both.

Physical Environment

Key (1986) found that groups arranged in a circle communicate more effectively between members and with the leader because each member has equal physical access to all other members. This design does not negate the impact of members who hold differing degrees of influence. The exercise environment, unlike other work environments, assumes mobility and flexibility of movement. Although usually a plus, this type of movement can have some disadvantages. For example, if members participate in activities in different parts of the facility, the instructor has to spend time at each location. To be more efficient and better monitor

class progress, the instructor may consider planning phases of activity to organize the class movement.

Status and Power

Every group has high-status and low-status members. Status is determined in a number of ways including role in the group, status outside the group, or technical knowledge. High-status members generally have a strong influence over the opinion of others (Kashyap, 1982). Both low- and high-status members focus more attention on high-status members (Hurwitz, Zander, & Hymovitch, 1968). Low-status members tend not to participate in the formal operations of a group for fear of criticism and devaluation. These members generally feel less and less a part of the group and defer to higher status members, at least publicly.

Exercise leaders can make use of status differences to promote exercise goal achievement and to enhance class involvement. People with greater exercise proficiency frequently group together as do those with less proficiency. The instructor should be aware of these patterns and promote mentoring and coaching by pairing high-status members with low-status members. The high-status member then feels important and useful and the low-status individual feels noticed and included.

General Group Factors

Bavelas (1950) and Shaw (1964) identified several trends of member behavior through group interaction studies:

■ The greater the degree of group participation, the higher the morale.

■ Groups in which communication is open tend to be inefficient. More participation leads to redundant, unproductive discussion, which requires additional time.

■ Greater efficiency exists in groups with a central leader who monitors progress in task functions. However, morale may decrease with centralized leadership.

■ Leaders of cohesive groups are most effective when they take a collaborative approach. Leaders of uncohesive groups are most effective when they are directive and task-oriented (Schreshum, 1980).

Understanding and Interpreting Group Communication

A classic model for awareness and interpretation of group behavior is the Johari Window. The model

	Known to self	Not known to self
Known to others	1 Open	2 Blind
Not known to others	3 Hidden	4 Unknown

Figure 9.6   Johari Window.

From *Group Processes: An Introduction to Group Dynamics* by Joseph Luft by permission of Mayfield Publishing Company. Copyright © 1984, 1970, and 1963 by Joseph Luft.

was developed in the 1960s by Joseph Luft and Harry Ingram, from whose first names "Johari" is derived. According to Luft (1969), the Johari Window recognizes the importance of self and of others and provides a structure for interpreting interpersonal transactions and changes in relationships (see Figure 9.6). This model can be easily used without extensive training in group behavior. The model is conceptually understandable and interpretable.

The Johari Window consists of four quadrants that represent the total person in relation to others:

Quadrant 1.   This quadrant comprises behavior, feelings, and motivations known to the individual and others. This area represents times when the public self is present.

Quadrant 2.   Quadrant 2 consists of behavior, feelings, and motivations known to others, but not to ourselves. This is called the "blind area." Through nonverbal behavior and various behavioral patterns, people unconsciously convey information about themselves. This nonverbal communication allows others to know more about a person than that person consciously knows.

Quadrant 3.   The hidden area represents the information about behavior, feelings, and motivations that the individual keeps private.

Quadrant 4.   The unknown area refers to behaviors, feelings, and motivations that are unknown to both ourselves and others.

In profiling a newly formed fitness group, Quadrant 1 of the Johari Window would be relatively small. Class or group members are initially concerned with appearances, being accepted, and fitting in. The "best foot forward" approach would necessitate disclosing as little as possible. A change in one quadrant affects the others. In this example, Quadrant 1 becomes smaller, Quadrant 3 becomes larger.

As members get to know each other, roles and norms become apparent and members feel more secure about their "place" in the group. At this juncture, members will likely begin to disclose things about themselves during class discussions or workout time. One member may share insecurities about physical appearance. Another may reveal a need to "outdo" the others in the class for recognition, while another member may disclose that she fears she is too hopeful about how much becoming fit can realistically change her life. All of these are examples of movement from Quadrant 3 to Quadrant 1, from the hidden to the known through self-disclosure.

Self-disclosure explains behavior and feelings that others may have observed but did not understand. As a result, others become more understanding of an individual's feelings and motivation and feel more trusting and open with the individual. The others can then give feedback to the individual, which provides the individual a glimpse of how others see him or her. Feedback reduces information known only to others and not known to oneself.

——— ■ ———

Maria, a member of a fitness class, discloses to the leader that she has not exercised since she was a high school athlete 10 years ago. She says she dreads facing the fact that she will never again be in the physical condition she was in at 18. The leader feels good about Maria's openness and also feels that she now has a better understanding of what Maria is going through. The leader gives Maria feedback about perseverance, discipline, and stamina that seem to come naturally to Maria. The leader also notices Maria's ease with other members and her ability to encourage them and joke with them in a pleasant way.

After several occurrences of receiving this new information about herself, Maria realizes that even though she is not 18 years old any longer, she has many valuable qualities now that she did not have then.

_____

A goal of both personal and group development is to increase the size of Quadrant 1 and decrease the size of Quadrants 2, 3, and possibly 4. The Johari Window is useful in any group setting in which interpersonal transactions occur and need to be understood.

GROUP CONFLICT AND PROBLEM SOLVING

Conflict is often interpreted as disagreement accompanied by tension, anxiety, and intense negative feelings. Conflicts are natural and predictable in ongoing relationships and in group interaction. Specialists in group work view conflict as an important vehicle for group development and problem solving.

Recent research has indicated that groups with dissenting members can achieve more than those without dissent, as long as the dissidence is supported and diversity is valued (Goddard, 1986). Dissonance can either stimulate creative problem-solving or become a source of intergroup competition, power struggles, and ultimately dysfunction.

Problem solving in interpersonal relationships and group interaction does not share the accurate, systematic, and often predictable processes enjoyed by other scientific disciplines. Interpersonal and intrapersonal dynamics continually bring into play influential factors of which the decision maker is often unaware.

This final section will consider the meaning, development, and causes of conflict and discuss the group dynamics involved. A general overview of problem solving will also be given. Lastly, this section will address the ultimate question of who decides.

Stages of Conflict

The word *conflict* is derived from the Latin word *conflictus*, which means a "striking together with force." In a group, conflict may arise at any time from numerous sources. Conflict is especially likely after a group has passed through the initial stages of foundation building and trust formation, and members are more willing to be forthright and candid. The needs to be liked and be part of the group are no longer primary concerns. Desire to work toward individual and group goals becomes a stronger need that stimulates members to clarify norms, set limits, and perform other task-related functions. The stages of conflict are disagreement, confrontation, escalation, de-escalation, and resolution (Forsyth, 1983). Although not all of the stages are present in every conflict, those that do occur do so sequentially.

Disagreement

During the exploration phase of a group, the individuality of members emerges. Similarities and differences between members are identified, and disagreements may arise. The group leader and member leaders should determine whether the disagreement is substantive or false (Deutsch, 1973). A false conflict arises from a misunderstanding or miscommunication. However, left unchecked, the result can be as damaging as a true conflict. For example, if a member unexpectedly breaks pace with the rest of the class, class members might assume he is showing off. After exploration, the leader discovers that the member has entered a race that is a few weeks away and requires a more rigorous training schedule. This situation left unexplained could easily have caused tension and resentment in the group.

Legitimate sources of conflict are often ignored in hopes that something will alleviate the problem. If the conflict continues, members must address the disagreement. As the main issues are identified, tangential conflicts are often revealed as well. Depending on the importance of the issues, the group will either attempt to resolve the problem or continue to ignore the conflict until it escalates and disrupts the group.

We will use the following case to describe the five stages of conflict from disagreement through resolution.

—————— ■ ——————

An exercise physiologist begins working in a cardiac rehabilitation unit. She soon notices a faction of the patient group that shows an undercurrent of resistance and resentment toward the staff, including herself. She learns by careful observation and by talking with other members that some of the patients are there voluntarily, while others are required by their physician to participate. Among the latter group are several vocal members who are disgruntled about being in the program.

During the initial stage of disagreement the group members fail to focus on the true source of conflict or clarify the problem situation. As members become familiar with each other, they begin to voice opinions and soon discover where and with whom the differences reside. The members are in fact resentful toward the cardiac specialist for requiring them to attend the class. They resent feeling out of control and are scared about their physical condition. They are angry with "fate" because this happened to them, and are experiencing the "why me?" reaction.

Frequently, the true source of conflict goes ignored or unrealized. The disgruntled members focused on external and environmental factors, such as dissatisfaction with the equipment, belief that the instructors were not competent, not wanting to be around sick people, and other artificial concerns. The true nature of group conflict can be camouflaged by external issues. Exercise leaders may miss what is happening if they do not understand the group dynamics.

Confrontation

During the confrontation phase, an incompatability between two or more members becomes evident. The ensuing dialogue is an attempt by each side to persuade the other to his or her point of view.

Group members who speak out in favor of a position will become increasingly more committed to the position as they talk. The intensity of commitment leads the participants to present supporting information in a biased way and to refute any disconfirming data. After a position has been taken, individuals frequently refuse to consider they may be mistaken and may distort information to make it conform to their belief.

As commitment increases, tension and anxiety increase as well. The interaction becomes less rational and more emotional (Fisher, 1980). Frequently, the disagreeing members persuade neutral members to take a stand, which polarizes the group (Gustafson, 1978).

———— ■ ————

The instructors decide to ignore the disruptive faction hoping they will settle down if no attention is paid to them. However, this approach fails and the group begins to verbally spar with others who disagree with them. The oppositional group becomes more adamant and intense in their complaints about the class, the instructors, and the activities.

Escalation

During this stage, the conflict frequently spirals into hostility and anger. Escalation is characterized by mistrust, frustration, and negative feelings. As frustration increases, the potential for aggression rises. The earlier goal of decision making or problem resolution fades and the previously passive group becomes hostile as well.

———— ■ ————

Passive members who have ignored the oppositional group become irritated because their class experience is being negatively affected. They begin dreading the class and feel they have to defend themselves against sarcastic and critical remarks. The instructors seem unable to resolve the conflict.

De-escalation

The tension, anxiety, and intensity of the escalation period cannot be sustained. As the arousal level drops, the factional members realize they are on a self-defeating course. Forsyth (1983) describes three components of de-escalation, which can be intentionally applied to reduce conflict.

Negotiation involves at least two people discussing potential solutions that would benefit the participants. Resolution may involve *distributive issues*, in which one group benefits if the other makes concessions, or *integrative issues*, in which both groups look for a mutually beneficial solution.

Trust in a group disintegrates when conflict arises. However, trust can be rebuilt if both groups consistently follow through on declared intentions (Lindskold, 1978).

Third-party intervention is the involvement of one or more people without a vested interest in the conflict, such as facilitators, mediators, advisors, negotiators, and others.

Rubin (1980) reviewed research focusing on the effectiveness of third-party interventions and determined the following:

■ Third parties can create a face-saving situation to facilitate reconciliation.

■ Most conventional intervention techniques are more effective when conflict intensity is low.

■ Occasionally, the oppositional groups will react negatively to the intervention and decide to settle the conflict themselves.

The cardiac rehabilitation class could de-escalate in one of two ways, depending on the skill level of the class instructors and their understanding of group dynamics. If the instructors understand the behavior of the oppositional group and realize that they are lashing out with misdirected anger, they could begin negotiation. Each group member would talk with the instructors privately. The instructors would be empathic and supportive, which would encourage the trust necessary for the members to reveal the real nature of their anger. After this debriefing and de-escalation, the members would meet as a group led by the instructors. The purpose of the meeting would be to disclose and give feedback about the members' experiences.

If the instructors are not skilled or prefer not to initiate the negotiation, a third party, preferably another exercise professional, could interview the members and instructors individually, facilitate a group meeting for self-disclosure and feedback, and make recommendations to the instructors.

Resolution

The return to a state of agreement can occur in various ways. Kriesburg (1973) identified five ways to reach resolution:

■ One of the adversaries withdraws demands for the sake of the group, but feels no true resolution or compromise.

■ One faction imposes its position on the larger group through a vote, proclamation, or authority.

■ A compromise is reached through negotiation. Each faction modifies their position to accommodate a need of the other group until they reach a mutually satisfying agreement.

■ One faction is persuaded to change positions and adopt the oppositional group's view.

■ The group disbands or one of the factions leaves the group.

The cardiac rehabilitation group is most likely to reach resolution by the oppositional group giving up their misdirected anger and adopting the positive viewpoint of the majority. Through discussion with the instructor, the factional group members can understand their emotions and resolve their feelings about being in cardiac rehabilitation. Once the true source of conflict is identified, the oppositional members would have no interpersonal resentment toward other group members.

Causes of Conflict

Group conflict is a natural stage in the development of a group. However, the group leader must know how to manage conflict to enable the group to work through the conflict and continue growing. The factors contributing to the creation of conflict in a group are complex and not fully understood. However, group dynamics research has focused on the nature of group conflict and the variables that seem to be consistent causal factors.

Interdependence is commonly described as an interpersonal dynamic in which the welfare or desires of one person somehow depend on the behavior of another. Although interdependence in itself does not foster healthy or unhealthy interactions, cooperation and competition greatly influence the outcome of interdependent relationships. Studies have indicated that when cooperation is fostered, conflict is low, and when competition is encouraged, conflict is high (Deutsch, 1973; Schelling, 1960).

Blake and Mouton (1970) investigated the impact of interpersonal style on conflict management. They identified the primary variables of interactive style as concern for people and concern for productivity or goal accomplishment. People concerned with productivity confront and overcome conflict without regard for the feelings of others, while those concerned with people avoid conflict with others to maintain harmony. There are, of course, various degrees and combinations of the two conflict management styles (see Figure 9.7). The significance of this factor is the way in which interpersonal style influences attitude and behavior in managing conflict.

Attribution theorists (Festinger, 1957; Heider, 1958; Jones & Nisbett, 1971) have noted that individuals tend to attribute the actions of others to personal motives rather than to situational factors. However, the same people will attribute their own actions primarily to situational factors rather than to personal motives. This hypothesis is termed *attribution bias*. When group conflict is low, the distorted attribution made by observers tends to be less pronounced than the distorted attribution made during a high level of conflict (Rosenberg & Wolfsfeld, 1977).

In the case of the cardiac rehabilitation group, the voluntary members (observers) attributed the behavior of the factional group to negative personal characteristics rather than to situational factors. The observers determined that the unhappy members were selfish, rude, disrespectful, and interested in sabotaging the class.

The members of the factional group, on the other hand, viewed themselves as victims of unfair circumstances who were being bossed around by doctors and staff. They interpreted their behaviors

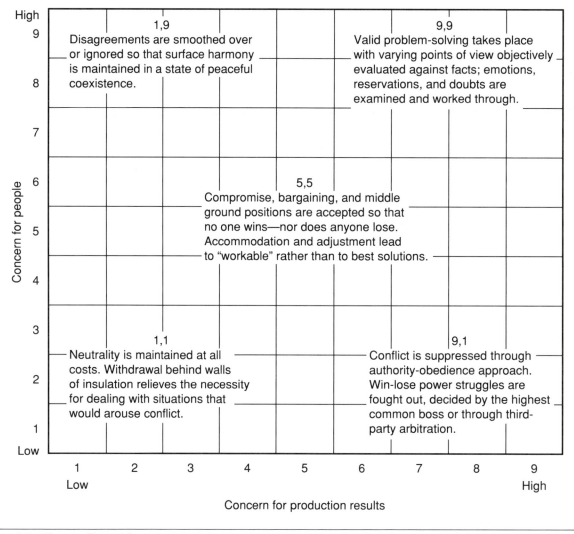

Figure 9.7   The conflict grid.

From ''The Fifth Achievement'' by R.R. Blake and J. Syrgley Mouton, *The Journal of Applied Behavioral Science,* **6**(4), p.418, 1970. Copyright 1970 by the NTL Institute.

as legitimate reactions to oppressive situational factors.

Problem Solving

Decision making is a normal process that occurs many times a day. Decision making is affected by so many factors, such as personal history, family influence, religion, socioeconomic status, education, and career, that it is difficult for theorists to predict with any certainty the influence of any one of these factors. In the case of group decision-making, the numbers of potential outcomes seems astronomical.

A six-stage procedure for group problem-solving (Napier & Gershenfeld, 1987) describes a logical means by which a problem may be addressed successfully.

Stage 1: Problem Identification

Problems can be identified by finding the source of tension and conflict. Although problems can often be identified readily, they may not be dealt with for several reasons. For example, individuals are sometimes afraid of appearing petty by identifying problems that are not yet out of control. It is also common for people in power to encourage feedback about problems, but then minimize or discount it. The lower ranking people fear this and do not want to be labeled as complainers. In organizations, problem identification is sometimes the last step rather than the first step in the process.

The following methods have been successful in overcoming problem identification obstacles:

■ Find out how widespread the problem is felt among the group.

■ Provide suggestion boxes, feedback forms, or questionnaires to periodically measure the groups' feelings and morale.

■ Identify specific factors that need to change to resolve the problem. How will the group know if the change has been made?

Stage 2: The Diagnostic Phase

The more successful method of diagnosing a problem involves describing the situation in relative rather than absolute terms. Statements that stress "either-or," "all or nothing," or "good or bad" symbolize a throwing down of the gauntlet and set the stage for a no-win situation. Relative statements that emphasize "less than optimal," "better or worse," or "needing improvement" open the door for negotiation.

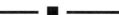

An aerobics instructor notices after the second session that the range of fitness and conditioning levels of the participants are somewhat varied. She does not see this as a problem, but soon notices frustration and irritation from members who are highly or moderately fit. After talking with the class members individually, the instructor finds that they all perceive the different levels of physical conditioning as a problem. They believe the solution is to create groups with similarly functioning people in them. However, this solution is not practical or feasible, and leaves no room for compromise. The instructor meets with the class and suggests redefining the problem. She believes the problem is that the class has not yet found a way to accommodate differences.

Options for a solution in this example should focus on ways to modify the class activity or organization to allow members to work at their own pace.

Once the problem is identified, the group must determine whether or not they can solve the problem within the group. A critical step in problem diagnosis is to decide whose problem it is. If the group does not accept ownership of the problem, resolution is doomed.

Critical questions that can help clarify a problem include:

■ Is there more than one problem? If so, what are the ancillary problems and what is the root problem?

■ What are the positive aspects of keeping the problem condition? Some problems are not easily resolved because there is some benefit to maintaining the problem. This benefit must be identified or it will sabotage the chosen solution. For example, a member of a cardiac rehabilitation course has received much attention and support because at the start of the class he was less capable and more afraid to exert himself than others were. He now feels greater confidence, but fears that if he shows this confidence, he will lose the sympathy and attention of others.

■ What solutions have already been tried and why did they fail? Consideration of this question is crucial to avoid repeating the same errors.

Stage 3: Generating Alternatives

Individuals tend to gravitate toward known behavioral approaches and familiar ways of thinking. As a result, solutions that have failed are often tried again. The old cliche "If at first you don't succeed, try, try again" might be more helpful if it were changed to "If at first you don't succeed, try something else."

The instructor and class members identify sources of frustrations for the highly and moderately fit members. The unsuccessful solution was to moderate the intensity of the high-level group and help the moderate-level group increase their pace. Rather than continuing with this solution, the group generates new ideas for reducing the incompatibilities. Suggestions include (a) modifying routines to accommodate people with moderate and high levels of conditioning; (b) the instructor demonstrating alternative aerobic movements, stretching, and toning exercises to match the exercise needs of the individual; and (c) some class members marching in place during difficult routines to continue participating.

Stage 4: Selecting Solutions

The "cost," or disadvantage, of implementing a solution is often overlooked. Just as people tend not to look at the benefits of a problem, they also tend to ignore the downside of a new alternative. The relief and optimism in finally making a group decision often outweighs the pragmatic aspect of acknowledging that no solution is problem free.

One last factor to consider is the group's anticipation of where the resistance to a resolution will reside. Resistance to a potential solution is not unusual. The group should expect this reaction, know from whom the reaction will come, and generate responses.

Stage 5: Implementation

Successful implementation is difficult for several reasons: (a) people with enough influence to sabotage a plan may not have been informed or included; (b) those recommending the new plan may not have developed a way to monitor the success of the solution; and (c) people in key positions to affect the success of the plan through every new phase may not have been included.

Once ideas for solutions have been generated, people often perceive the work as being done. A successful leader ensures the ideas are implemented to give the solution a good chance to work.

Stage 6: Evaluation

Evaluation, more than any other phase of problem solving, tends to be omitted. Reluctance to give negative feedback or critique another person's ideas, and feeling uncertain about the feedback are frequent reasons for avoiding evaluation. However, without evaluating the planned solution, small snags can turn a good idea in need of small corrections into a plain bad idea. Evaluation can identify a small problem early enough to save the larger plan.

Who Makes the Decisions?

We have discussed the process of decision making and several factors involved in making decisions. A different aspect of this process is the question of who decides. Which situations lend themselves to leader decision-making? If the group decides, how is the decision reached? Napier and Gershenfeld (1987) described various means of determining who decides.

The group leader must decide whether to make a unilateral decision or to involve the group. A popular approach is to keep the options open and handle each circumstance discriminately. The price for this approach is that (a) the group will probably not feel any investment in the success of the leader's decision, (b) the group may try to sabotage the leader's decision, and (c) the leader's

motives will be suspect because of the unwillingness to play by clearly defined rules.

The effective leader should clearly define which decisions will be made by the leader and which decisions will be made by the group. The leader loses some flexibility in the approach, but gains credibility.

The following approaches are frequently used when the group is making the decision.

Majority Rule

This method works best when most of the group agrees and the majority vote can be a show of solidarity. This method is also effective when a relatively inconsequential decision needs to be taken care of. A majority vote is ineffective when 25% to 49% of the members disagree about an important decision. The large minority will be disgruntled and uncommitted, and may even sabotage the decision.

Two-Thirds Majority

Approval by a two-thirds majority lends greater credibility to a decision than does a simple majority. Psychologically, the minority members can more easily accept a decision with a two-thirds ratio than if only 51% agree.

Consensus

Many people misunderstand "consensus" to mean that all members share the same thinking. In most cases, a consensus is reached when those who disagree willingly defer to the rest of the group. Although their thinking has not changed, they have decided to put aside differences to resolve the problem.

Occasionally, a consensus vote is taken without proper cultivation of the group members. When this happens, the consensus effectively forces the dissenting members to change their minds, drop out of the group, or become inactive in the group. Leaders and member leaders who invest the time necessary to build a consensus, can extract a strong commitment from group members.

Delegated Decisions

This method works well when groups are too large to make a decision together. The group at large must trust the designated decision makers for the decisions to hold credibility. Routine decisions are easier to delegate than those that are very important. Important decisions need input from the whole group.

SUMMARY

Group dynamics is a complex set of concepts important to the fitness professional. This chapter has reviewed several principles of group dynamics that are particularly applicable to the fitness setting.

Leadership is an elusive concept, and leadership styles vary depending on the circumstances. Leadership theory initially focused on traits, such as physical attributes or personality. However, theorists soon realized that leadership is not one dimensional.

Models, including contingency, participation, multidimensional, and normative, integrate the interactional and reciprocal aspects of the leader's characteristics. Situational conditions greatly influence leadership styles. The multidimensional models of Fiedler, Vroom, Chelladurai, and Lewin rest on the premise that leadership effectiveness depends on leader characteristics and situational factors. Task and maintenance roles differentiation emerged naturally from these leadership models. They remain as the most effective and applicable means of describing leadership roles.

Group theorists have consistently identified stages through which a group evolves. This development generally includes a beginning, transitory, working, and termination stage. Through group development, norms for both individual and group behavior emerge. Norms provide a blueprint for the formation of group characteristics.

Group conflict is a naturally occurring phenomenon. Studies of group conflict have identified common stages of conflict, such as disagreement, confrontation, escalation, de-escalation, and resolution. Competitive groups are more likely to experience recurring conflict than cooperative groups. The leader concerned with productivity overcomes conflict to reach the group goals, and the leader concerned with relationships avoids conflict at all costs. These styles are identified and assessed in the conflict management grid (see Figure 9.7). The resolution of conflict is a six-stage procedure of (1) identifying the problem, (2) diagnosing the problem, (3) generating alternatives, (4) selecting solutions, (5) implementing a solution, and (6) evaluating the solution. This section also describes how decisions can be made.

GROUP DYNAMICS EXERCISES

These exercises enable the reader to apply the theories and principles espoused in this chapter. Each exercise highlights aspects of group interaction and leadership that will be relevant to the fitness professional's environment. To promote honesty and a high comfort level, perform the activities in small groups. For each exercise, read the objective and follow the instructions under "Task" and "Discussion." Note that a time limit is suggested for each exercise.

Leadership

Exercise 1: Understanding Leadership Perspectives

Objective: To understand the functions of leadership by applying leadership characteristics to a personalized work role.

Task: The group divides into subgroups of five or six. Each person envisions a leadership role that he or she has held. List and describe the practical ways in which Stogdill's 11 perspectives on leadership apply to that role.

Discussion: The group members share their responses. What are some ways in which these perspectives could be misused? How could they strengthen a leadership position?

Time: 45 minutes

Exercise 2: Personalizing Leadership

Objective: To understand ways in which our individuality and personality can affect leadership style.

Task: The group divides into subgroups of four to six. Subgroup members identify what they believe to be their most salient personality characteristics.

Discussion: Members discuss how they believe their leadership ability as a fitness professional will be affected by each characteristic, positively and negatively.

Variation: The group members may identify other members' positive personality characteristics and describe how the characteristics can be helpful.

Time: 30 minutes

Exercise 3: Decision Making

Objective: To understand and be able to apply decision-making methods to actual problems.

Task: Individuals form groups of five or six and identify a leadership problem that each has recently dealt with. Then each member applies the problem attributes and questions as they appear on Vroom's decision tree to the identified problem.

Discussion: Each group discusses the differences between the solutions they reached in their original decision and the solutions reached through the decision tree. Would the decisions have been different had this method of assessment been used?

Time: 30 minutes

Exercise 4: Characteristics of Power

Objective: To better understand the relationship between characteristics of power and effective leadership.

Task: Members form groups of five or six. Each member identifies several people they believe to be effective leaders and lists the characteristics that contribute to those leaders' effectiveness.

Discussion: Each member applies the sources of power identified by French and Raven (see pp. 178 to 179 in this text) to the individuals selected as effective leaders. Which sources of power can be attributed to these individuals and how do they combine different sources of power to increase their influence?

Time: 45 minutes

Exercise 5: Personalized Use of Power

Objective: To apply types of power to one's own role and setting.

Task: Individuals divide into groups of four to six. Members identify specific roles and specific settings in which they hold some form of leadership responsibility.

Discussion: Members discuss the types of power as identified by French and Raven that they believe they exercise. In what settings are these kinds of power used and how might the members' effectiveness be improved?

Time: 30 minutes

Structure

Exercise 6: The Influence of Norms

Objective: To understand the impact of norms on a group and on individual members.

Task: Members in groups of five or six think back to high school years. They list and describe norms of dress and behavior.

Discussion: The group discusses the behaviors and modes of dress that were "in" and those that were "out." Members discuss their conformity or nonconformity to the norms.

Time: 45 minutes

Exercise 7: Individual Role and Participation Within Different Groups

Objective: To identify differences in roles, involvement, and interaction of individuals in different groups.

Task: In groups of four to six, individuals identify and describe two different groups of which they are members.

Discussion: Members discuss how they participate differently in each group based on (1) who they talk to and how much they talk, (2) the degree of member responsibility, (3) the role they play, and (4) feelings of belonging.

Time: 45 minutes

Exercise 8: Awareness of the Operation of Group Norms

Objective: To observe informal norms in a group.

Task: Class members observe a selected class or group to which they belong. Observers notice and record the group leaders' reactions to deviations from the norm in such areas as class members arriving late, being unprepared, leaving early, being distracting, talking in class, or exhibiting attention-getting behaviors.

Discussion: Each member discusses his or her observations.

Time: 30 minutes observing and 45 minutes for discussion

Group Communication

Exercise 9: Self-Disclosure and Feedback Communication Process

Objective: To gain greater understanding of individual behavior and feelings within the context of a group.

Task: In groups of five or six, individuals draw their own Johari Windows (see Figure 9.6) according to how they see themselves in social and work settings.

Discussion: Individuals discuss (a) which experiences and beliefs were influential in forming the Johari pattern, (b) in which direction the member would like to change, and (c) in which direction would it be easier to change and in which would it be harder?

Time: 15 minutes for leader to explain the Johari Window and 30 minutes for task and discussion

Exercise 10: Increasing the Effectiveness of Group Communication

Objective: To identify and implement communication factors that enhance effectiveness.

Task: Individuals recall two groups in which they participated regularly: one that was effective in group communication and one that was ineffective. Members list and identify characteristics of each. Each group should be considered in terms of Napier and Gershenfeld's influential factors in group communication (see pages 186 to 187).

Discussion: Members discuss how the identified groups compare on these dimensions.

Time: 45 minutes

Group Conflict

Exercise 11: Conflict Management Style

Objective: To better understand management styles in times of group conflict.

Task: Members divide into groups of four to six. They identify individuals who have handled conflict situations and list characteristics of these individuals.

Discussion: Members discuss which style on the conflict management grid (see Figure 9.7) best describes them and how effective their management style would be.

Time: 10 minutes for leader to explain conflict grid and 30 minutes for task and discussion

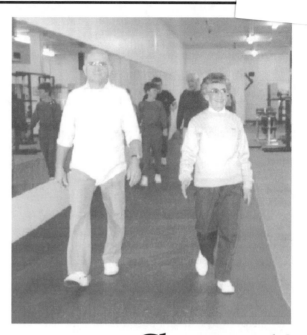

Chapter 10
Exercise and Special Groups

In this chapter we shall look at the psychological implications of exercise for certain special populations as well as important implications for the exercise professional. The special groups we will address include people with heart disease, obese people, the elderly, children, and people with physical disabilities. As medical personnel become more knowledgeable of the benefits of exercise and increasingly recommend it for their patients, the exercise practitioner can expect to see more people with special needs. Exercise can make a significant contribution to the health and quality of life of people in these groups. Moreover, positive psychological effects are a significant part of the overall benefits of physical activity.

PEOPLE WITH CORONARY HEART DISEASE

Coronary heart disease is the leading cause of death in North America and in most other industrialized nations. Thousands of people suffer from the effects of heart disease each year. Many of these people are placed in group programs that feature exercise as one of the primary modes of rehabilitation. In this section, we shall discuss the psychological impact of coronary heart disease and the role of exercise in the emotional and physical rehabilitation of the patient. This discussion applies not only to the rehabilitation of myocardial infarction patients but also to those recovering from coronary bypass surgery.

Despite a 30% drop in mortality attributed to coronary heart disease since 1968, it remains the Number 1 killer in the United States (Oldridge, 1988b). This encouraging decline in mortality has been associated with decreases in risk factors and changes in lifestyles. Risk factors are classified as either primary or secondary. Primary risk factors are those believed to have a major influence on the progression of atherosclerotic disease but that can be controlled or altered (Hall, 1984). Hypertension, hyperlipidemia, and smoking are examples of primary risk factors. Secondary risk factors may or may not be under an individual's control. The secondary factors that can be modified are exercise and obesity, while age, gender, and heredity are obviously beyond an individual's control. At the present it is generally believed that there is no way to remove or reduce the risk associated with the secondary factor of diabetes, even when the diabetes is treated (Hall, 1984).

In recent years, the contributions of psychological risk factors to coronary heart disease have been debated extensively. The debate has centered on the relationship between Type A behavior and coronary heart disease. Although there is considerable evidence to support this relationship, several recent studies have failed to corroborate the relationship between global measures of Type A behavior and coronary heart disease (Costa et al., 1987). However, some specific components of Type A behavior have been found to relate to coronary heart disease. Irritability, anger, and cynicism have been associated with coronary heart disease, whereas global Type A scores and subcomponents, such as ambition and hurrying, may not be related to coronary heart disease (Costa et al., 1987).

Psychological Implications of Myocardial Infarction

The psychological impact of experiencing a myocardial infarction is considerable. Many people who experience chest pains and other symptoms of myocardial infarction often discount or minimize their discomfort and may delay treatment for several hours. The typical reaction to symptoms of a myocardial infarction is disbelief and denial. A person experiencing denial consciously or unconsciously repudiates all or part of the meaning of an event to lessen fear, anxiety, or other unpleasant effects (Soloff & Bartel, 1979). Denial is thought to significantly alter the recognition of symptoms and their seriousness, and apparently is unaffected by previous experience (Hall, 1984). Despite this, denial helps many patients cope with anxiety and fear during the acute phase of post-infarction care. However, if denial is carried over into convalescence, the patient may not comply with rehabilitation. Such patients often disregard dietary restrictions, fail to take prescribed medications, or refuse to cooperate with other treatment recommendations. Deniers are prime candidates for not attending or dropping out of cardiac rehabilitation programs.

Approximately three to five days after the infarction, the patient usually moves into a second stage of psychological distress. Denial and feelings of desperation give way to an acknowledgment of what has occurred and the considerable implications of the event. The fact of having to live with a damaged heart is a serious blow to one's self-esteem and often leads to a period of depression. The perception of no longer being healthy and vigorous and the resulting loss of self-confidence, independence, and self-direction along with the fear of losing one's earning power and sexual prowess causes an inevitable sense of despair. Because depression is a serious barrier to recovery, the patient is encouraged to express these feelings as well as feelings of anger and frustration (Hall, 1984). However, there is some evidence that encouraging patients to express feelings of anxiety and fear only works for patients who do not adopt denial as a coping mechanism (Gentry & Haney, 1975). Deniers tend to show more stress when encouraged to express these feelings. Depression often continues well after the patient returns home. Many people are totally unprepared for the physical limitations they experience upon their release from the hospital (Wishnie, Hackett, & Cassem, 1971). Physical weakness prevents a quick return to a normal routine and may cause despair and depression for up to 6 months or a year. High percentages of coronary heart disease patients report feelings of anxiety, depression, insomnia, and weakness. Among the most common fears are pain, dyspnea (difficulty getting sufficient oxygen), and having another infarction. Again, patients are encouraged to work through these normal emotional processes until they have accepted the situation. Failure to accept one's condition may lead to either denial or cardiac invalidism. As mentioned earlier, denial at this stage is associated with failure to comply with rehabilitation procedures. Cardiac invalids, on the other hand, habitually allow themselves to be overprotected and pampered. Establishing a program of rehabilitation and returning to a stable psychological state are crucial to the coronary heart disease patient resuming some degree of normalcy (Hall, 1984).

A myocardial infarction also affects people other than the patient. At the very least, family life is disrupted, and at worst, the family structure may undergo major alterations. Often, financial woes are at the center of the family crisis. One study found that 9 out of 24 patients had to make major changes in their living arrangements, including four patients who were forced to sell their homes (Wishnie et al., 1971). Family members in this study also experienced significant anxiety about the patient's recuperation and their role in the process. Wives in particular tended to be overprotective, sometimes to the point of hindering the patient's recovery. This overprotectiveness had a deleterious effect on the marriage as well. Conflicts between patients and family members were found to occur even in marriages that were stable before the myocardial infarction. Not surprisingly, long-standing marital problems tended to worsen as well. Interpersonal friction was often related to misunderstanding the nature of coronary disease and misinterpreting the physician's instructions.

The spouse should be involved in the cardiac rehabilitation program for several reasons. They are a major source of social support for the patient, and spouses need emotional support themselves. Because they will be involved with the patient's efforts to live a healthier lifestyle, spouses need to understand the doctor's recommendations and why they are important (Anderson, 1983). Spouses can be involved in classes or lectures, in a support group of other cardiac spouses, or even in counseling when necessary.

A dramatic way of demonstrating the patients' capabilities to their spouses is to involve the spouses in the diagnostic stress test. A study that compared 10 wives who were uninvolved, 10 who observed their husband's stress test, and 10 who observed and then participated in the test themselves showed clear perceptual differences (Taylor, Bandura et al., 1985). Wives' confidence ratings in their husbands' physical capabilities were significantly higher for those who also performed the test than for the two groups who did not. This method was viewed as a good way to reassure spouses about their partner's capacity for safely resuming normal physical activities.

The Efficacy of Cardiac Rehabilitation

Cardiac rehabilitation programs that feature exercise have increased considerably in recent years. The major objectives of cardiac rehabilitation include increased functional capacity, improved quality of life, and reduced mortality and morbidity (Oldridge, 1988b). Not long ago, the myocardial infarction patient was assigned to bed for a month or more. Now the trend is for the patient to become ambulatory as soon as possible. Cardiac rehabilitation programs vary greatly. Some programs use exercise only, while others tackle other contributing factors, such as smoking, obesity and nutritional problems, psychological disorders, and stress. The wide range of programs probably reflects the relative newness of the field. After more and better research, the most effective programs will be implemented more universally (Peterson, 1983).

Psychological and behavioral changes are important parts of the rehabilitation program. The rehabilitation program that includes exercise, proper eating, smoking cessation, and ways to cope with stressors involves changing old behaviors and beginning new ones. The success of a cardiac rehabilitation program, therefore, depends on its ability to foster these behavioral changes in its patients. The program leadership must provide a setting that will foster behavioral change. The enthusiasm, concern, and optimism of the staff as well as the support of other patients are important components of the behavioral change process (Anderson, 1987).

Most cardiac rehabilitation programs are based on the assumption that post-infarction exercise training yields physiological and psychological outcomes that improve the patient's long-term prognosis. However, some skeptics suggest that these programs unnecessarily put patients at risk, are expensive, and promise little proven benefit. Indeed, cardiac rehabilitation has not yet been universally accepted as the treatment of choice for coronary heart disease.

Blackburn (1974) presented a negative position on exercise rehabilitation. Point by point, he refuted findings that are most often used to justify exercise programs. He evaluated the evidence of changes in cardiovascular functioning resulting from exercise training as minor, equivocal, or absent. Another aspect of the controversy centers on the lack of knowledge of the criteria used to select patients for rehabilitation and how to properly prescribe exercise. Indications, contraindications, and eligibility criteria for exercise training are not firm, and individual exercise prescriptions are difficult to determine, administer, or control. Moreover, there is little professional knowledge and experience in this area and few medical facilities available to conduct exercise therapy. According to Blackburn, there is little evidence that exercise reduces coronary risk factors, primarily because of weaknesses in the research involving selection biases and confounding effects of therapeutic changes. In summary, Blackburn cautions against the hasty adoption of an unproven and costly therapeutic regimen. Instead, he recommends that patients be encouraged to adopt a new way of life that includes a gradual increase in exercise in the form of walking and changes in eating, smoking, and drinking habits.

In a controlled study of English postmyocardial infarction patients, Mayou (1980) found that the exercise treatment group performed significantly better on a bicycle ergometer test than subjects in a regular treatment control group or a counseling placebo group. However, their superior performance was attributed to increased confidence rather than to a physiological training effect. Mayou also observed that, despite considerable enthusiasm for exercise in the experimental group, there were no psychological benefits from participating in the exercise rehabilitation program. He suggested that due to the high cost of rehabilitation, only high-risk patients be offered the more intensive program of exercise rehabilitation. Mayou's recommendation for the "best possible aftercare" was to offer a basic program of advice, discussion, and booklets, along with systematic monitoring of indicators of progress.

In contrast to the previously discussed findings, the medical and psychological literature does contain considerable support for the effectiveness of exercise rehabilitation following myocardial infarction or heart surgery. Although Haskell (1974) acknowledged the lack of evidence for the influence of physical activity on cardiovascular morbidity or mortality, he reviewed the existing evidence on several additional claims associated with exercise rehabilitation. Haskell concluded that through proper patient selection, exercise prescription, program supervision, and periodic re-evaluation, postmyocardial infarction patients can safely increase their levels of physical activity. Moreover, his assessment of the substantiated benefits of increased activity included fewer complications than associated with bed rest and an increased symptom-free working capacity resulting from improved blood circulation and metabolic function. In addition, a more successful psychological adjustment and a more frequent and earlier return to employment were noted.

Results of a study of 651 postmyocardial infarction patients in a 3-year randomized clinical trial of the effects of prescribed exercise generally favored exercise training (L.W. Shaw, 1981). Although not statistically significant, the 3-year mortality rate was 7.3% for the control group and 4.6% for the exercise group. The rate for recurrent myocardial infarction was 7.0% and 5.3%, respectively. Although this study provided some support for exercise rehabilitation, the evidence was not convincing. A study with a much larger sample was called for to provide more definitive answers about exercise program efficacy.

A follow-up study of patients 9 years after their participation in an exercise rehabilitation program shed some light on the question of program efficacy (Prosser et al., 1985). Although there was no difference in mortality between the exercise group and nonparticipants, the exercise group was more likely to be symptom free and less likely to have experienced another myocardial infarction. In addition, exercise positively correlated with cardiovascular and general health and negatively correlated with angina. The results of the study encouraged continuing the program and finding ways to help outpatients keep exercising.

One of the major problems in making the case for cardiac rehabilitation has been the lack of randomized clinical research studies demonstrating that exercise does have an effect on mortality and morbidity. Oldridge, Guyatt, Fisher, and Rimm (1988) pooled the results of 10 published randomized controlled trials of mortality and morbidity and found that cardiac rehabilitation significantly reduced all-cause mortality by 24% and cardiovascular mortality by 25%. For reasons that are unclear, there was no significant difference in groups in nonfatal recurrent myocardial infarction. The researchers identified several possible mechanisms that may explain the lower mortality in rehabilitation patients including improved cardiovascular revascularization, protection against fatal dysrhythmias, decreased risk factors, improved cardiovascular fitness, and increased patient surveillance by the medical staff.

Despite the lack of overwhelming evidence that cardiac rehabilitation prevents the recurrence of myocardial infarction, reduces mortality, and improves quality of life, it is without question a treatment approach that is here to stay. Wilson (1988) sees an extension of the expertise developed in cardiac rehabilitation programs to other dysfunctions such as diabetes, chemical dependency, and psychiatric disorders. According to Wilson, future programs will include a great deal more than exercise. Multifaceted programs that offer a variety of educational services will become the standard. A comprehensive program will include nutrition, smoking termination, relaxation skills, stress reduction, and vocational rehabilitation. Emphasis will be placed on a healthy lifestyle and a lifetime commitment to all aspects of the program.

Several professional groups have supported exercise training after myocardial infarction. The American College of Sports Medicine, the American Heart Association, the American College of

Cardiology, and the American Association of Cardiovascular and Pulmonary Rehabilitation are the main organizations providing leadership for cardiac rehabilitation in the United States (Wilson, 1988). These organizations train and certify personnel and disseminate information. It is unlikely that these organizations would invest precious resources in cardiac rehabilitation if they did not believe in the efficacy of the treatment. One can only conclude that convincing supporting evidence will be forthcoming.

Psychological Benefits of Cardiac Rehabilitation

According to Anderson (1983, p. 120), "the psychologically therapeutic effects of general program participation on reactive emotional states can be characterized as a nonmedical tranquilizer and antidepressant."

A major advantage of participation in a cardiac rehabilitation program is the improved morale and general outlook of the patient. While still in the hospital, a patient can begin to engage in light exercises. The ability to perform even low-level exercises gives the patient hope, not only for survival but also for a good future (Hackett & Cassem, 1978). Being able to perform exercises at this stage also proves to the patient that recovery is possible and helps dispel fears of invalidism.

Another advantage of early physical conditioning is that it can prevent homecoming depression. By raising self-esteem and promoting a sense of independence, physical conditioning may be one of the most important aspects of convalescence in terms of controlling depression (Hackett & Cassem, 1973). A conditioning program during convalescence also provides structure. Rather than watching TV or sitting around, exercise gives the patient something worthwhile to do. As Hackett and Cassem (1973) noted, in a life filled with "don'ts" (don't smoke, don't rush, don't eat ice cream), physical conditioning stands out as a positive affirmation.

Research on the psychological effects of participation in rehabilitation programs has generally yielded positive results. McPherson and associates (1967) were among the first to explore this relationship. They found that patients who exercised experienced more psychological changes after 24 weeks of an exercise program than those who did not exercise. An improved sense of well-being, increased self-confidence and optimism,

and reduced anxiety and tension were observed in the exercise participants. Favorable short-term mood changes were noted as well. Prosser and colleagues (1981) also observed increased confidence following exercise rehabilitation. Subjects randomly assigned to an exercise program for 3 months had morale scores that correlated positively with work capacity and had significantly lower anxiety scores than control subjects. Researchers in the Netherlands received similar results (Erdman, Hugo, & Duivenvoorden, 1983). In this study, subjects randomly assigned to the exercise rehabilitation group scored lower on anxiety and had fewer feelings of social inadequacy than subjects assigned to a physician-encouraged home rehabilitation program. Self-esteem scores were also higher for the exercise rehabilitation participants.

A study of the effects of long-term participation in exercise rehabilitation found a significant reduction in depression scores (Kavanagh et al., 1977). The decrease in depression was associated with exercise compliance. Subjects who failed to meet the participation standard of 60% of the exercise sessions showed no change in depression scores. Similar results were observed in a study of 106 postmyocardial infarction patients that compared the effectiveness of exercise therapy with group counseling (Stern, Gorman, & Kaslow, 1983). In addition to increasing work capacity and decreasing fatigue, exercise participation reduced anxiety and depression, and promoted independence and sociability.

Although exercise testing soon after myocardial infarction is widely used to determine prognosis and establish guidelines for subsequent exercise, the use of exercise testing for shaping patients' expectations and attitudes has been largely overlooked (Ewart et al., 1983). This study demonstrated that increases in self-efficacy for activities similar to treadmill exercises, such as walking, stair climbing, and running, were greatest following treadmill exercise. In contrast, self-efficacy for dissimilar activities, such as lifting weights or sexual intercourse, were greatest after the test results were explained by a physician or nurse. Additionally, the patients' physical activity at home was correlated with self-efficacy following treadmill testing and counseling. A follow-up study found that the adoption of novel activities was governed by highly specific self-perceptions (Ewart et al., 1986). Circuit weight training yielded greater gains in strength and endurance than volleyball, and subjects who did weight training had increased self-efficacy for similar activities. It was suggested that exercise programs designed to increase self-efficacy should expose participants to a variety of activities with carefully graduated performance goals. Such programs would have a greater psychological and motivational impact than those that emphasize a single task, such as walking or jogging.

The effects of cardiac rehabilitation on mood states also appear to be quite positive (Shephard, Kavanagh, & Klavora, 1985). A group of 317 myocardial infarction patients involved in an exercise program for 1 year showed improvement in five of the six dimensions of the Profile of Mood States. Decreases were noted in tension and anxiety, depression and dejection, anger and hostility, and confusion. An increase in vigor was also observed. However, there was no evidence that psychological gains were related to improvements in physiological conditioning. It was suggested that the period of observation should be longer than 1 year to observe correlations between changes in mood and gains in physiological function.

In spite of the considerable research that generally supports the psychological benefits of cardiac rehabilitation, not all studies have corroborated these findings. For example, the National Exercise and Heart Disease Project compared 651 myocardial infarction patients randomly assigned to either exercise or control conditions at 6 months, 1 year, and 2 years (Stern & Cleary, 1982). No group differences were observed on any of three psychosocial measures at any of the testing periods. The researchers offered several explanations for these results, including an adherence rate of only 48%, a concern about the intensity level of the exercise program, and questions about the sensitivity of the psychological instruments used. The point we want to make is the need for continued research on the psychological effects of cardiac rehabilitation programs.

For the exercise practitioner, most of the suggestions made in chapter 2 concerning the promotion of exercise adherence, techniques for motivation, and behavioral change strategies apply to patients with coronary heart disease. Of special importance with this group, however, is the heightened need for social support, especially from one's spouse. Also not to be overlooked is the importance of support and encouragement from program leaders and other group members. Additional recommendations for working with coronary heart disease patients are to provide them with authoritative counseling about specific details of their exercise prescription and give frequent feedback on progress (Falk, 1986).

THE OBESE

One of the more common complaints that the exercise practitioner encounters in working with clients is the need to lose weight. In this section, we shall review the nature and extent of obesity and the psychosocial problems associated with it. We will then consider the role of exercise in ameliorating the condition and make suggestions for working with obese clients.

Obesity and Health

A person is obese when fat makes up a greater than normal fraction of total body weight (Bray, 1976). At age 18, approximately 15% to 18% of a man's body weight is fat, while for 18-year-old women fat approximates 20% to 25% of body weight. A general guide for determining obesity is body fat content of more than 25% for men and 30% for women. A distinction is usually made between obesity and being "overweight," the latter being defined in relation to standards of desirable weight such as the tables prepared by life insurance companies. An obese person is always overweight but an overweight individual is not necessarily obese.

Between 10% and 20% of children in the United States are obese, and the percentage is rising (Price, Galli, & Slenker, 1985). Because obese children tend to become obese adults, the future looks rather bleak unless something is done to reverse this trend. The situation is no better for adults. The incidence of obesity among adults in the United States has been estimated to be as high as 34% (Heston, 1983). Consider these figures from Dintiman and Greenberg (1983):

■ 50% of men ages 30 to 39 are at least 10% overweight;

■ 60% of men ages 50 to 59 are at least 10% overweight and 33% are at least 20% overweight;

■ the percentage of overweight women under 40 is lower than that of men;

■ the percentages of overweight men and women ages 40 to 49 are identical; and

■ the percentage of overweight women over 49 is greater than that of men.

Obesity is associated with several health risks. Moreover, maladies of almost every body function occur more frequently among the obese than among people of normal weight (Jeffrey & Lemnitzer, 1981). Obese people have a higher incidence of cardiovascular disease including strokes, arteriosclerosis, hypertension, and varicose veins. Susceptibility to these diseases increases 30% for every 10% increase above ideal weight (Jeffrey & Lemnitzer, 1981). The obese also have a higher incidence of respiratory difficulties. They have more problems with arthritis and back pain, as well as hip, knee, and ankle difficulties. Furthermore, obese people suffer more from gall bladder diseases, diabetes, and cancer than people of normal weight. And deaths due to all causes occur at an earlier age for obese people. Mortality rates for men who are markedly overweight are 70% higher than for men of normal weight, and even for moderately overweight men mortality rates are 42% higher. For women the rates are 61% and 42%, respectively (Jeffrey & Lemnitzer, 1981).

Causes of Obesity

Obesity can be caused by several factors, including excessive food consumption, too little exercise, psychological problems, social and cultural influences, physiological imbalances, and heredity (Price et al., 1985). Some people discount organic factors and base the cause for obesity squarely on the law of conservation of energy—that is, to lose weight a person must take in fewer calories than are used up (Mendelson, 1966). In contrast to this rather simplistic point of view, some people believe that obesity may also be attributed to interactions among two or more of the factors cited earlier. Studies of the roles of heredity or environment in obesity have revealed that children with parents of normal weight are obese in only about 7% to 8% of the cases studied. However, when one parent is obese this figure jumps to 40%, and when both parents are obese it rises to 80% (Dintiman and Greenberg, 1983). Studies of identical twins separated at birth and raised separately in different environments also tend to indicate the greater influence of genetic factors over environment in determining obesity. However, this does not mean that environment is inconsequential. Early eating habits are thought to carry over into later life. The parent who insists that a child finish all the food on the plate may establish habits of overeating that could be a factor in the child being overweight or obese later in life.

Another possible cause of obesity is *external cue sensitivity*. External cue sensitivity refers to eating behavior that is largely controlled by environmental cues that are unrelated to the physiological state of hunger. However, an extensive review of the research on aspects of this theory has yielded equivocal results (Leon & Roth, 1977).

Classification Systems

Several classification systems for obesity have been developed. One approach divides obese people into three groups. The first group consists of people who are *naturally* overweight and whose weight has no relation to emotional problems (Mendelson, 1966). The second group, described as the *reactively* obese, is composed of individuals who overeat in times of psychological stress or deprivation. The reactively obese overeat to reduce feelings of tension, loneliness, or as a substitute gratification in unpleasant life situations. The third group, called the *developmentally* obese, are people who have been obese all their lives and for whom being overweight has been an integral part of their growth and development. Concern with size and weight and an inability to tolerate frustration or delay in gratification are central to their development (Mendelson, 1966). Another classification scheme is based on the age of the person at the onset of obesity. *Juvenile obesity* refers to people who first became obese in childhood or adolescence. *Adult obesity* refers to people who first became obese after adolescence.

Mendelson (1966) devised a continuum characterized by increasing emotional instability to conceptualize the complex psychological components of obesity. At the low end of the continuum are those who are emotionally stable, about 20% to 25% of the obese. Farther along the continuum are those who eat for emotional reasons. At this point on the continuum, hyperphagia (extreme overeating) may occur only at certain levels of intensity or may occur sporadically at times of considerable stress. At the high end of the continuum are individuals whose eating disorders are central issues in their lives. A preoccupation with food at every hour of the day is typical of this group.

Psychosocial Implications of Obesity

Obese people are devalued by society, which often results in self-devaluation. Society perceives obese people as inadequate, unattractive, weak-willed, and less intelligent (Price et al., 1985). Obesity is also associated with social position. One study revealed a striking relationship between socioeconomic status of origin and obesity (Moore,

Stunkard, & Srole, 1962). In this study, the prevalence of obesity was 7 times greater among women raised in the lowest social class than for women reared in the highest social class.

Prejudice against obese people begins in childhood and continues throughout life. Obese children are teased and ridiculed and often left out of social and athletic activities. This alienation often leads to withdrawal. The cycle of rejection and isolation often causes the obese child to substitute eating for acceptance. Overweight adults typically face difficulties in interpersonal relationships and career progress. Perceptions that obese people are less competent, less productive, indecisive, mentally lazy, and lacking in self-discipline make potential employers wary of hiring these people (Price et al., 1985).

Given these social difficulties, one might assume obese people would experience a disproportionate share of psychological problems. However, there is some controversy on this point. After reviewing the research, Hayes and Ross (1986) concluded that there was no evidence that being overweight increased psychological distress. This conclusion was corroborated by their own research on a community sample that demonstrated that being overweight did not decrease psychological well-being. This result was consistent across all income groups.

However, some researchers believe that dieting increases the likelihood of emotional disturbance. According to Wilson and Brownell (1980), depression, anxiety, fatigue, irritability, or similar symptoms occur in at least 50% of all dieters. Such disturbances may be the emotional response to inability to control eating habits or signs of psychological distress stemming from movement away from one's biologically natural weight.

After summarizing the literature on the effects of obesity on emotions, Storlie (1984) found studies in which obese people were characterized as more troubled, frustrated, overwrought, and submissive as well as prone to exhibit higher levels of anxiety, repression, and defensiveness. Low self-esteem, body-image disturbances, and poor communication skills were also associated with obesity. Storlie pointed out that although these affective characteristics may apply to the obese as a whole, not all obese people manifest these disturbances.

Personality does not appear to be a factor in obesity. Although considerable effort has gone into the psychological appraisal of obese clients, no one has identified a typical personality or behavioral structure (Storlie, 1984). A study on the prevalence of neuroticism and psychiatric disturbance among obese people found that the incidence of these disturbances was no greater among obese people than among people of normal weight (Silverstone, 1968). Similarly, a study that used the MMPI to detect an obese "profile" found diverse behavior patterns among the obese (Johnson, Swenson, & Gastineau, 1976). A review by Hallstrom and Noppa (1981) found no definite relationships between obesity and mental illness. In a community study involving 401 subjects, Hayes and Ross (1986) also found obesity to be unrelated to psychological distress.

The locus-of-control construct has shown some promise in the treatment of obesity (Pemberton, 1984). There is some evidence that the locus of control may predict success in dieting. People with an internal locus of control are more likely to succeed in programs that emphasize self-direction and self-reinforcement, while externally controlled people may require more attention, reinforcement, and direction from a clinician. There is some evidence that locus of control may change as a result of weight reduction and exercise training (Speaker, Schultz, Grinker, & Stern, 1983). In a study of obese adolescent boys who attended a 7-week summer camp that offered a program of increased physical activity and controlled diet there were weight losses averaging 29.3 pounds and decreases in body fat of 11.5%. The boys' loci of control became significantly more internal over the course of the program. The researchers suggested that the experience of seeing their efforts pay off in increased physical performance and weight loss may have led to the change to a more internal locus.

Body-Image Disturbances

Body-image disturbances are relatively common among the obese, particularly among the juvenile obese. *Body image* refers to the concept a person has of his or her body as an object in space, independent of all other objects (Stunkard & Mendelson, 1961). The body image develops during infancy and childhood and changes radically during adolescence. Under normal circumstances, body image is a natural part of our existence. However, when this image is disturbed, it can strongly affect a person's life. Among the obese, body-image disturbances usually take the form of an overwhelming preoccupation with being overweight. Obese people often perceive their bodies as grotesque and loathsome and believe that others can see them only with horror and contempt (Stunkard & Mendelson, 1961).

Mendelson (1966) reported that almost half of juvenile obese medical patients he studied had severely disturbed body images and self-concepts with accompanying impairments in interpersonal and heterosexual adjustment. However, in a group of obese adults, none of the people had the same degree of body-image disturbance. Statements of subjects with disturbed body image are characterized by extreme self-loathing and disgust, while those without body-image disturbances seem almost unaware of their extreme condition.

Three factors seem to predispose the development of a disturbed body-image: (a) age at the onset of obesity, (b) the presence of neurosis, and (c) the parental evaluation of the obese person (Stunkard & Mendelson, 1961). As noted previously, body-image disturbance occurs almost exclusively among those who became obese during childhood or adolescence. Secondly, a disturbed family environment and the development of emotional problems predispose one to body-image disturbances. Finally, in a disturbed family environment, the child's obesity often becomes the focus of parental hostility and contempt, which the child internalizes. It is interesting to note that gender, degree of obesity, and intelligence have not been found to be important factors in body-image disturbance (Stunkard & Mendelson, 1961).

Although intensive psychotherapy can modify body-image disturbances, this approach is generally available only to a few. The more beneficial approach would be to emphasize prevention (Stunkard & Mendelson, 1961). The prevention of obesity would likely reduce the occurrence of body-image disturbance and the associated emotional distress.

Treatment of Obesity

Despite the pervasiveness of the problem and the extensive research devoted to the treatment of obesity in the past 2 decades, successful weight loss and maintenance of the loss over time remain elusive, perplexing, and frustrating. As one researcher has observed, if one defines successful treatment as a return to ideal body weight and maintenance for 5 years, a person is more likely to recover from almost any form of cancer than to successfully conquer obesity (Brownell, 1982).

Although this pessimistic view may discourage the practitioner, one should remember that there are some success stories. If these few people can be successful, perhaps we can learn to duplicate their success with other clients. An awareness of the current treatment methods would seem a desirable place to start. There are numerous approaches to the treatment of obesity, many of which are of questionable value. Jordan (1987) has reviewed these methods, which we shall briefly summarize.

Drugs

The use of appetite-suppressant drugs is based on the belief that overeating is the result of uncontrolled hunger. Although amphetamines were initially used as appetite suppressants, phenylpropanolamine has increasingly been used for this purpose and is found in at least 64 over-the-counter products. There is almost no evidence that these medications are of long-term value in controlling weight. Moreover, there are many reports of negative side effects.

Hormones have also been used to treat obesity, most notably human chorionic gonadotrophin (HCG) hormone. HCG is administered in daily injections and is usually used in combination with a restrictive diet. However, controlled studies have shown no advantage of HCG over placebo injections and its popularity is diminishing.

Also somewhat popular for treatment of obesity are drugs that interfere with the absorption of certain nutritional elements. The most common of these are the so-called starch blockers. Despite a lack of evidence to support their effectiveness, many thousands are still being sold.

Surgery

A rather drastic approach to the treatment of obesity is surgery. The first surgical technique used for this purpose was the ileojejunal bypass operation. This surgical technique creates a malabsorption syndrome by surgically rearranging portions of the gastrointestinal tract to bypass large segments of the small intestine. Although weight loss was often dramatic after this procedure, long-term adverse side effects has led to the development of new techniques that alter the anatomy of the stomach. However, even the newer procedures to reduce stomach size have experienced failure rates of about 50%.

Jaw Wiring

A slightly less drastic procedure is jaw wiring in which the teeth are wired together to prevent normal eating. Although this technique has been effective in producing weight loss, most people gain the weight back when the wires are removed.

Purging

Many people with eating disorders use emetics and purgatives to control their weight. Agents of this sort produce vomiting or the rapid movement of food through the gastrointestinal tract. The use of purgatives and laxatives to control weight should be discouraged because of the potential medical danger as well as the lack of effectiveness of treatment.

Dieting

The most universal intervention for obesity is to diet. People who are anxious to lose weight are even willing to try outlandish, unsafe diets. The DuPont Diet, The Drinking Man's Diet, Dr. Stillman's Quick Weight Loss Diet, Dr. Atkin's Diet Revolution, The Scarsdale Diet, The Cambridge Diet, and The Beverly Hills Diet are just a few of the famous diets of the last 3 decades (Stern, 1983). Almost all of these fad diets have used a basic formula: capitalize on a person's fear of being obese and promise an effortless, instant, and painless cure—often without feeling hungry or having to exercise. Most fad diets forego scientific research on their effectiveness and therefore the scrutiny of peer review, relying instead on testimonials of people who reportedly have had success with the diet (Stern 1983).

Stern (1983) identified four criteria for evaluating a diet program:

■ Does the information provided go beyond personal observation?

■ Have the observations been evaluated using adequate scientific controls in a double-blind design?

■ Is the diet safe?

■ Is the diet effective in promoting fat loss?

Although a nutritionally balanced and calorically restricted diet is important in the treatment of obesity, the success rate for even medically sound dieting is very low. Dieting should be just a part of a comprehensive program tailored to the individual's needs and lifestyle.

Behavioral Approaches to Treatment

Most of the behavioral change techniques discussed in chapter 7 apply to the treatment of obesity. Indeed, a wide range of behavior therapies have been employed in obesity research. Although results of these studies have not been impressive, the record of success with behavioral methods is about as good as with any other treatment method (Wilson & Brownell, 1980).

Exercise and Obesity

It is probably no accident that obesity has soared as the necessity to exert physical effort has declined. The penchant for doing things the easy way and labor-saving devices have produced a generation of children and adults with poor muscle tone and poor cardiovascular fitness. Moreover, the incidence of obesity in the United States is higher now than early in this century, yet the per capita caloric intake is approximately 5% less now than it was in 1910 (Stern, 1983). In this section, we shall look at the relationship between exercise and obesity from two perspectives: first, lack of exercise in the development of obesity and second, exercise in the treatment of obesity.

Exercise and the Development of Obesity

Several prominent researchers believe that physical inactivity rather than diet is the major contributor to obesity. In studies of adolescent girls and young babies, Jean Mayer (1968) found inactivity to be the major cause of fatness rather than food intake. In fact, obese girls seemed to eat slightly less than girls of normal weight, but they also exercised considerably less. Fat babies also ate less and were less active, while thin babies took in considerably more food and were very active.

The role of energy expenditure in the development of obesity is not as straightforward as it might appear. There is some evidence that obese children are just as active as their nonobese peers, while obese adults seem to be less active than adults of normal weight (Brownell & Stunkard, 1980). This inconsistency suggests that inactivity is more a consequence of obesity than a cause. Other studies have found that obese adults often eat no more than people of normal weight, but they also exercise a great deal less. A review of the role of activity level and caloric intake in the development of obesity concluded that the relationship between the two factors was unclear, due primarily to methodological limitations of the research (Thompson, Jarvie, Lahey, & Cureton, 1982).

Exercise in the Treatment of Obesity

Physical activity produces a complex series of metabolic consequences that can affect body weight, body composition, and basal metabolism. Although lean body mass increases with physical activity, because lean tissue is more dense than the fat it replaces, body weight may not change much. A study of 11 obese women who progressively increased daily walking over a year or more with no dietary restrictions found weight loss to be slow and much less than anticipated (Gwinup, 1975). An analysis of exercise and weight loss studies using meta-analytic techniques also found weight loss due solely to exercise to be quite small when compared to other forms of weight control (Epstein & Wing, 1980).

Slow progress and modest weight losses are often disappointing to people who have exercised vigorously for a long time. However, exercise may still play an important role in the treatment of obesity (Brownell & Stunkard, 1980). In summing up the rationale for including exercise in a weight loss program, Brownell and Stunkard concluded that even though the immediate effects of exercise are limited, the cumulative effects of even small increases in physical activity may be beneficial over the long term. They also concluded that the loss of lean body mass during weight reduction is minimized when both diet and exercise are used together as compared to dieting alone. They also noted that exercise often decreases appetite, particularly among the more obese subjects. An increase in basal metabolism accompanying regular exercise can also promote weight loss and help counteract a decrease in metabolic rate produced by restricted caloric intake. Caloric restriction alone typically reduces basal metabolic rate by 15% to 30%, which hampers or even prevents further weight loss.

It is not clear why more people do not choose exercise as a primary means of losing weight. Many people apparently believe that dieting is easier and less disruptive to their lives (Dwyer, Feldman, & Mayer, 1970), and some people mistakenly believe that they are not inactive. But the best approach to losing weight seems to be to combine exercise with caloric restriction. This approach accelerates the rate of weight loss produced by either exercise or diet alone (Stern, 1983). Some experienced clinicians believe that no weight control program can be successful without regular exercise. For long-term success, exercise must become a permanent part of a new lifestyle (Altschul, 1987).

Implications for the Practitioner

Exercise practitioners should study the methods used in successful weight loss programs to learn what works. One such program started with 11 female subjects and grew to include 100 women (Kindl & Brown, 1976). Subjects involved in the program for 6 months to a year averaged weight losses of 26 pounds and a decrease in body fat of 41% to 29%. This program had three major

components: exercise, diet counseling, and group interaction. The exercise component was designed to be enjoyable and included flexibility, aerobic, relaxation, and aquatic activities. Music and rhythmic activities were regular program features and clients were instructed in ways to incorporate physical activity into their lifestyles.

Epstein and associates demonstrated the superiority of lifestyle exercise over programmed exercise in maintaining weight loss among obese children (Epstein, Wing, Koeske, Ossip, & Beck, 1982; Epstein, Wing, Koeske, & Valoski, 1985). They used a point system based upon metabolic equivalents for both lifestyle and programmed exercise groups. Programmed exercise group members were required to pick one aerobic exercise from a list provided and do it daily, while the lifestyle group members were encouraged to earn their exercise points in any way they wanted by choosing from a list of common childhood activities. Lifestyle subjects were given considerable flexibility in the choice of activities, scheduling, and intensity of exercise as compared to the programmed group. Although both groups lost weight and improved fitness during the 6-month treatment phase, only the lifestyle subjects continued to lose weight and maintain their improved fitness levels during the maintenance phase of 11 months. The researchers suggested that the lifestyle program provided opportunities for changes that were better incorporated into a person's routine than a rigid schedule of exercise. Other possible reasons for the differences included the greater fatigue and soreness associated with programmed exercise, the need to set aside blocks of time, and the necessity of traveling to special sites to participate.

A recent study of an exercise program for overweight women offered some interesting insights into factors that contribute to program success (Bain, Wilson, & Chaikind, 1989). The researchers offered several practical suggestions for working with obese clients:

■ Because many obese people feel self-conscious and embarrassed about exercising in public, separate classes for overweight beginners can help minimize this concern.

■ A successful exercise class for overweight people requires attention to the needs and concerns of the participants. A qualified instructor who is nonjudgmental is the most critical factor.

■ Creating a climate of social support is also important to program success. Maintaining group stability and providing ample opportunities for discussion of common problems are crucial.

■ Because overweight people are particularly put off by "hard-core" exercisers, sensitive to people observing their arrival and departure, and self-conscious of people watching their exercise sessions, classes should be scheduled to minimize these types of exposure.

■ The goals and content of the program should be appropriate for the group. Rigid or unrealistic goals should be discouraged because of the likelihood of failure.

■ A climate in which participants feel free to offer suggestions about the content and conduct of the program can contribute to its success. An atmosphere of collaboration permits shared goals and communicates respect for the clients.

Some helpful techniques for maintaining gains made in treatment programs include the continued monitoring of key behaviors, frequent phone contacts with therapists, and peer-group support (Perri, Lauer, McAdoo, McAllister, & Yancey, 1986). Social pressure in the form of phone calls and follow-up letters are suggested ways of preventing attrition as well as the use of the group as a source of approval or disapproval of attendance patterns (Hagen, Foreyt, & Durham, 1976). Requiring program participants to deposit personal items of some value for return at the end of the program was also observed to be an effective means of preventing attrition in the Hagen et al. (1976) study.

Support from family members is also important to successful weight loss and maintenance. Matson (1977) demonstrated the effectiveness of praise from a spouse in helping reduce and maintain weight loss over 90 weeks. Epstein and colleagues (1984) observed that including parents in the treatment of the child was helpful. Training spouses has also been reported to be effective not only in a weight-loss program but also in maintaining long-term weight loss (Brownell, Heckerman, Westlake, Hayes, & Monti, 1978). A spouse is likely to check dietary transgressions and, perhaps more importantly, to provide strong, immediate reinforcement for appropriate eating behavior.

THE ELDERLY

Sometimes referred to as the "graying" of America (Ostrow, 1984), the North American population is aging. According to the U.S. Census Bureau, in July 1988 the number of Americans ages 35 to 59

surpassed the number of citizens ages 18 to 34 for the first time in history (DiMambro & Wolfe, 1989). Americans 60 and older now outnumber children under 10 and teenagers (ages 13 to 19). In a culture that has long had a youthful orientation, there is certain to be greater attention to issues and interests of older citizens. Because health is a major concern of older people, an increased focus on preventing disease and improving quality of life is inevitable. Exercise is one way to improve quality of life for older citizens. Although regular exercise may not enable a person to live longer, the active senior has more energy and leads a vigorous, independent life. In this section, we shall address the issues of aging that are most important to the exercise professional.

Not only is America aging, it is aging quickly. From 1980 to 1985 the number of older Americans incrased by 11%, while the population below 65 increased only 4%. By the year 2000 the over-65 group is expected to represent 13% of the population. This percentage is predicted to climb to 21% by the year 2030, representing an estimated 64.6 million people (Ostrow, 1984).

Older people are also living longer. In 1985, there were 8.8 million people between the ages of 75 and 84 and 2.7 million people over 85. Compared to 1900, the number of people in the 75 to 84 group is 11 times larger, and the number of people over 85 is 22 times larger. These longer life spans can be attributed to control of communicable diseases, improved health care, better nutrition, improved sanitary conditions, advances in occupational safety, greater knowledge of hygienic principles, and better child-care practices (Ostrow, 1984).

The trend toward a more mature populace has not gone unnoticed by government or industry. In the 1970s, The Older Americans Act directed the Administration on Aging to encourage the development of services to help older Americans attain and maintain physical and mental well-being through exercise and physical activity (Conrad, 1976). More recently, the International Racquet Sports Association, an organization of professional fitness clubs, identified the over-40 age group as an important area of potential growth and suggested that marketing be directed to this segment of the population (DiMambro & Wolfe, 1989).

Misconceptions about aging abound. Many believe that most people over 65 are senile, institutionalized, in poor health, and live in poverty, loneliness, and isolation (McPherson, 1986). In actuality, a majority of seniors are independent, live in the community, and lead active lives. Only 4% of people over 65 are institutionalized and, even more remarkably, only 17% of people over 85 live in institutions (Ostrow, 1984). Most seniors can participate in physical activity programs as long as proper safeguards are maintained.

The Aging Process

Aging happens to different people at different rates. Although the government and most businesses stipulate 65 as the age at which one is officially considered "old," this is little more than an arbitrary method for deciding when a person is no longer productive. To fix old age at a given point ignores the difference between chronological age and physiological or biological age. Two 60-year-old people may be vastly different physically, mentally, and emotionally. Biological age is much more representative of an individual's physical capabilities (Smith, 1984). Gerontologists have divided people over 65 into two groups: those who are 65 to 74, which is considered early old age, and people who are 75 and above, which is considered advanced old age (Butler & Lewis, 1977). These two groups are sometimes referred to as the "young-old" and the "old-old" (Ostrow, 1984, p. 2).

We will now look at the typical pattern of aging and see how exercise can affect the process. Sedentary people reach the peak of their physiological capabilities around age 30. These capabilities then begin to decline on an average of between .75% and 1% per year. Between the ages of 30 and 70, maximal work capacity decreases 25% to 30% (Smith, 1984). During this period, cardiac output declines due to decreases in stroke volume and maximum heart rate; vital capacity declines 40% to 50%; and metabolic rate decreases 8% to 12%. Decreases in the number and size of muscle fibers result in strength loss of 25% to 30%, and reduced nerve conduction velocity of 10% to 15% increases reaction time and slows movement (Smith, 1984).

Other areas of decline include a decrease in flexibility and a loss of bone strength, and a reduction in flexibility of 20% to 30% due primarily to connective tissue changes in muscles, tendons, and joints. The decreased strength of bones is caused by the depletion of minerals. This condition is particularly troublesome for women. A decline in renal function of 30% to 50% and a reduction of total body water of 10% to 15% are also common between ages 30 and 70 (Smith, 1984).

Psychology of Aging

Many people assume that aging entails memory loss, the lack of ability to learn or perform new tasks, and the lack of capacity for self-help, decision making, and problem solving (Saul, 1974). In reality, healthy seniors can maintain mental abilities, such as practical reasoning and good vocabulary, with very little decline as long as they remain interested, active, and involved.

In the psychological and emotional experiences of older people, loss is a predominant theme. The elderly are inevitably confronted by multiple losses: death of a spouse; death of friends and relatives; decline of physical health and a loss of one's own illusions of immortality; loss of status, prestige, and social participation; and, for many, lower living standards, cultural devaluation, and neglect (Butler & Lewis, 1977). Dealing with these losses requires strength, stamina, and the ability to adjust to changes.

The most common emotions in old age are grief, guilt, loneliness, depression, anxiety, helplessness, and rage (Butler & Lewis, 1977). As a time of reflection and reminiscence, old age may also evoke feelings of guilt and remorse. Widows and widowers often feel guilty that they did not do more for their spouses. Loneliness and an increasing sense of isolation are common among the elderly as they outlive family members and friends and see their social network reduced (Butler & Lewis, 1977). Feelings of helplessness and impotence are often experienced as is a sense of rage at real or imagined indignities and neglect by a society that once valued their capabilities. Rage may also be a reaction to the inevitability of aging and death (Butler & Lewis, 1977).

Depression is a prevalent affective disorder of the elderly. An estimated 15% to 20% of older adults experience depression severe enough to require psychiatric intervention, yet only about 15% of these people actually receive treatment (Shamoian, 1983). Many elderly people accept depression as part of being old and do not seek treatment. Although the many losses accompanying old age often trigger the onset of depression, depression may also be a symptom of an undiagnosed medical illness. Among the usual signs of depression are unexplained dysphoria, prolonged unhappiness, insomnia, weight loss, fatigability, loss of self-esteem, and a preoccupation with death (Shamoian, 1983).

Another common disorder of aging is anxiety, which in the elderly is usually associated with an anticipated or imagined fear of loss and separation. However, anxiety may also be a manifestation of an undiagnosed medical illness. Some of the more common symptoms of anxiety are palpitations, abdominal spasms, diarrhea, dizziness, urinary frequency, excessive sweating, and clammy hands. Anxiety in the elderly may also be a sign of underlying depression or incipient dementia (Shamoian, 1983).

Suicide is a major problem associated with aging. Accounting for about one-fourth of all suicides in the United States each year, the highest suicide rate is among white males in their eighties. At high risk is the elderly person who lives alone, who has a chronic illness, who has a history of alcohol or drug abuse, or whose spouse has recently died (Shamoian, 1983). Suicide attempts among the elderly are usually successful. Suicide is sometimes done "subintentionally" by purposely not eating, failing to take medication, taking physical risks, or delaying medical treatment (Butler & Lewis, 1977).

Exercise and Aging

Although aging is inevitable, much of the physiological decline associated with aging is attributable to disuse and atrophy and may be reversed through physical activity (Smith, 1984). Because as much as 50% of physiological decline may be due to lack of use and deconditioning, regular exercise may promote a high level of phyisological functioning even into the 7th and 8th decades. Exercise is an inexpensive lifestyle intervention that can provide substantial benefits to older adults (Spirduso, 1986).

While the physiological benefits of exercise in young adults has been well documented in recent years, research with older adults is comparatively rare. However, there is some evidence that healthy older adults are as trainable as young people (deVries, 1981). One of the more significant and consistent findings from research with seniors has been that work capacity increases with exercise training. Improved cardiovascular and neuromuscular functioning, increased flexibility, and better joint mobility are among the benefits realized by older adults through exercise. Increases have also been observed in bone density and strength due to exercise (Smith, 1984).

Some of the more encouraging research has been done on psychomotor performance. There is some evidence that individuals who are physically active seem to maintain psychomotor speed (Spirduso, 1986). Investigators have found that seniors who exercise consistently have faster simple and complex reaction time than their sedentary peers. Researchers speculate that regular exercise improves psychomotor speed by improving general overall speed of the perceptual and motor system (Spirduso, 1986). Daily endurance

training has been shown to prevent the attrition of slow- and fast-twitch muscle fibers. Fast-twitch fibers help maintain the capacity for vigorous movement. By stimulating blood flow, exercise also enhances contractility and permeability of blood vessels, thereby reducing local ischemia (insufficient blood supply). Healthy circulation also stabilizes temperatures in the extremities, which helps maintain normal nerve conduction. Regular exercise may also counteract negative changes in neurotransmitters associated with aging (Spirduso, 1986).

Seniors now routinely compete in track and field, swimming, and other sports. Even sports that require high levels of stamina attract large numbers of older participants. Several years ago, the New York City Marathon had 1,302 participants in their 50s, 217 in their 60s, and 19 over 70. At age 85, one participant was running in the event for the fifth consecutive time (Ward, 1984).

Although more seniors are participating in physical activity, the majority remain inactive. In 1980, one of the national health objectives set by the U.S. Public Health Service was that 50% of adults 65 and older would be engaged in appropriate physical activity by 1990. A midcourse review of this objective found that only 7.5% of this group reached this goal (Casperson, Christenson, & Pollard, 1986). Much of the inactivity is due to cultural influences, lack of knowledge about fitness, and inaccurate beliefs about exercise.

Evidence is accumulating to support the notion that society expects people to become less physically active as they get older (Ostrow & Dzewaltowski, 1986; Ostrow, Jones, & Spiker, 1981). Some common misconceptions that older people have about exercise are that their need for exercise diminishes and eventually disappears as they get older; that vigorous exercise is risky; that light, sporadic exercise is beneficial; and that they are less capable than they really are (Conrad, 1976).

The exercise practitioner must counter these misconceptions about exercise, involve seniors in exercise appropriate for their physiological status, and help them maintain physical activity. To counter the cultural imperative to "slow down," the practitioner should identify and employ older adults who exercise as role models. By prominently displaying pictures of older adults enjoying various types of physical activity, using older adults in advertising and promotions, and encouraging the elderly to exercise the practitioner can communicate the message that exercise is desirable and beneficial for people of all ages.

Exercise Psychology and Aging

In this section, we will examine the psychological effects of exercise on older people. Because the general topic of psychology and exercise was examined in detail in chapter 3, we shall concentrate on how exercise uniquely affects the elderly.

Exercise and Cognition

A particularly important concern in old age is the maintenance of mental functioning. Several researchers have examined how exercise affects the mental processes of older adults. In one of the earlier studies, eight subjects averaging 70 years of age received 3 months of fitness training and were examined for changes in cognition as well as in other psychological and motor fitness variables (Barry, Steinmetz, Page, & Rodahl, 1966). Despite improvements in several areas, no significant changes occurred in cognition. Although there were improvements on an imaging task and in one of three visual discrimination tasks, no differences were observed in six other cognitive tasks. Another investigation of the effects of exercise on fluid intelligence (intellectual development attributable to biological factors) revealed no significant differences betweeen exercisers and nonexercisers, although subjects who exercised did score slightly higher on the fluid intelligence measure than sedentary subjects (Powell & Pohndorf, 1971). Elsayed, Ismail, and Young (1980) also found fluid intelligence to be related to physical fitness and age. Highly-fit subjects scored higher in fluid intelligence than unfit subjects in both young and old categories. In contrast, scores on crystallized intelligence (intelligence related to collective learning and acculturation) were unaffected by either age or physical condition.

In other research results have also been mixed. A 14-week walk-jog program for 23 subjects averaging 65 years of age failed to show improved memory as measured by the Rey Verbal Learning Task (Perri & Templer, 1985). However, a study that compared an experimental aerobic training group, an exercise control group that engaged in strength and flexibility exercises, and a nonexercise control group revealed several significant improvements in cognitive functioning (Dustman, Ruhling, Russell, & Shearer, 1984). While the aerobically trained subjects demonstrated significantly greater improvements on the test battery than either of the other groups, the strength and flexibility group showed some improvements while the nonexercise group showed no improvement. The

results seemed to support the position that physically unfit seniors can exercise at an intensity sufficient to significantly improve their physical fitness level as well as their mental functioning. The researchers suggested that the improved neuropsychological performance in the aerobically trained subjects was due to enhanced cerebral metabolic activity attributable to exercise.

Several researchers have examined the effects of exercise on elderly subjects with either cognitive deficits or psychiatric problems. A particularly interesting study looked at the effects of acute exercise on the cognitive functioning of 15 subjects over 60. Six of the subjects had Parkinson's disease and nine were outpatients for memory impairment (Molloy, Beerschoten, Borrie, Crilly, & Cape, 1988). Using a battery of neuropsychological tests, improvement was noted in six of the eight tests of cognitive function following 20 minutes of aerobic exercise. However, despite group improvements in the cognitive tests, no significant clinical improvements were observed in individual patients after exercise.

A study of institutionalized geriatric mental patients found that exercise therapy resulted in significant cognitive improvements (Powell, 1974). Thirty subjects ranging in age from 59 to 89 were randomly assigned to exercise therapy, social therapy, or a control group. The exercise therapy lasted 12 weeks and consisted of brisk walking, calisthenics, and rhythmic activities. The social therapy included arts and crafts, social interaction, and music. Improvements on the Progressive Matrices Test and Wechsler Memory Scale were significant for the exercise group but not for the other two groups. Other studies of psychogeriatric groups have noted relationships between exercise and improvements in some cognitive functions (Diesfeldt & Diesfledt-Groenendijk, 1977; Stamford, Hambacher, & Fallica, 1974).

There is insufficient evidence at present to support the contention that exercise favorably affects cognitive functioning in the elderly. On the other hand, such a relationship has not been disproven, and, in our opinion, the current evidence slightly favors a positive relationship.

Exercise and Subjective Well-Being

Subjective well-being has been the object of much research since the mid-1940s (Horley, 1984). *Subjective well-being* is broadly defined as a "self-perception of positive feeling or state" (Horley, 1984). Concepts often linked to subjective well-being are life satisfaction, happiness, and morale. Researchers have been greatly interested in which factors are important to the subjective well-being of older adults. Much of the research has been based on the activity theory of aging, which essentially maintains that a positive relationship exists between the older individual's level of participation in social activity and life satisfaction (Knapp, 1977).

Although several studies have addressed the relationship between life satisfaction and leisure activities in general, very few have investigated the role of exercise in subjective well-being and morale. However, a national survey of over 2,000 retired men provided some support for the activity theory (Beck & Page, 1988). This study measured psychological well-being with the Bradburn Affect Balance Scale, which contains subscales for positive and negative affect. Ten types of activities, ranging from sports and hobbies to reading, volunteering, and attending meetings, were found to be related to higher levels of psychological well-being, particularly in terms of positive affect and emotional balance. The most beneficial activity was helping friends or neighbors without pay, which seemed to reinforce feelings of competence and usefulness. In a study of older women, leisure activity emerged as the strongest contributing factor to life satisfaction (Riddick & Daniel, 1984). The researchers suggested that active leisure was important for successful aging and positive mental health in later years. A similar conclusion was reached in a study of male and female retirees (Russell, 1987). Although the frequency of participation in recreation was unrelated to life satisfaction, the degree of satisfaction with recreation was significantly related to life satisfaction.

Whether exercise is a factor in the subjective well-being of the elderly remains unclear. Sidney and Shephard (1976) failed to find changes in life-satisfaction scores of older adults following a 14-week conditioning program, although 83% of the subjects reported improvements in well-being. A cross-sectional study found no differences between the perceived well-being of 30 women ages 55 to 81 who participated in a variety of aerobic and flexibility exercises and 30 sedentary women in the same age group (Coleman, Washington, & Price, 1985).

A comparison of adults over 60 who participated in an exercise program for 12 weeks and an inactive control group found no differences in morale (Ray, Gissal, & Smith, 1982). The researchers speculated that morale scales may not be sensitive enough to detect personal changes after short-term intervention. In contrast, a survey of men and women averaging 63 years of age who had been active in a formal exercise program for over two years found that participation in the program contributed significantly to perceptions of physical well-being (Stones, Kozma, & Stones, 1987).

The inconsistencies in the subjective well-being research are attributable in large part to a lack of consistent terminology as well as to inappropriate or incomplete measurements (Horley, 1984). Until these and other issues, such as global versus multilevel assessment, are resolved, the relationship between exercise and subjective well-being for the elderly will remain unclear.

Exercise and Depression in the Elderly

Although research with seniors has not been extensive, several studies have addressed the relationship between exercise and depression in this group. Valliant and Asu (1985) observed that a 12-week structured exercise program produced significant results. In this study subjects who selected exercise rather than social activities or no exercise tended to be more depressed and fearful initially but showed marked improvement with the exercise program. It was speculated that exercise was viewed as a means of coping with negative perceptions associated with the aging process.

In a study of 38 senior adults averaging 75 years of age, subjects were randomly assigned to an 8-week program of flexibility, general muscle toning, and balance exercises. Significant improvement in depression scores was found for exercise participants but not for the control subjects involved in social activities (Bennett, Carmack, & Gardner, 1982). Similar results were observed in a study of older adults who participated in a 14-week aerobic exercise program (Perri & Templer, 1985). Although depression scores were not significant, improvement in depression was observed in the exercise but not in the control group.

Not all studies have shown exercise to be effective in reducing levels of depression in older people. Dustman and associates (1984) failed to find differences in depression as measured by either the Beck Depression Inventory or the Zung Self-Rating Depression Scale between an experimental aerobic exercise group, a nonaerobic exercise control group, and a nonexercise control group. This result may be due to the low initial depression scores of subjects in this study. Individuals with good mental health have less room to improve than subjects who begin a program with high levels of depression. A study of the acute effects of aerobic exercise on psychological functioning concluded that a single bout of exercise had no effect on depression as measured by the Geriatric

Depression Scale (Molloy et al., 1988). Blumenthal and colleagues (1982) also found no change in depression scores in a group of older subjects after an 11-week aerobic exercise program, although 40% of the subjects indicated that they felt healthier, more self-confident, and happier than when they began the program. The researchers speculated that older subjects may require longer intervals of training to achieve psychological changes.

Other Psychological Effects

The research on the psychological effects of exercise in the elderly has been very limited. While many observations made regarding the psychological effects of exercise discussed in chapter 3 may be appropriate for older individuals, many may not be. Until there is considerably more psychological research on older subjects, generalizations about the effects of exercise on mood, anxiety, self-concept, and related topics will be impossible. We shall now briefly review the few studies that do address these topics.

Two studies that examined the effects of exercise on mood states generally failed to note differences attributable to exercise. With the exception of a decrease in anger, Blumenthal and colleagues (1982) observed no changes in scores on the Profile of Mood States after an exercise program in which subjects rode bicycle ergometers. Similarly, a second study of the acute effects of exercise recorded no changes in mood after subjects engaged in one session of light aerobic exercise (Molloy et al., 1988).

Sidney and Shephard (1976) observed an overall decline in anxiety following an exercise program using the Taylor Manifest Anxiety Scale and a section of the Cornell Medical Index. Subjects also increased their perceptions of activity as a relief from tension. Another study showed improvement in anxiety scores following exercise, but the results were not statistically significant (Perri & Templer, 1985). Elderly subjects who identified themselves as having anxiety and tension reduced their tension levels significantly more following an exercise bout that involved walking at a heart rate of 100 beats per minute than after receiving meprobamate (deVries & Adams, 1972).

Studies on the effects of exercise on self-concept, self-esteem, and body image have generally shown exercise to be beneficial. Although a study by Perri and Templer (1985) noted enhanced self-concept after exercise, Sidney and Shephard (1976) observed no self-concept changes attributable to conditioning except for in those subjects who trained the hardest.

Parent and Whall (1984) found self-esteem scores to be related to participation in an activity program, while another study found changes in self-esteem related to exercise only in male subjects (Valliant & Asu, 1985). Hogan and Santomier (1984) observed changes in the self-efficacy of older adults after 5 weeks of swimming instruction. Compared to a control group, the swim group scored significantly higher in swimming self-efficacy. Moreover, 78% of the experimental group indicated a change in feelings concerning their ability to perform in other areas, which was interpreted as general enhancement of self-efficacy.

As research accumulates, we are likely to see more definitive conclusions emerging. In the meantime, we know that exercise produces highly beneficial physiological results. Moreover, the psychological results that have been demonstrated are generally encouraging. At the very least, there has been no evidence that exercise is psychologically harmful to the elderly. We would therefore conclude that exercises designed to meet the unique capacities and needs of seniors should become a significant part of fitness and health programming.

CHILDREN AND YOUTH

The current physical condition and future health of children and youth are a major concern. The extremely poor performance of children on physical fitness tests and the high incidence of overweight, sedentary young people have led to calls for programs to turn this trend around. There are many reasons why children are becoming less active including the increase in single-parent families and the "latchkey" phenomenon, concerns about child safety, cutbacks in school physical education programs, poorly run physical education programs, and increased interest in sedentary activities such as watching television and playing video games.

In this section, we shall briefly address the state of fitness among children and youth and how physical activity may affect their psychological functioning. We will limit our discussion to the research on the psychological implications of exercise and noncompetitive, nonskill-oriented physical activity on children and adolescents. Although there is extensive literature on the psychological effects of competitive sports for children, this research is beyond the scope of the present work. Although the remaining research is admittedly meager, this lack of research should point out the need to know more about the exercise behaviors of children and youth and their physical and psychological effects.

The State of Children's Fitness

Undoubtedly the best time to instill beneficial health practices is in childhood, especially because lifestyle factors are responsible for 53% of the potential years of life lost before age 65 (Powell, 1988). The prevalence of known risk factors for chronic diseases among children is particularly disturbing. Risk factors such as smoking, obesity, hypertension, hyperlipidemia, diabetes, stress, and Type A behaviors are all too common among children and youth (Dishman & Dunn, 1988).

Major health and fitness goals for children and adolescents include promoting optimal physical growth and development, developing interest in and skills for an active lifestyle, reducing risk factors of coronary heart disease, and fostering good psychological adjustment (Haskell, Montoye, & Orenstein, 1985). These researchers recommend activities that emphasize large-muscle, dynamic exercise; moving the body over distance and against gravity; some heavy resistive activity; and flexibility exercises. Activities should be of moderate to vigorous intensity, last for at least 30 minutes, and be performed daily.

Information from the Public Health Service (1989) regarding health priorities for the year 2000 and related objectives for increasing physical activity and fitness follow. Where available, estimated baseline data is cited.

In the area of risk reduction the following has been proposed:

■ Increase to 90% the proportion of children and adolescents ages 6 to 17 who participate in moderate physical activities three or more times a week for 20 minutes or more. (78% in 1984)

■ Increase to at least 75% the proportion of children and adolescents who participate in vigorous physical activities that promote the development and maintenance of cardiovascular fitness three or more times a week for 20 minutes or more. (66% in 1984)

■ Increase to at least 75% the proportion of children and adolescents ages 6 to 17 who regularly perform physical activities that maintain muscular strength, muscular endurance, and flexibility. (Baseline data unavailable)

■ Reduce the percentage of overweight adolescents ages 12 to 17 to less than 15%. (15% in 1976-1980)

■ Increase to 75% the percentage of overweight adolescents ages 12 and older who have adopted sound dietary practices combined with physical activity to lose weight. (Baseline data unavailable)

In the area of services and protection, the following goals have been proposed:

■ Increase to at least 45% the proportion of children and adolescents in grades 1 to 12 who participate in daily school physical education programs. (36% in 1984-1986)

■ Increase to 70% the proportion of physical education teachers who spend 30% or more of class time on skills and activities that promote lifetime physical activity participation. (Baseline data unavailable)

The Public Health Service has also set goals that address public knowledge and awareness of fitness, the effects of exercise on fitness, primary health providers who assess and counsel their patients about physical activity, community-based participation in physical activity, and community fitness facilities.

Although a majority of students are enrolled in physical education, these programs seem to have little effect on the fitness levels of children and on developing lifelong physical activity skills (Iverson, Fielding, Crow, & Christenson, 1985). As evidence of this, performance on the AAHPERD Youth Fitness test showed no gains for boys and only slight gains for girls between 1965 and 1975. More recently, the 1984 Amateur Athletic Union/Nabisco physical fitness program reported that approximately 74% of the youth tested failed to meet standards for their age and sex on basic motor fitness tests (Iverson et al., 1985).

In an observational study of 24 children in grades 3 to 6, each child was observed for 2 days and had all activities recorded from 7:00 a.m. until 7:00 p.m. (Baranowski, Hooks, Tsong, Cieslik, & Nader, 1987). Observers detected no instances of aerobic activity as defined by nationally accepted criteria in 48 days of observation. Using a much less stringent criterion of 14 minutes of trunk movement through space with only 1 interval of stationary behavior, only half of the children engaged in physical activity on any one day. These results seem to contradict the common perception that children are very active. In this study, children's activity tended to occur in short spurts rather than in longer periods that might be expected to produce a training effect. Although the results of this study cannot be generalized to all children, they do not engender hope that our children are getting sufficient exercise for normal growth and development.

Unless school programs can be improved to meet the nation's fitness needs, other agencies, both public and private, will have to fulfill this responsibility. For the nonschool exercise practitioner, this community need may turn into a significant professional opportunity.

Psychological Effects of Exercise on Children

We shall now turn our attention to the psychological implications of exercise and fitness in children and youth.

Participation Motives

Very few studies have addressed children's motives for exercise involvement. A study of junior high students revealed that boys wanted to have fun, whereas girls sought the benefits of looking better (Godin & Shephard, 1986). These researchers found that students with high intentions to exercise have strong beliefs about the consequences of exercise and evaluated these consequences as beneficial, while students with low intentions to exercise held more neutral beliefs about these consequences and were less convinced of the benefits of exercise. Beliefs about the consequences of exercise were stable across all three grades, with the exception of a decrease in the belief that exercise is fun as students moved from the 7th to 9th grade. The findings also supported the promotion of early life experiences in physical activity because attitudes and current exercise habits were strongly influenced by past experience.

Research on the participation motives of young athletes may provide some valuable insights for youth fitness programming. One review of youth-sport participation showed that fun was an important motive for almost every athlete (Passer, 1982). It was speculated that fun is closely tied to other major participation motives, such as skill development, excitement, success and status, fitness, energy release, and affiliation, which is related to team atmosphere and friendship. Passer (1982) made the important point that children become involved and stay involved for multiple reasons.

In a study of the factors contributing to the enjoyment of soccer, hockey, and baseball among 822 boys ages 7 to 14, Wankel and Kreisel (1985) found that intrinsic factors (excitement of the sport, personal accomplishment, improving one's skills,

and testing one's skills against others) were more important than extrinsic factors (pleasing others, winning rewards, and winning the game). In a subsequent study, Wankel and Sefton (1989) investigated factors that affected the boy and girls' perceptions of fun over the course of an entire season. Postgame positive affect, how well one played, and challenge were consistently found to be the best predictors of fun.

It would appear that people who organize fitness activities for children should include a strong component of fun. Activities should also be challenging and improve skill and fitness levels. In addition, opportunities for making friends and achieving recognition for fitness improvements also seem to foster the desire to participate. Because of the importance of participation motives for entering and remaining in a fitness program, such motives should be a priority for future research.

Exercise and Self-Concept

As discussed in chapter 4, although most research on the effects of exercise on self-concept has design weaknesses, exercise participation seems to have a positive effect on self-concept. The same observations are appropriate with respect to research on children and self-concept.

In a comprehensive analysis of research on physical activity and self-esteem development in children, Gruber (1986) found that 53 of 65 studies claimed that play and physical activity contribute to development in the affective domain. After examining only controlled experimental studies, overall results supported the position that participation in directed play and physical education programs influences the development of self-concept in children. An interesting observation was that children who were emotionally disturbed, mentally handicapped, economically disadvantaged, and perceptually handicapped showed greater gains in self-concept than normal children. This was attributed to the increased attention which students receive in enrichment programs and feelings of increased importance and success, which lead to significant improvements in self-concept.

This study also observed the importance of specific activities to self-concept changes. Physical fitness and aerobic activities were far superior to learning sport skills or creative and perceptual-motor activities in improving self-concept. It was speculated that the immediate feedback one gets from meeting fitness goals that do not require complex skills and the feeling of body mastery as one successfully meets the demands of fitness activities may account for this difference.

Exercise and Emotional Changes

Exercise can improve the emotional states of both children and adults. Shipman (1984) demonstrated this point in a study that incorporated running into a treatment program for emotional and behavioral disorders. The 12-week program included 56 children between the ages of 6 and 13 who participated voluntarily. Although objective results were minimal, subjective results such as the development of a sense of cohesion and increased enthusiasm were significant. It was also noted that the more a child ran, the less psychotropic medication he or she required.

Miller (1979) found jogging to be an effective technique for improving communication and rapport with inner-city children. He observed that during a jog students felt free to discuss their concerns and relationships as well as their aspirations and goals. Miller speculated that the jogging program was successful for several reasons: Jogging took students away from a negative environment; it served as a calming agent for highly active students; it involved the completion of a task, which was reinforced; and the teacher was viewed as a friend.

Jogging was also used successfully to reduce disruptive behaviors in a class of 12 boys who were learning handicapped (Allen, 1980). The boys jogged at the beginning of the day before commencing the normal academic program. Allen found that the fewest behavioral problems occurred in the hour immediately following jogging, and that overall daily behavioral disruptions were reduced by one half.

Other Psychological Effects

Stress is a part of growing up, and adolescence is especially stressful due to the many physical, social, and psychological changes taking place. In a cross-sectional study of 220 adolescent females, Brown and Lawton (1986) investigated whether exercise can favorably affect the physical and emotional distress accompanying periods of high stress. Using self-report measures of life events, physical illness, mood, and exercise, subjects who were identified as low exercisers experienced significantly more stress and concomitant ill effects than subjects who adhered to a regimen of vigorous physical activity.

A study that compared body-image scores of high school female athletes in gymnastics, basketball, and track to the scores of nonathletes revealed some interesting differences (Snyder & Spreitzer, 1976). Overall, the athletes' body-image scores and perceived energy levels were significantly higher than those of the nonathletic group. The researchers hypothesized that the more favorable body images of athletes were due to their childhood participation in sport or factors that induced their participation in sport. Seventy percent of the gymnasts considered themselves to be "very feminine," while only 44% of basketball players perceived themselves in this way. Track athletes and nonathletes had percentages of 56 and 58, respectively, on the femininity dimension. The findings indicated that socialization into sport begins in childhood and continues into high school, with considerable encouragement being received from significant others. It was also observed that the stigma associated with female athletes was perhaps declining.

The effect of exercise on locus of control was explored in a study of children ages 6 to 14 who attended an 8-week fitness day camp (Duke, Johnson, & Nowicki, 1977). The camp program consisted of daily participation in aquatics, track and field events, distance running and interval training, tumbling and gymnastics, conditioning activities, and games. A comparison of pre-camp and post-camp locus-of-control scores indicated significant changes from external to internal. Significant improvements were also noted on six physical fitness dimensions. Although causality cannot be inferred from this study, some interesting possibilities were suggested regarding the role of fitness, the group experience with peers, and reinforcement from camp leaders.

The same camp setting was used in a study of the relationship between physical fitness and social status of children (Gross, Johnson, Wojnilower, & Drabman, 1985). Significant improvements in physical fitness and social status were observed at the end of the program for both boys and girls. Although considered an exploratory study, the results suggested a role for physical fitness in social skills training programs for children with low social status.

PEOPLE WITH PHYSICAL DISABILITIES

Participation of the physically disabled in various forms of physical activity has grown dramatically in recent years. Wheelchair athletes train and compete in a variety of individual and team sports in local, national, and international competitions. The Paralympics follow the Olympic Games every 4 years and attract the best physically disabled athletes from around the world. At the local level, many road races have wheelchair divisions that extend opportunities for competition to thousands more disabled individuals. Many physically disabled persons would participate in noncompetitive forms of exercise if opportunities were provided. Indeed, it is our premise that the disabled have the same fitness needs and interests as other people, and it is incumbent on the exercise professional to see that these needs are met and their interests accommodated. The impairments we associate with physical disability most often are the result of traumatic brain injury, amputation, spinal cord damage, cerebral palsy, or stroke—all of which affect motor functioning.

Various terms have been used to describe impaired or limited functioning. The term *disability* usually refers to some limitation in function that directly results from an impairment of a specific organ or body system (Wright, 1983). The term *handicap* refers to the obstacles that a person encounters in the pursuit of life goals. A major point here is that the source of obstacles and difficulties are not always entirely attributable to the disability. For example, a person confined to a wheelchair may be a perfectly capable accountant in terms of having the skills and knowledge required for the job. However, if no one will hire this person or if this person cannot negotiate the stairs to the office, he or she is handicapped by these factors as well. On the other hand, this person would be minimally handicapped if he or she were operating in a barrier-free situation. By the same token, a person with a disability is not necessarily handicapped, while a person who is handicapped may or may not have a disability. What is regarded as a disability or handicap depends on the requirements and expectations in a given situation, and one should not automatically equate a disability with a handicap (Wright, 1983). As a rule, the term *disabled* is preferable to *handicapped* because the latter suggests a more pronounced need for assistance (Adams & McCubbin, 1991).

Psychosocial Factors in Physical Disability

There are considerable individual differences in how disabled people react to their condition. One's personal response to disability may vary at any given time from denial of its existence to exaggeration of its consequences (Marinelli & Orto, 1984). Much of this fluctuation is undoubtedly attributable to psychological characteristics and ability and willingness to adjust to the disability. Following a severe spinal cord injury, the usual psychological progression is shock, denial, depression, and adaptation. The injured person usually moves from a defensive reaction to recognition and accommodation of the disability (Caplan, 1987).

This psychological progression is often characterized by frustration and prolonged bitterness and grief. Some disabled people show evidence of maladjustment, retarded emotional development, social alienation, self-pity, depression, excessive submissiveness, and other undesirable characteristics (Shephard, 1990). Following a spinal cord injury, emotional problems are expected. Anxiety and depression are probably the most common problems, but alcohol and drug abuse are also prevalent, and, to a much lesser extent, self-destructive behavior and suicide (Caplan, 1987).

The impact of a traumatic event such as a spinal cord injury has far-reaching effects. There is no doubt that it affects the entire family. Nevertheless, there is some evidence that paraplegia does not seriously impair marital functioning nor does it significantly affect the divorce rate of those involved. However, a change in emotional tone of a marriage often does occur, characterized by a sense of loss and feelings of sadness (Caplan, 1987). Of course, the success of rehabilitation largely determines whether the person is able to live independently, return to productive employment, and enjoy leisure time.

A summary of research on societal attitudes toward disabilities identified several recurring themes:

■ interaction strain, which involves uncertainty about what to say or how to act with a disabled person;

■ rejection of intimacy, or unwillingness to be involved in a close relationship;

■ generalized rejection, which reflects the belief that the severely disabled should be segregated from the rest of society;

■ authoritarian virtuousness, which is a form of patronizing benevolence;

■ inferred emotional consequences, which assumes that a disabled person is likely to have been emotionally damaged by the experience;

■ distressed identification, or feeling sadness and pity for the disabled person; and

■ inferred functional limitations, or the assumption that a person is extremely limited in what he or she is able to do (Caplan, 1987).

Benefits of Exercise

A common consequence of physical disability attributable to a sedentary lifestyle is a degenerative process resulting in decreased lean body mass, lowered aerobic capacity, osteoporosis, and renal dysfunction (Cowell, Squires, & Raven, 1986). According to these researchers, the physically disabled are also at an increased risk of atherosclerosis, which is a leading factor in reduced life expectancy for this group. Reviewing the literature on the effects of exercise training on paraplegics, Cowell and associates (1986) observed that physically disabled people responded to prolonged exercise in basically the same manner as able-bodied individuals. They recommend swimming, wheelchair basketball, and long-distance wheelchair races for cardiovascular training because of the use of many muscle groups and the ability to vary the intensity and duration of the activities. Modified weight training and flexibility exercises were also recommended.

Psychological Effects of Exercise and Fitness Activities

Research on the psychological effects of exercise on physically disabled people is extremely limited at present. In one of the few existing studies, hemiplegic patients who participated in a physical conditioning program showed significant improvements in self-concept, physical fitness, and functional status after training for 12 weeks on a bicycle ergometer (Brinkman & Hoskins, 1979). Similarly, a clinical report noted improvements in mood of a paraplegic man diagnosed with congenital spina bifida (Katz, Adler, Mazzarella, & Ince, 1985). The subject in this study participated in a 12-week program of exercise using a hand ergometer. Significant improvements were noted in heart rate, blood pressure, and oxygen uptake. Moreover, the man showed reduced tension and depression and increased vigor as measured by the Profile of Mood States.

Because of the extremely sparse literature on psychological implications of exercise and fitness training, we decided to see if extrapolations could be made from the literature on competitive sports for the disabled. Opportunities for the disabled to participate in sports have grown dramatically since World War II. Local, regional, national, and even international competitions are held in a variety of sports, including track and field, swimming, archery, table tennis, softball, tennis, road racing, soccer, and skiing. The increase in competitive events for disabled participants is seen as a very positive sign that disabled people are discovering the same emotional and mental benefits from sport as able-bodied competitors (Bernhardt, 1985). It is also believed that the growth of special sports programs and the increased visibility of disabled athletes has created a greater awareness and appreciation of special populations in our society.

Despite the dramatic growth in sports participation for disabled people, we were again disappointed by the small amount of information available on psychological effects of sports involvement. Asken and Goodling (1986) noted the neglect of disabled athletes by sport psychology researchers and practitioners. Nevertheless, the effect of participation in competitive sports on self-concept and self-esteem of wheelchair athletes has been the subject of at least three studies. A study of 87 wheelchair athletes showed that these athletes had high levels of self-esteem and high occupational aspirations (Hopper & Santomier, 1984/1985). Ten novice wheelchair athletes were evaluated on self-concept and acceptance of disability before a major competition and again 5 months later (Patrick, 1986). Significant improvements were noted on both dimensions. These results supported sports competition as a powerful positive influence on self-concept and acceptance of disability, both of which are considered important to the rehabilitation process.

A comparison of disabled athletes with disabled nonathletes showed that the athletes had higher levels of self-esteem, life satisfaction, and happiness (Valliant, Bezzubyk, Daley, & Asu, 1985). The researchers suggested that the psychosocial functioning of disabled people might be enhanced through sports participation.

A study of personality characteristics of wheelchair athletes and moderately active paraplegics revealed several interesting findings (Goldberg & Shephard, 1982). Body-image scores of the disabled subjects were lower than test norms of able-bodied subjects, and the disabled subjects also tended to have an external locus of control. Differences noted on the Cattell 16PF included higher apprehension scores for subjects with severe spinal lesions. Wheelchair athletes were observed to be more intelligent, adventuresome, and tough-minded than normative subjects. With the exceptions of significantly higher scores on pursuit of vertigo and exercise as an ascetic experience, attitudes toward physical activity were similar to those of able-bodied subjects., These results seemed to confirm the abnormal psychological profile of the paraplegic. However, it was suggested that certain aspects of mood, attitude, and body image may be increased through a physical training program.

Considerably different results were obtained in a study of attitudes toward physical activity in a group of 165 elite athletes with cerebral palsy (Cooper, Sherrill, & Marshall, 1986). In this study, pursuit of vertigo and exercise as an ascetic experience received the lowest scores. Overall the subjects were found to have positive attitudes toward the total concept of physical activity and felt favorably toward physical activity as a social experience, as a way to release tension, as an aesthetic experience, and for health and fitness.

A comparison of psychological profiles of wheelchair athletes and able-bodied athletes showed little difference (Henschen, Horvat, & French, 1984). Scores on the Profile of Mood States (POMS) of wheelchair athletes conformed to the familiar "iceberg" pattern, while scores on the Trait-State Anxiety Inventory revealed low trait anxiety and average levels of state anxiety. A second study using the POMS found that elite athletes with cerebral palsy selected for international competition did not differ from other elite competitors except on vigor (Canabal, Sherrill, & Rainbolt, 1987). Athletes who competed internationally scored significantly higher on this dimension.

Summarizing available research, DePauw (1988) observed more similarities than differences between disabled and able-bodied athletes on psychological factors. Mood profiles, anxiety scores, and responses to success and failure of wheelchair athletes were quite comparable to those of able-bodied athletes.

Implications for the Practitioner

The exercise practitioner who has the opportunity to work with physically disabled people will no doubt find the experience rewarding. Physically disabled people are generally motivated clients who will probably try to put the practitioner at ease. The basic rule of interacting with a disabled person is to be oneself. Practitioners should talk in the same manner as they would with anyone else. They should be helpful but not overprotective. Emphasis should be placed on what a person is able to do rather than on what he or she cannot do, which means individualizing the program

more than usual. Exercise practitioners will probably be challenged to think of ways to help disabled clients accomplish their exercise goals, but creative problem solving can be interesting and extremely rewarding. Coming up with an adaptation, either in an exercise or in a piece of equipment, is the sort of professional challenge that most practitioners welcome.

Reluctance to work with disabled clients can be overcome with experience. The more practitioners are around disabled people, the more they will perceive them not as disabled but as "regular" people. Practitioners should also keep in mind that disabled people need exercise as much as, if not more than, anyone else. As helping professionals, practitioners must see that disabled clients have opportunities to meet their fitness goals. For practitioners who would like to gain experience working with disabled people, most communities provide ample opportunities to volunteer in programs such as wheelchair sports or adapted physical education. Books and videotapes can also prepare practitioners for this experience.

SUMMARY

In this chapter, we have discussed five subgroups of the population that exercise professionals will undoubtedly encounter. Exercise has considerable physiological and psychological benefits for all these groups, regardless of specific limitations. Individuals recovering from coronary heart disease or bypass surgery find exercise helpful in overcoming emotional as well as physical symptoms. Anxiety, depression, and loss of self-confidence are improved as gradual increases in exercise duration and intensity show that recovery is possible and that the person can return to some semblance of normalcy. Lack of exercise has been identified as a major factor in the development of obesity. It is also considered one of the more effective treatments for obesity, especially when combined with a sound diet program. As people age, exercise can slow the physiological aging process, especially aspects of aging associated with inactivity and disuse. Exercise may also increase feelings of well-being and self-efficacy and help to relieve anxiety and depression in the elderly. The desirablity of establishing good exercise habits in childhood is based on the premise that skills and knowledge developed when one is young carry over into adulthood. In addition to reducing risk factors for chronic diseases and contributing to a child's growth and development, exercise is a positive factor in the development of the child's self-esteem and body image. Finally, disabled people respond positively to exercise and experience essentially the same physiological and psychological benefits as able-bodied people.

This book has provided an enormous amount of information and suggestions to help exercise professionals become more effective. The challenges ahead are enormous. As a new profession, exercise science has a great deal of work to do in promoting exercise and a healthy lifestyle to a largely sedentary culture. Moreover, professionals will be challenged to extend exercise and health promotion programs to segments of society that have been excluded primarily due to lack of program access or financial limitations. However, we are optimistic for the future. We expect nothing less than eventual success in extending opportunities to all who wish to participate in exercise. We also anticipate the continued development of exercise science as a significant discipline of research and exercise leadership as an important helping profession in the years ahead.

References

Adams, R.C., & McCubbin, J.A. (1991). *Games, sports, and exercises for the physically disabled* (4th ed.). Philadelphia: Lea & Febiger.

Adams, T.B., & Landgreen, M.A. (1988). Noncompliance in corporate health and fitness programs. *Fitness in Business,* **2**(4), 142-144.

Adamson, B.J., & Wade, K.J. (1986). Predictors of sport and exercise participation among health science students. *Australian Journal of Science and Medicine in Sport,* **18**(4), 3-10.

Agnew, R., & Levin, M.L. (1987). The effect of running on mood and perceived health. *Journal of Sport Behavior,* **10**(1), 14-27.

Ajzen, I. (1985). From intentions to actions: A theory of planned behavior. In J. Kuhl & J. Beckman (Eds.), *Action control: From cognition to behavior* (pp. 11-39). New York: Springer-Verlag.

Ajzen, I., & Fishbein, M. (1980). *Understanding attitudes and predicting social behavior.* Englewood Cliffs, NJ: Prentice Hall.

Ajzen, I., & Madden, T.J. (1986). Prediction of goal directed behavior: Attitudes, intentions, and perceived behavioral control. *Journal of Experimental Social Psychology,* **22**, 453-474.

Alderman, M.K. (1980). Self-responsibility in health care/promotion: Motivational factors. *Journal of School Health,* **50**, 22-25.

Alderman, R.B., & Wood, N.L. (1976). An analysis of incentive motivation in young Canadian athletes. *Canadian Journal of Applied Sport Sciences,* **1**, 169-175.

Alexy, B. (1985). Goal setting and health risk reduction. *Nursing Research,* **34**, 263-288.

Allen, J.I. (1980). Jogging can modify disruptive behaviors. *Teaching Exceptional Children,* **12**(3), 66-70.

Allen, L.D., & Iwata, B.A. (1980). Reinforcing exercise maintenance using existing high rate activities. *Behavior Modification,* **4**, 337-354.

Allison, K., & Coburn, D. (1985). Explaining low levels of exercise amongst blue collar workers. *Canadian Association for Health, Physical Education, and Recreation Journal,* **51**(7), 34-37.

Allison, M.G., & Ayllon, T. (1980). Behavioral coaching in the development of skills in football, gymnastics, and tennis. *Journal of Applied Behavior Analysis,* **13**, 297-314.

Altschul, A.M. (1987). Energy balance. In A.M. Altschul (Ed.), *Weight control: A guide for counselors and therapists* (pp. 37-51). New York: Praeger.

American Association for Counseling and Development (1981). *Ethical standards.* Alexandria, VA: Author.

American Association of Marriage and Family Therapy. (1981). *Code of professional ethics.* Clairmont, CA: Author.

American Psychological Association. (1981). *Ethical principles of psychologists* (rev. ed.). Washington, DC: Author.

Anderson, M.P. (1983). Psychological aspects of cardiovascular disorders and rehabilitation. In L.H. Peterson (Ed.), *Cardiovascular rehabilitation: A comprehensive approach* (pp. 94-117). New York: Macmillan.

Anderson, M.P. (1987). Psychological issues in cardiovascular rehabilitation. In J.W. Elias & P.H. Marshall (Eds.), *Cardiovascular disease and behavior* (pp. 151-178). Washington, DC: Hemisphere.

Andrew, G.M., Oldridge, N.B., Parker, J.O., Cunningham, D.A., Rechnitzer, N.L., Jones, N.L., Buck, C., Kavanagh, T., & Shephard, R.J.

(1981). Reasons for dropout from exercise programs in post-coronary patients. *Medicine and Science in Sports and Exercise,* **13**(3), 164-168.

Andrew, G.M., & Parker, J.O. (1979). Factors related to dropout of post myocardial infarction patients from exercise programs. *Medicine and Science in Sports,* **11**(4), 376-378.

Anthony, W.A., & Vitalo, R.L. (1982). Human resource development model. In E.K. Marshall, P.D. Kurtz, & Associates (Eds.) *Interpersonal helping skills: A guide to training methods, programs, and resources* (pp. 59-92). San Francisco: Jossey-Bass.

Asken, M.J., & Goodling, M.D. (1986). Sport psychology: An undeveloped discipline from among the sport sciences for disabled athletes. *Adapted Physical Activity Quarterly,* **3**, 312-319.

Association for Specialists in Group Work. (1989). *Ethical guidelines for group counselors.* Alexandria, VA: Author.

Atkinson, J.W. (1978). *An introduction to motivation.* Princeton, NJ: D. Van Nostrand.

Bahrke, M.S. (1981). Alterations in anxiety following exercise and rest. In F.J. Nagle & H.J. Montoye (Eds.), *Exercise in health and disease* (pp. 291-297). Springfield, IL: Charles C. Thomas.

Bahrke, M.S., & Morgan, W.P. (1978). Anxiety reduction following exercise and meditation. *Cognitive Therapy and Research,* **2**(4), 323-333.

Bain, L.L. (1985). A naturalistic study of students' responses to an exercise class. *Journal of Teaching in Physical Education,* **5**, 2-12.

Bain, L.L., Wilson, T., & Chaikind, E. (1989). Participant perceptions of exercise programs for overweight women. *Research Quarterly for Exercise and Sport,* **60**(2), 134-143.

Bales, R.F. (1950). *Interaction process analysis: A method for the study of small groups.* Reading, MA: Addison-Wesley.

Bandura, A. (1969). *Principles of behavior modification.* New York: Holt Rinehart & Winston.

Bandura, A. (1977a). Self-efficacy: Toward a unifying theory of behavioral change. *Psychological Review,* **84**(2), 191-215.

Bandura, A. (1977b). *Social learning theory.* Englewood Cliffs, NJ: Prentice Hall.

Bandura, A. (1982). Self-efficacy mechanism in human agency. *American Psychologist,* **37**(2), 122-147.

Bandura, A. (1986). *Social foundations of thought and action: A social cognitive theory.* Englewood Cliffs, NJ: Prentice Hall.

Bandura, A., & Adams, N.E. (1977). Analysis of self-efficacy theory of behavioral change. *Cognitive Therapy and Research,* **1**, 287-308.

Bandura, A., & Walters, R.H. (1963). *Social learning and personality development.* New York: Holt Rinehart & Winston.

Bannister, D., & Francella, F. (1971). *Inquiring man.* New York: Penguin Books.

Baranowski, T., Hooks, P., Tsong, Y., Cieslik, C., & Nader, P.R. (1987). Aerobic physical activity among third to sixth grade children. *Developmental and Behavioral Pediatrics,* **8**(4), 203-206.

Barnstuble, J.A., Klesges, R.C., & Terbizan, D. (1986). Predictors of weight loss in a behavioral treatment program. *Behavior Therapy,* **17**, 288-294.

Barry, A.J., Steinmetz, J.R., Page, H.F., & Rodahl, K. (1966). The effects of physical conditioning on older individuals. II. Motor performance and cognitive function. *Journal of Gerontology,* **21**, 192-199.

Bass, B.M. (1981). *Stogdill's handbook of leadership.* New York: Free Press.

Baun, W.B., Bernacki, E.J., Riggins, N., & Landgren, M.L. (1983). Influence of biologic variables on exercise adherence. *Medicine and Science in Sports and Exercise,* **15**, 120-121.

Bavelas, A.. (1950). Communication patterns in task oriented groups. *Journal of the Acoustical Society of America,* **22**, (725-730).

Beck, A.T. (1967). Depression: Clinical, experimental, and theoretical aspects. New York: Hoeber.

Beck, A.T. (1976). *Cognitive therapy and the emotional disorders.* New York: International University Press.

Beck, A.T., Rush, A.J., Shaw, B.F., & Emery, G. (1979). *Cognitive therapy of depression.* New York: Guilford.

Beck, R.C. (1978). *Motivation: Theory and principles.* Englewood Cliffs, NJ: Prentice Hall.

Beck, S.H., & Page, J.W. (1988). Involvement in activities and the psychological well being of retired men. *Activites, Adaptation & Aging,* **11**(1), 31-47.

Becker, M.H., & Maiman, B.A. (1975). Sociobehavioral determinants of compliance with health and medical care recommendations. *Medical Care,* **13**(1), 10-24.

Belisle, M., Roskies, E., & Levesque, J.M. (1987). Improving adherence to physical activity. *Health Psychology,* **6**(2), 159-172.

Benne, K.D., & Sheats, P. (1948). Functional roles of group members. *Journal of Social Issues,* **4**(2), 41-49.

Bennett, J., Carmack, M.A., & Gardner, V.J. (1982). The effect of a program of physical exercise on depression in older adults. *Physical Educator*, **39**(1), 21-24.

Berger, B.G. (1984). Running strategies for women and men. In M.L. Sachs & G.W. Buffone (Eds.), *Running as therapy: An integrated approach* (pp. 23-62). Lincoln, NE: University of Nebraska Press.

Berger, B.G., Friedman, E., & Eaton, M., (1988). Comparison of jogging, the relaxation response, and group interaction for stress reduction. *Journal of Sport and Exercise Psychology*, **10**, 431-447.

Berger, B.G., & Owen, D.R. (1988). Stress reduction and mood enhancement in four modes: Swimming, body conditioning, Hatha yoga, and fencing. *Research Quarterly for Exercise and Sport*, **59**(2), 148-159.

Berger, B.G., & Owen, D.R. (1983). Mood alteration with swimming—swimmers really do feel better. *Psychosomatic Medicine*, **45**(5), 425-433.

Berkman, L.F., & Syme, S.L. (1979). Social networks, host resistance, and mortality: A nine-year follow-up study of Alameda County residents. *American Journal of Epidemiology*, **109**, 186-204.

Bernhardt, D.B., (1985). The competitive spirit. *Physical and Occupational Therapy in Pediatrics*, **4**(3), 77-83.

Bernstein, D.A., & Borkovec, T.D. (1973). *Progressive relaxation training: A manual for the helping professions*. Champaign, IL: Research Press.

Berscheid, E., Walster, E., & Bohrnstedt, G. (1973). The happy American body: A survey report. *Psychology Today*, **7**, 119-131.

Best, J.A. (1980). Mass media, self-management, and smoking modification. In P.O. Davidson & S.M. Davidson (Eds.), *Behavioral medicine: Changing health lifestyles* (pp. 371-390). New York: Brunner/Mazel.

Biddle, S., & Bailey, C. (1985). Motives for participation and attitudes towards physical activity of adult participants in fitness programs. *Perceptual and Motor Skills*, **61**, 831-834.

Bird, C. (1940). *Social psychology*. New York: Appelton-Century.

Birdwhistell, R.L. (1970). *Kinesics and context*. Philadelphia: University of Pennsylvania Press.

Blackburn, H. (1974). Disadvantages of intensive exercise therapy after myocardial infarction. In F.J. Ingelfinger, R.V. Ebert, M. Finland, & A.S. Relamn (Eds.), *Controversy in internal medicine* (Vol. 2, pp. 162-172). Philadelphia: Saunders.

Blair, S.N., Mulder, R.T., & Kohl, H.W. (1987). Reaction to "Secular trends in adult physical activity: Exercise boom or bust?" *Research Quarterly for Exercise and Sport*, **58**(2), 106-110.

Blake, R.R., & Mouton, J.S. (1970). The fifth achievement. *Journal of Applied Behavioral Science*, **6**, 413-426.

Blittner, M., Goldberg, J., & Merbaum, M. (1978). Cognitive self-control factors in the reducing of smoking behavior. *Behavior Therapy*, **9**, 553-561.

Blumenthal, J.A., Emery, C.F., Walsh, M.A., Cox, D.K., Kuhn, C.M., Williams, R.B., & Williams, R.S. (1988). Exercise training in healthy Type A middle aged men: Effects on behavioral and cardiovascular responses. *Psychosomatic Medicine*, **50**, 418-433.

Blumenthal, J.A., O'Toole, L.C., & Chang, J.L. (1984). Is running an analogue of anorexia nervosa? *Journal of the American Medical Association*, **252**(4), 520-523.

Blumenthal, J.A., Rose, S., & Chang, J.L. (1985). Anorexia nervosa and exercise: Implications from recent findings. *Sports Medicine*, **2**, 237-247.

Blumenthal, J.A., Williams, R.S., Wallace, A.G., Williams, R.B., & Needles, T.L. (1982). Physiological and psychological variables predict compliance to prescribed exercise therapy in patients recovering from myocardial infarction. *Psychosomatic Medicine*, **44**(6), 519-527.

Blumenthal, J.A., Williams, R.S., Williams, R.B., & Wallace, A.G. (1980). Effects of exercise on the Type A (coronary prone) behavior pattern. *Psychosomatic Medicine*, **42**(2), 289-296.

Borgatta, E.F., Couch, A.S., & Bales, R.F. (1954). Some findings relevant to the great man theory of leadership. *American Sociological Review*, **19**, 755-759.

Boylan, J.C., Malley, P.B., & Scott, J. (1988). *Practicum and internship: Textbook for counseling and psychotherapy*. Muncie, IN: Accelerated Development.

Bray, G.A. (1976). *The obese patient*. Philadelphia: Saunders.

Briggs, C.S., Sandstrom, E.R., & Nettleton, B. (1979). An approach to prediction of performance using behavioral and physiological variables. *Perceptual and Motor Skills*, **49**, 843-848.

Brinkman, J.R., & Hoskins, T.A. (1979). Physical conditioning and altered self-concept in rehabilitated hemiplegic patients. *Physical Therapy*, **59**(7), 859-865.

Brody, N. (1988). *Personality: In search of individuality*. San Diego: Academic Press.

Brooks, C. (1988). A causal modeling analysis of sociodemographics and moderate to vigorous physical activity behavior of American adults. *Research Quarterly for Exercise and Sport, 59*(4), 328-338.

Brown, J.D., & Lawton, M. (1986). Stress and well-being in adolescence: The moderating role of physical exercise. *Journal of Human Stress, 12*(3), 125-131.

Brown, J.D., & Siegel, J.M. (1988). Exercise as a buffer of life stress: A prospective study of adolescent health. *Health Psychology, 7*(4), 341-353.

Brownell, K.D. (1982). Obesity: Understanding and treating a serious, prevalent, and refractory disorder. *Journal of Consulting and Clinical Psychology, 50*, 820-840.

Brownell, K.D., Heckerman, C.L., Westlake, R.J., Hayes, S.C., & Monti, P.M. (1978). The effect of couples training and partner cooperativeness in the behavioral treatment of obesity. *Behavior, Research, and Therapy, 16*, 323-333.

Brownell, K.D., Marlatt, G.A., Lichtenstein, E., & Wilson, G.T. (1986). Understanding and preventing relapse. *American Psychologist, 41*, 765-782.

Brownell, K.D., & Stunkard, A.J. (1980). Physical activity in the development and control of obesity. In A.J. Stunkard (Ed.), *Obesity* (pp. 300-324). Philadelphia: Saunders.

Brownell, K.D., Stunkard, A.J., & Albaum, J.M. (1980). Evaluation and modification of exercise patterns in the natural environment. *American Journal of Psychiatry, 137*, 1540-1545.

Bruce, E.H., Frederick, R., Bruce, R.A., & Fisher, L.D. (1976). Comparison of active participants and dropouts in CAPRI cardiopulmonary rehabilitation programs. *American Journal of Cardiology, 37*, 53-60.

Brunner, B.C. (1969). Personality and motivating factors influencing adult participation in vigorous physical activity. *Research Quarterly, 3*, 464-469.

Butler, R.N., & Lewis, M.I. (1977). *Aging and mental health*. St. Louis: Mosby.

Canabal, M.Y., Sherrill, C., & Rainbolt, W.J. (1987). Psychological mood profiles of elite cerebral palsied athletes. In M.E. Berridge & G.R. Ward (Eds.), *International perspectives on adapted physical activity* (pp. 157-164). Champaign, IL: Human Kinetics.

Caplan, B. (1987). *Rehabilitation psychology desk reference*. Rockville, MD: Aspen.

Carkhuff, R.R. (1969). *Helping and human relations Vol. I: Selection and training*. New York: Holt Rinehart & Winston.

Carkhuff, R.R., Pierce, R.M., & Cannon, J.R. (1977). *The art of helping (Vol. 3)*. Amherst, MA: Human Resource Development Press.

Carlson, B.R., & Petti, K. (1989). Health locus of control and participation in physical activity. *American Journal of Health Promotion, 3*(3), 32-36.

Carmack, M.A., & Martens, R. (1979). Measuring commitment to running: A survey of runner's attitudes and mental states. *Journal of Sport Psychology, 1*, 25-42.

Carnwath, T., & Miller, D. (1986). *Behavioural psychotherapy in primary care: A practice manual*. London: Academic Press.

Carron, A.V. (1984). *Motivation: Implications for teaching and coaching*. London, ON: Sports Dynamics.

Carron, A.V., Widmeyer, W.N., & Brawley, L.R. (1985). The development of an instrument to assess cohesion in sport teams: The Group Environment Questionnaire. *Journal of Sport Psychology, 7*(3), 244-266.

Carron, A.V., Widmeyer, W.N., & Brawley, L.R. (1988). Group cohesion and individual adherence to physical activity. *Journal of Sport and Exercise Psychology, 10*, 127-138.

Carter, R. (1977). Exercise and happiness. *Journal of Sports Medicine and Physical Fitness, 17*, 307-313.

Cartwright, D., & Zander, A. (1968). *Group dynamics* (3rd ed.). New York: Harper & Row.

Cash, T.F., Winstead, B.A., & Janda, L.H. (1986). The great American shape-up. *Psychology Today, 20*, 30-37.

Caspersen, C.J., Christenson, G.M., & Pollard, R.A. (1986). Status of the 1990 physical fitness and exercise objectives—evidence from NHIS 1985. *Public Health Reports, 101*(6), 587-592.

Caspersen, C., Powell, K.E., & Christenson, G.M. (1985). Physical activity, exercise and physical exercise: Definitions and distinctions for health related research. *Public Health Reports, 100*(2), 126-130.

Cattell, R. (1951). New concepts for measuring leadership in terms of group syntality. *Human Relations, 4*, 161-184.

Cattell, R.B. (1960). Some psychological correlates of physical fitness and physique. In S.C. Staley (Ed.), *Exercise and fitness* (pp. 138-151). Chicago: Athletic Institute. (A collection of papers presented at the colloquium on exercise and fitness)

Cattell, R.B., & Eber, H.W. (1964). *Handbook for the Sixteen Personality Factor Questionnaire*. Champaign, IL: Institute for Personality and Ability Testing.

Cavanaugh, M.E. (1982). *The counseling experience*. Pacific Grove, CA: Brooks/Cole.

Chalip, L., Csikszentmihalyi, M., Kleiber, D., & Larson, R. (1984). Variations of experience in formal and informal sport. *Research Quarterly for Exercise and Sport*, **55**(2), 109-116.

Chalmers, J., Catalan, J., Day, A., & Fairburn, C. (1985). Anorexia nervosa presenting as morbid exercising. *The Lancet*, **1**(8423), 286-287.

Chelladurai, P. (1985). *Sport management*. London, ON: Sports Dynamics.

Chung, K.H. (1977). *Motivational theories and practices*. Columbus, OH: Grid.

Clarke, H.H. (1973, May). National adult physical fitness survey. *President's Council on Physical Fitness and Sports Newsletters*.

Clough, P., Shephard, J., & Maughan, R. (1989). Motives for participation in recreational running. *Journal of Leisure Research*, **21**(4), 297-309.

Coleman, M., Washington, M.A., & Price, S. (1985). Physical exercise, social background, and the well-being of older adult women. *Perceptual and Motor Skills*, **60**, 737-738.

Collingwood, T.R., Bernstein, I.H., Hubbard, D., & Blair, S.N. (1983). Canonical correlation analysis of clinical and psychologic data in 4,351 men and women. *Journal of Cardiac Rehabilitation*, **3**, 706-711.

Collis, M.L. (1977). *Employee fitness*. Ottawa: Minister of State for Fitness and Amateur Sport.

Combs, A.W. (1971). Self-concept: Product and producer of experience. In A.W. Combs, D.L. Avila, & W.W. Purkey (Eds.). *Helping relationships: Basic concepts for the helping professions* (pp. 39-61). Boston: Allyn & Bacon.

Condiotte, M.M., & Lichtenstein, E. (1981). Self-efficacy and relapse in smoking cessation programs. *Journal of Consulting and Clinical Psychology*, **49**, 648-658.

Conrad, C.C. (1976). When you're young at heart. *Aging*, **258**, 11-13.

Cooper, K.H. (1970). *The new aerobics*. New York: Bantam.

Cooper, M.A., Sherrill, C., & Marshall, D. (1986). Attitudes toward physical activity of elite palsied athletes. *Adapted Physical Activity Quarterly*, **3**, 14-21.

Corey, G. (1985). *The theory and practice of group counseling* (2nd ed.). Pacific Grove, CA: Brooks/Cole.

Cormier, W.H., & Cormier, L.S. (1990). *Intervening strategies for helpers: Fundamental skills and cognitive behavioral interventions* (2nd ed.). Pacific Grove, CA: Brooks/Cole.

Costa, P.T., Krantz, D.S., Blumenthal, J.A., Furberg, C.D., Rosenman, R., & Shekelle, R.B. (1987). Task force 2: Psychological risk factors in coronary artery disease. *Circulation*, **76**(1), 145-149.

Cowell, L.L., Squires, W.G., & Raven, P.B. (1986). Benefits of aerobic exercise for the paraplegic: A brief review. *Medicine and Science in Sports and Exercise*, **18**(5), 501-508.

Cowen, E.L. (1982). Help is where you find it. *American Psychologist*, **37**, 385-395.

Cox, M.H. (1984). Fitness and life-style programs for business and industry: Problems in recruitment and retention. *Journal of Cardiac Rehabilitation*, **4**, 136-142.

Cox, T. (1978). *Stress*. Baltimore: University Park Press.

Crews, D.J., & Landers, D.M. (1987). A meta-analytic review of aerobic fitness and reactivity to psychosocial stressors. *Medicine and Science in Sports and Exercise*, **19**(5), S114-120.

Crossman, J., Jamieson, J., & Henderson, L. (1987). Responses of competitive athletes to layoffs in training: Exercise addiction or psychological relief. *Journal of Sport Behavior*, **10**(1), 28-37.

Csikszentmihalyi, M. (1975). Play and intrinsic rewards. *Journal of Humanistic Psychology*, **15**(3), 41-63.

Cummings, C., Gordon, J.R., & Marlatt, G.A. (1980). Relapse: Prevention and prediction. In W.R. Miller (Ed.), *The addictive disorders: Treatment of alcoholism, drug abuse, smoke, and obesity* (pp. 291-322). Elmford, NY: Pergamon Press.

Danielson, R.R., & Wanzel, R.S. (1977). Exercise objectives of fitness program dropouts. In D.M. Landers & R.W. Christina (Eds.), *Psychology of motor behavior and sports* (pp. 310-320). Champaign, IL: Human Kinetics.

Dannenmaier, W.E. (1978). *Mental health: An overview*. Chicago: Nelson-Hall.

De Charms, R. (1968). *Personal causation: The internal affective determinants of behavior*. New York: Academic Press.

Deci, E.L. (1975). *Intrinsic motivation*. New York: Plenum Press.

Deci, E.L. (1977). Intrinsic motivation: Theory and application. In D.M. Landers, & R.W. Christina (Eds.), *Psychology of motor behavior and sport* (pp. 388-396). Champaign, IL: Human Kinetics.

Deci, E.L., & Ryan, R.M. (1985). The general causality orientations scale: Self-determination in personality. *Journal of Research in Personality,* **19**, 109-134.

DePauw, K.P. (1988). Sport for individuals with disabilities: Research opportunities. *Adapted Physical Activity Quarterly,* **5**, 80-89.

De Rivera, J. (1984). Development and the full range of emotional experience. In C.Z. Malatesta & C.E. Izard (Eds.), *Emotion in adult development* (pp. 45-63). Beverly Hills, CA: Sage.

Desharnais, R., Bouillon, J., & Godin, G. (1987). Self-efficacy and outcome expectations as determinants of exercise adherence. *Psychological Reports,* **59**, 1155-1159.

Deutsch, M. (1973). *The resolution of conflict.* New Haven, CN: Yale University Press.

deVries, H.A. (1968). Immediate and long term effects of exercise upon resting muscle action potential level. *Journal of Sports Medicine and Physical Fitness,* **8**, 1-11.

deVries, H.A. (1981). Functional fitness for older Americans. In *President's Council on Physical Fitness and Sports: A synopsis of the National Conference on Fitness and Aging* (pp. 27-28). Washington, DC: President's Council on Physical Fitness and Sports.

deVries, H.A., & Adams, G.M. (1972). Comparison of exercise response in old and young men: 1. The cardiac effort/total body effort relationship. *Journal of Gerontology,* **27**(3), 344-348.

Dienstbier, R.A. (1984). The effects of exercise on personality. In M.L. Sachs & G.W. Buffone (Eds.), *Running as therapy* (pp. 253-272). Lincoln, NE: University of Nebraska Press.

Diesfeldt, H., & Diesfeldt-Groenendijk, H. (1977). Improving cognitive performance in psychogeriatric patients: The influence of physical exercise. *Age and Aging,* **6**, 58-64.

DiMambro, K., & Wolfe, D. (January, 1989). Forty plus. *Club Business International,* pp. 45-59.

Dintiman, G.B., & Greenberg, J.S. (1983). *Health through discovery* (2nd ed.). New York: Random House.

Dishman, R.K. (1981). Biologic influences on exercise adherence. *Research Quarterly for Exercise and Sport,* **52**(2), 143-159.

Dishman, R.K. (1982). Compliance/adherence in health-related exercise. *Health Psychology,* **1**(3), 237-267.

Dishman, R.K. (1985). Medical psychology in exercise and sport. *Medical Clinics of North America,* **69**(1), 123-143.

Dishman, R.K. (1986). Mental health. In V. Seefeld (Ed.), *Physical activity and well being* (pp. 304-

341). Reston, VA: American Association for Health, Physical Education, Recreation and Dance.

Dishman, R.K., & Dunn, A.L. (1988). Exercise adherence in children and youth: Implications for adulthood. In R.K. Dishman (Ed.), *Exercise adherence: Its impact on public health* (pp. 155-200). Champaign, IL: Human Kinetics.

Dishman, R.K., & Gettman, L.R. (1980). Psychobiologic influences on exercise adherence. *Journal of Sport Psychology,* **2**, 295-310.

Dishman, R.K., & Ickes, W. (1981). Self-motivation and adherence to therapeutic exercise. *Journal of Behavioral Medicine,* **4**(4), 421-438.

Dishman, R.K., Ickes, W., & Morgan, W.P. (1980). Self-motivation and adherence to habitual physical activity. *Journal of Applied Social Psychology,* **10**(2), 115-132.

Doan, R.E., & Scherman, A. (1987). The therapeutic effect of physical fitness on measures of personality: A literature review. *Journal of Counseling and Development,* **66**, 28-36.

Dobson, K.S., & Block, L. (1988). Historical and philosophical bases of the cognitive-behavioral therapies. In K.S. Dobson (Ed.), *Handbook of cognitive behavioral therapies* (pp. 3-34). New York: Guilford Press.

Dotson, C.O., & Stanley, W.J. (1972). Values of physical activity perceived by male university students. *Research Quarterly,* **43**(2), 148-156.

Doyne, E.J., Chambliss, D.L., & Beutler, L.E. (1983). Aerobic exercise as a treatment for depression in women. *Behavior Therapy,* **14**, 434-440.

Doyne, E.J., Ossip-Klein, D.J., Bowman, E.D., Osborn, K.M., McDougall-Wilson, I.B., & Neimeyer, R.A. (1987). Running versus weight lifting in the treatment of depression. *Journal of Consulting and Clinical Psychology,* **55**(5), 748-754.

Driscoll, R. (1976). Anxiety reduction using physical exertion and positive images. *Psychological Record,* **26**, 87-94.

Duke, M., Johnson, T.C., & Nowicki, S. (1977). Effects of sports fitness camp experience on locus of control orientation in children ages 6 to 14. *Research Quarterly,* **48**(2), 280-283.

Dunbar, J.M., Marshall, G.D., & Hovell, M.F. (1979). Behavioral strategies for improving compliance. In R.B. Haynes, D.W. Taylor, & D.L. Sackett (Eds.), *Compliance in health care* (pp. 174-190). Baltimore: Johns Hopkins University Press.

Dupont, H. (1978). Affective development: Stage and sequence. In R.L. Mosher (Ed.), *Adolescents' development and education* (pp. 163-183). Berkeley, CA: McCutchon.

Durbeck, D.C., Heinzleman, F., Schacter, J., & Haskell, W. (1972). The National Aeronautics and Space Administration-US Public Health Service health evaluation and enhancement program. *American Journal of Cardiology, 30*, 784-790.

Dustman, R.E., Ruhling, R.O., Russell, E.M., & Shearer, D.E. (1984). Aerobic exercise training and improved neurophysical function of older adults. *Neurobiology of Aging, 5*, 35-42.

Dwyer, J.T., Feldman, J.J., & Mayer, J. (1970). The social psychology of dieting. *Journal of Health and Social Behavior, 11*, 269-287.

Dyer, J.B., & Crouch, J.G. (1988). Effects of running and other activities on moods. *Perceptual and Motor Skills, 67*, 43-50.

Dzewaltowski, D.A. (1989). Toward a model of exercise motivation. *Journal of Sport and Exercise Psychology, 11*, 251-269.

Egan, G. (1984). People in systems: A comprehensive model of psychosocial education and training. In D. Larson (Ed.), *Teaching psychological skills: Models for giving psychology away* (pp. 133-150). Monterey, CA: Brooks/Cole.

Egan, G. (1986). *The skilled helper: A systematic approach to effective helping* (3rd ed.). Pacific Grove, CA: Brooks/Cole.

Ellis, A. (1962). *Reason and emotion in psychology.* New York: Lyle Stuart.

Ellis, A. (1977). Psychotherapy and the value of a human being. In A. Ellis & R. Grieger (Eds.), *Handbook of rational-emotive therapy.* New York: Springer.

Ellis, A. (1984). Rational-emotive therapy. In R. Corsini (Ed.), *Current psychotherapies* (3rd ed.). Itasca, IL: T.E. Peacock.

Elsayed, M., Ismail, A.H., & Young, R.J. (1980). Intellectual differences of adult men related to age and physical fitness before and after an exercise program. *Journal of Gerontology, 35*(3), 383-387.

Employee Fitness and Lifestyle Project. (1978). Toronto: Minister of State, Fitness, and Amateur Sport.

Epstein, L.H., Koeske, R., & Wing, R.R. (1984). Adherence to exercise in obese children. *Journal of Rehabilitation, 4*, 185-195.

Epstein, L.H., & Wing, R.R. (1980). Aerobic exercise and weight. *Addictive Behaviors, 5*, 371-388.

Epstein, L.H., Wing, R.R., Koeske, R., Ossip, D., & Beck. S. (1982). A comparison of lifestyle change and programmed aerobic exercise on weight and fitness changes in obese children. *Behavior Therapy, 13*, 651-665.

Epstein, L.H., Wing, R.R., Koeske, R., & Valoski, A. (1985). A comparison of lifestyle exercise, aerobic exercise, and calisthenics on weight loss in obese children. *Behavior Therapy, 16*, 345-356.

Epstein, L.H., Wing, R.R., Thompson, J.K., & Griffin, W. (1980). Attendance and fitness in aerobics exercise: The effects of contract and lottery procedures. *Behavior Modification, 4*(4), 465-479.

Erdman, R.A.M., Hugo, M.S., & Duivenvoorden, H.J. (1983). Psychologic evaluation of a cardiac rehabilitation program: A randomized clinical trial in patients with myocardial infarction. *Journal of Cardiac Rehabilitation, 3*, 696-704.

Erickson, E.L., McEvoy, A., & Colucci, N.D. (1984). *Child abuse and neglect: A guidebook for educators and community leaders* (2nd ed.). Homes Beach, FL: Learning Publications.

Erikson, E.H. (1963). *Childhood and society* (2nd ed.). New York: Norton.

Erling, J., & Oldridge, N.B. (1985). Effect of a spousal support program on compliance with cardiac rehabilitation. *Medicine and Science in Sports and Exercise, 17*, 284.

Ewart, C.K., Stewart, K.J., Gillian, R.E., & Keleman, M.H. (1986). Self-efficacy mediates strength gains during circuit weight training in men with coronary artery disease. *Medicine and Science in Sports and Exercise, 18*(5), 531-540.

Ewart, C.K., Taylor, C.B., Reese, L.B., & DeBusk, R.F. (1983). Effects of early postmyocardial infarction exercise testing on self-perception and subsequent physical activity. *American Journal of Cardiology, 51*, 1076-1080.

Eysenck, H.J. (1959). *Manual of the Maudsley personality inventory.* London: University of London Press.

Eysenck, H.J., & Eysenck, S.G.B. (1964). *The Eysenck personality inventory.* London: University of London Press.

Falk, J.R. (1986). Psychology of exercise. In A.R. Leff (Ed.), *Cardiopulmonary exercise testing* (pp. 233-256). New York: Grune & Stratton.

Feeling fat in a thin society. (1984, February). *Glamour, 46*, 198-201.

Festinger, L.A. (1957). *A theory of cognitive dissonance.* Evanston, IL: Row, Peterson.

Fiedler, F.E. (1967). *A theory of leadership effectiveness.* New York: McGraw-Hill.

Fiedler, F.E. (1978). The contingency model and the dynamics of the leadership process. In L. Berkowitz (Ed.), *Advances in experimental social psychology.* New York: Academic Press.

Fiedler, F.E. (1981). Leadership effectiveness. *American Behavioral Scientist, 24*, 619-632.

Fishbein, M., & Ajzen, I. (1975). *Belief, attitude, intention, and behavior.* Reading, MA: Addison-Wesley.

Fisher, B.A. (1980). *Small group decision-making* (2nd ed.). New York: McGraw-Hill.

Fitness Ontario. (1981). *Those who know but don't do (Research Report).* Toronto: Ministry of Culture and Recreation.

Fitness Ontario. (1983). *Physical activity patterns in Ontario-II.* Toronto: Ministry of Tourism and Recreation.

Folkins, C.H. (1976). Effects of physical training on mood. *Journal of Clinical Psychology, 32*(2), 385-388.

Folkins, C.H., & Sime, W.E. (1981). Physical fitness training and mental health. *American Psychologist, 36*(4), 373-389.

Folkins, C.H., & Wieselberg-Bell, N. (1981). A personality profile of ultramarathon runners: A little deviance may go a long way. *Journal of Sport Behavior, 4*(3), 119-127.

Forsterling, F. (1980). Attribution aspects of cognitive behavior modification: A theoretical approach and suggestions for technique. *Cognitive Therapy and Research, 4*, 27-37.

Forsyth, D.R. (1983). *An introduction to group dynamics.* Pacific Grove, CA: Brooks/Cole.

Fox, K.R., & Corbin, C.B. (1989). The physical self-perception profile: Development and preliminary validation. *Journal of Sport and Exercise Psychology, 11*, 408-430.

Fox, K.R., Corbin, C.C., & Couldry, W.H. (1985). Female physical estimation and attraction to physical activity. *Journal of Sport Psychology, 7*(2), 125-136.

Frank, J.D. (1973). *Persuasion and healing* (2nd ed.). Baltimore: Johns Hopkins University Press.

Franken, R.E. (1982). *Human motivation.* Monterey, CA: Brooks/Cole.

Franklin, B.A. (1978). Motivating and educating adults to exercise. *Journal of Physical Education and Recreation, 49*(6), 13-17.

Franklin, B.A. (1984). Exercise program compliance. In J. Storlie & H.A. Jordan (Eds.), *Behavioral management of obesity* (pp. 105-135). New York: Spectrum Press.

Franklin, B.A. (1986). Clinical components of a successful adult fitness program. *American Journal of Health Promotion, 1*(1), 6-13.

Franklin, B.A. (1988). Program factors that influence exercise adherence: Practical adherence skills for the clinical staff. In R.K. Dishman (Ed.), *Exercise adherence: Its impact on public health* (pp. 237-258). Champaign, IL: Human Kinetics.

Frazier, S.E. (1988). Mood state profiles of chronic exercisers with differing abilities. *International Journal of Sport Psychology, 19*, 65-71.

Fremont, J., & Craighead L.W. (1987). Aerobic exercise and cognitive therapy in the treatment of dysphoric moods. *Cognitive Therapy and Research, 11*(2), 241-251.

French, J.R., Jr., & Raven, B. (1959). The bases of social power. In D. Cartwright (Ed.), *Studies in social power* (pp. 150-167). Ann Arbor, MI: Institute for Social Research.

Friedman, E.H., & Hellerstein, H.K. (1973). Influence of psychosocial factors on coronary risk and adaptation to a physical fitness evaluation program. In J. Naughton & H.K. Hekkerstein (Eds.), *Exercise testing and exercise training in coronary heart disease* (pp. 225-251). New York: Academic Press.

Friedman, H.S., & Booth-Kewley, S. (1987). The disease prone personality. *American Psychologist, 42*(6), 539-555.

Friedman, M., & Rosenman, R.H. (1974). *Type A behavior and your heart.* New York: Knopf.

Fujimura, L.E., Weis, D.M., & Cochran, F.R. (1985). Suicide: Dynamics and implications for counseling. *Journal of Counseling and Development, 63*, 612-625.

Gale, J.B., Eckhoff, W.T., Mogel, S.F., & Rodnick, J.E. (1984). Factors related to adherence to an exercise program for healthy adults. *Medicine and Science in Sports and Exercise, 16*(6), 544-549.

Garner, D.M., Garfinkel, P.E., Schwartz, D., & Thompson, M. (1980). Cultural expectations of thinness in women. *Psychological Reports, 47*, 483-491.

Gatchel, R.J., & Baum, A. (1983). *An introduction to health psychology.* New York: Random House.

Gauvin, L. (1989). The relationship between regular physical activity and subjective well being. *Journal of Sport Behavior, 12*(2), 107-114.

Gavin, J. (1988). *Body moves: The psychology of exercise.* Harrisburg, PA: Stackpole Books.

Gazda, G.M. (1973). *Human relations development: A manual for educators.* Needham Heights, MA: Allyn & Bacon.

Gazda, G.M. (1984). Multiple impact training: A life skills approach. In D. Larson (Ed.), *Teaching psychological skills: Models for giving psychology away* (pp. 87-103). Monterey, CA: Brooks/Cole.

Gazda, G.M. (1989). *Group counseling: A developmental approach* (4th ed.). Needham Heights, MA: Allyn & Bacon.

Gazda, G.M., Asbury, F.R., Balzer, F.J., Childers, W.C., & Walters, R.P. (1984). *Human relations development: A manual for educators* (3rd ed.). Boston: Allyn & Bacon.

Gazda, G.M., Childers, W.C., & Brooks, D.K., Jr. (1987). *Foundations of counseling and human services*. New York: McGraw-Hill.

Gazda, G.M., Childers, W.C., & Walters, R.R. (1982). *Interpersonal communication: A handbook for health professionals*. Rockville, MD: Aspen System Corporation.

Gentry, W.D., & Haney, T. (1975). Emotional and behavioral reaction to acute myocardial infarction. *Heart and Lung, 4*(5), 738-745.

Gentry, W.D., & Kobasa, S.C. (1979). Social and psychological resources mediating stress illness relationships in humans. In R.B. Haynes, D.W. Taylor, & D. Sackett (Eds.), *Compliance in health care* (pp. 87-116). Baltimore: Johns Hopkins University Press.

Gettman, L.R., Pollock, M.L., & Ward, A. (1983). Adherence to unsupervised exercise. *The Physician and Sportsmedicine, 11*(10), 56-66.

Gibb, C.A. (1969). Leadership. In G. Lindzey & E. Aronson (Eds.), *The handbook of social psychology* (Vol. 4, 2nd ed.) (pp. 205-282). Reading, MA: Addison-Wesley.

Gillett, P.A. (1988). Self-reported factors influencing exercise adherence in overweight women. *Nursing Research, 37*(1), 25-29.

Girdano, D.A., Everly, G.S., & Dusek, D.E. (1990). *Controlling stress and tension: A holistic approach* (3rd ed.). Englewood Cliffs, NJ: Prentice Hall.

Gladding, S.T. (1988). *Counseling: A comprehensive profession*. Columbus, OH: Merrill.

Gladstein, G.A., & Feldstein, J.C. (1983). Using film to increase counselor empathic experiences. *Counselor Education and Supervision, 23*, 125-131.

Glasser, W. (1976). *Positive addiction*. New York: Harper & Row.

Goddard, R.W. (1986). The healthy side of conflict. *Management World, 15*(5), 8-12.

Godin, G. (1987). Importance of the emotional aspect of attitude to predict intention. *Psychological Reports, 61*, 719-723.

Godin, G., Cox, M.H., & Shephard, R.J. (1983). The impact of physical fitness evaluation on behavioral intentions towards regular exercise. *Canadian Journal of Applied Sport Science, 8*(4), 240-245.

Godin, G., & Shephard, R.J. (1985). Psycho-social predictors of exercise intentions among spouses. *Canadian Journal of Applied Sport Science, 10*(1), 36-43.

Godin, G., & Shephard, R.J. (1986). Importance of type of attitude to the study of exercise behavior. *Psychological Reports, 58*(3), 991-1000.

Godin, G., Shephard, R.J., & Colantino, A. (1986). The cognitive profile of those who intend to exercise but who do not. *Public Health Reports, 101*(5), 521-526.

Godin, G., Valois, P., Shephard, R.J., & Desharnais, R. (1987). Prediction of leisure-time exercise behavior: A path analysis (LISREL V) model. *Journal of Behavioral Medicine, 10*(2), 145-158.

Goldberg, G., & Shephard, R.J. (1982). Personality profiles of disabled individuals in relation to physical activity patterns. *Journal of Sports Medicine, 22*, 477-484.

Goldfarb, L.A., & Plante, T.G. (1984). Fear of fat in runners: An examination of the connection between anorexia nervosa and distance running. *Psychological Reports, 55*, 296.

Goldwater, B.C., & Collins, M.L. (1985). Psychologic effects of cardiovascular conditioning: A controlled experiment. *Psychosomatic Medicine, 47*(2), 174-181.

Gondola, J.C., & Tuckman, B.W. (1982). Psychological mood state in "average" marathon runners. *Perceptual and Motor Skills, 55*, 1295-1300.

Goodrick, G.K., Hartung, G.H., Warren, D.R., & Hoepfel, J.A. (1984). Helping adults to stay physically fit: Preventing relapse following aerobic exercise training. *Journal of Physical Education, Recreation and Dance, 55*(2), 48-49.

Gould, D., & Horn, T. (1984). Participation motives in young athletes. In J.M. Silva & R.S. Weinberg (Eds.), *Psychological foundations of sport* (pp. 359-370). Champaign, IL: Human Kinetics.

Graham, L.E., Taylor, C.B., Hovell, M.F., & Siegel, W. (1983). Five year follow-up to a behavioral weight loss program. *Journal of Consulting and Clinical Psychology, 51*, 322-323.

Greist, J.H., Klein, M.H., Eischens, R.R., & Faris, J.T. (1978). Running out of depression. *The Physician and Sportsmedicine, 6*(12), 49-51.

Gross, A.M., Johnson, T.C., Wojnilower, D.A, & Drabman, R.S. (1985). The relationship between sports fitness training and social status in children. *Behavioral Engineering, 9*(2), 58-65.

Gruber, J.J. (1986). Physical activity and self-esteem development in children: A meta-analysis. *American Academy of Physical Education Papers, 19*, 30-48.

Gruen, W. (1975). Effects of brief psychotherapy during the hospitalization period on the recovery process in heart attacks. *Journal of*

Consulting and Clinical Psychology, 43, 223-232.

Gustafson, J.P. (1978). Schismatic groups. *Human Relations, 31*, 139-154.

Gwinup, G. (1975). Effect of exercise alone on the weight of obese women. *Archives of Internal Medicine, 135*, 676-680.

Haaga, D.A., & Davison, G.C. (1986). Cognitive change methods. In F.H. Kanfer & A.P. Goldstein (Eds.), *Helping people change: A textbook of methods* (pp. 236-282). New York: Pergamon Press.

Hackett, T.P., & Cassem, N.H. (1973). Psychological adaptation to convalescence in myocardial patients. In J. Naughton & H.K. Hellerstein (Eds.), *Exercise testing and exercise training in coronary heart disease* (pp. 253-262). New York: Academic Press.

Hackett, T.P., & Cassem, N.H. (1978). Psychological factors related to exercise. *Cardiovascular Clinics, 9*, 223-231.

Hagen, R.L., Foreyt, J.P., & Durham, T.W. (1976). The drop-out problem: Reducing attrition in obesity research. *Behavior Therapy, 7*, 463-471.

Hall, C.S., & Lindzey, G. (1978). *Theories of learning.* New York: Wiley.

Hall, L.K. (1984). Psychological concerns of the cardiac patient. In L.K. Hall & G.L. Meyer (Eds.), *Cardiac rehabilitation: Exercise testing and prescription* (pp. 107-121). New York: SP Medical.

Hallstrom, T., & Noppa, H. (1981). Obesity in women in relation to mental illness, social factors and personality traits. *Journal of Psychosomatic Research, 25*(2), 75-82.

Hannaford, C.P., Harrell, E.H., & Cox, K. (1988). Psychophysiological effects of a running program on depression and anxiety in a psychiatric population. *Psychological Record, 38*, 37-48.

Harper, N.L., & Askling, L.R. (1980). Group communication and quality of task solution in a media production organization. *Communication Monographs, 49*, 77-100.

Harris, D.V. (1970). Physical activity history and attitudes of middle-aged men. *Medicine and Science in Sports, 2*(4), 203-208.

Harris, M.B. (1981a). Runners' perceptions of the benefits of running. *Perceptual and Motor Skills, 52*, 153-154.

Harris, M.B. (1981b). Women runners' views of running. *Perceptual and Motor Skills, 53*, 395-402.

Haskell, W.L. (1974). Physical activity after myocardial infarction. *American Journal of Cardiology, 33*, 776-783.

Haskell, W.L. (1984). Overview: Health benefits of exercise. In J.D. Matarrazzo, S.M. Weiss, J.A.

Herd, W.E. Miller, & S.M. Weiss (Eds.), *Behavioral health: A handbook of health enhancement and disease prevention* (pp. 409-423). New York: Wiley.

Haskell, W.L., Montoye, H.J., & Orenstein, D. (1985). Physical activity and exercise to achieve health related physical fitness components. *Public Health Reports, 100*(2), 202-211.

Hathaway, S.R., & McKinley, J.C. (1948). *Minnesota Multiphasic Personality Inventory.* New York: Psychological Corporation.

Hayden, R.M., Allen, G.J., & Camaione, D.N. (1986). Some psychological benefits resulting from involvement in an aerobic fitness program from the perspectives of participants and knowledgeable informants. *Journal of Sports Medicine, 26*, 67-76.

Hayes, D., & Ross, C.E. (1986). Body and mind: The effect of exercise, overweight, and physical health on psychological well-being. *Journal of Health and Social Behavior, 27*, 387-400.

Hayman, P.M., & Covert, J.A. (1986). Ethical dilemmas in college counseling centers. *Journal of Counseling and Development, 64*, 318-320.

Heider, F. (1958). *The psychology of interpersonal relations.* New York: Wiley.

Heinzelmann, F., & Bagley, R.W. (1970). Response to physical activity programs and their effects on health behavior. *Public Health Reports, 85*(10), 905-911.

Heitmann, H.M. (1986). Motives of older adults for participating in physical activity programs. In B.D. McPherson (Ed.), *Sport and aging* (pp. 199-204). Champaign, IL: Human Kinetics.

Henning, A.D. (1987). Exercise at work? I don't have time. *Fitness in Business, 2*(2), 68-69.

Henschen, K., Horvat, M., & French, R. (1984). A visual comparison of psychological profiles between able bodied and wheelchair athletes. *Adapted Physical Activity Quarterly, 1*, 118-124.

Hersey, P., & Blanchard, K.H. (1977). *Management of organizational behavior. Utilizing human resources* (3rd ed.). Englewood Cliffs, NJ: Prentice Hall.

Heston, M.L. (1983). Childhood obesity: Implications for physical education. *Physical Educator, 40*(3), 145-149.

Hilyer, J.C., Wilson, D.G., Dillon, C., Caro, L., Jenkins, C., Spencer, W.A., & Booker, W. (1982). Physical fitness training and counseling as treatment for youthful offenders. *Journal of Counseling Psychology, 29*(3), 292-303.

Hindi-Alexander, M.C., & Throm, J. (1987). Compliance or noncompliance: That is the question. *American Journal of Health Promotion*, **1**(4), 5-11.

Hinton, E.R., & Taylor, S. (1986). Does placebo response mediate runner's high? *Perceptual and Motor Skills*, **62**, 789-790.

Hobson, C.J., Hoffman, J.J., Corso, L.M., & Freismuth, P.K. (1987). Corporate fitness: Understanding and motivating employee participation. *Fitness in Business*, **2**(3), 80-85.

Hoepfel-Harris, J.A. (1980). Rehabilitation of the cardiac patient: Improving compliance with an exercise program. *American Journal of Nursing*, **80**, 449-450.

Hogan, P.I., & Santomier, J.P. (1984). Effect of mastering swim skills on older adults' self-efficacy. *Research Quarterly for Exercise and Sport*, **55**(3), 294-296.

Holland, R.L. (1977). *The self-directed search*. Palo Alto, CA: Consulting Psychologists Press.

Hopper, C., & Santomier, J. (1984/1985). Self-esteem and aspirations of wheelchair athletes. *Humboldt Journal of Social Relations*, **12**(1), 24-35.

Horley, J. (1984). Life satisfaction, happiness and morale: Two problems with the use of subjective well-being indicators. *The Gerontologist*, **24**(2), 124-127.

Horn, T.S. (1984). Expectancy effects in the interscholastic athletic setting: Methodological considerations. *Journal of Sport Psychology*, **6**(4), 60-76.

Hughes, J.R., Casal, D.C., & Leon, A.S. (1986). Psychological effects of exercise: A randomized cross-over trial. *Journal of Psychosomatic Research*, **30**(3), 355-360.

Hummel, D.L., Talbutt, L.C., & Alexander, M.D. (1985). *Law and ethics in counseling*. New York: Van Nostrand Reinhold.

Hurwitz, J., Zander, A., & Hymovitch, B. (1968). Some relations among group members. In D. Cartwright and A. Zander (Eds.), *Group dynamics* (3rd ed.) (pp. 291-297). New York: Harper & Row.

Iverson, D.C., Fielding, J.E., Crow, R.S., & Christenson, G.M. (1985). The promotion of physical activity in the United States population: The status of programs in medical, worksite, community, and school settings. *Public Health Reports*, **100**(2), 214-224.

Jablenski, A. (1985). Approaches to the definition and classification of anxiety and related disorders in European psychiatry. In A.H. Tuma & J.D. Maser (Eds.), *Anxiety and the anxiety disorders* (pp. 735-758). Hillsdale, NJ: Erlbaum.

Jacobson, E. (1938). *Progressive relaxation*. Chicago: University of Chicago Press.

Janz, N.K., & Becker, M.H. (1984). The health belief model: A decade later. *Health Education Quarterly*, **11**(1), 1-47.

Jarvie, G.J., & Thompson, J.K. (1985). Appropriate use of stationary exercycles in the natural environment: The failure of instructions and goal setting to appreciably modify exercise patterns. *Behavior Therapist*, **8**(9), 187-188.

Jasnoski, M.L., Cordray, D.S., Houston, B.K., & Osness, W.H. (1987). Modification of Type A behavior through aerobic exercise. *Motivation and Emotion*, **11**(1), 1-17.

Jasnoski, M.L., & Holmes, D.S. (1981). Influence of initial aerobic fitness, aerobic training and changes in aerobic fitness on personality functioning. *Journal of Psychosomatic Research*, **25**(6), 553-556.

Jasnoski, M.L., Holmes, D.S., & Banks, D.L. (1988). Changes in personality associated with changes in aerobic and anaerobic fitness in women and men. *Journal of Psychosomatic Research*, **32**(3), 273-276.

Jeffrey, D.B., & Lemnitzer, N. (1981). Diet, exercise, obesity, and related health problems: A macroenvironmental analysis. In J.M. Ferguson & C.B. Taylor (Eds.), *The comprehensive handbook of behavioral medicine* (Vol. 2, pp. 47-93). New York: Spectrum Books.

Jenkins, C.D. (1976). Recent evidence supporting psychologic and social risk factors for coronary disease. *New England Journal of Medicine*, **294**, 987-994.

Johnsgard, K. (1983 January). Why do you do it? *Running Times*, **1**, 38-39.

Johnsgard, K. (1985a). The motivation of the long-distance runner: I. *Journal of Sports Medicine*, **25**, 135-139.

Johnsgard, K. (1985b). The motivation of the long distance runner: II. *Journal of Sports Medicine*, **25**, 140-143.

Johnson, S.F., Swenson, W.M., & Gastineau, C.F. (1976). Personality characteristics in obesity: Relation of MMPI profile and age of onset of obesity to success in weight reduction. *American Journal of Clinical Nutrition*, **29**, 626-632.

Jones, E.E., & Nisbett, R.E. (1971). *The actor and observer: Divergent perceptions on the causes of behavior*. Morristown, NJ: General Learning Press.

Jordan, H.A. (1987). Obesity treatment. In J. Storlie & H.A. Jordan (Eds.), *Evaluation and treatment of obesity* (pp. 1-21). Champaign, IL: Life Enhancement.

Joseph, P., & Robbins, J.M. (1981). Worker or runner? The impact of commitment to running and work on self-identification. In M. Sacks &

M. Sachs (Eds.), *Psychology of running* (pp. 131-149). Champaign, IL: Human Kinetics.

Jourard, S.M., & Secord, P.F. (1955). Body-cathexis and the ideal female figure. *Journal of Abnormal Social Psychology, 50*, 243-246.

Kagan, D.M., & Squires, R.L. (1985). Addictive aspects of physical exercise. *Journal of Sports Medicine, 25*, 227-237.

Kagan, N. (1973). Can technology help us toward reliability in influencing human interaction? *Educational Technology, 13*, 44-51.

Kane, J.E. (1970). Personality and physical abilities. In G.S. Kenyon (Ed.), *Contemporary psychology of sport* (pp. 131-141). Chicago: Athletic Institute.

Kanfer, F.H. (1970). Self-regulation: Research issues and speculations. In C. Neuringer & J.L. Michael (Eds.), *Behavior modification in clinical psychology* (pp. 178-220). New York: Appleton-Century-Crofts.

Kanfer, F.H., Cox, L.E., Gruner, J.M., & Karoly, P. (1974). Contracts, demand characteristics, and self-control. *Journal of Personality and Social Psychology, 30*, 605-619.

Kanfer, F.H., & Gaelick, L. (1986). Self-management methods. In F.H. Kanfer & A.P. Goldstein (Eds.), *Helping people change: A textbook of methods* (pp. 283-345). New York: Pergamon Press.

Kaplan, R.M., Atkins, C.J., & Reinsch, S. (1984). Specific efficacy expectations mediate exercise compliance in patients with COPD. *Health Psychology, 3*(3), 223-242.

Karoly, P., & Harris, A. (1986). Operant methods. In F.H. Kanfer & A.P. Goldstein (Eds.), *Helping people change: A textbook of methods* (pp. 111-144). New York: Pergamon Press.

Kashyap, A. (1982). Differential efficacy of power base in opinion change in group discussion. *Journal of Psychological Research, 26*, 9-12.

Katz, J.F., Adler, J.C., Mazzarella, N.J., & Ince, L.P. (1985). Psychological consequences of an exercise training program for a paraplegic man: A case study. *Rehabilitation Psychology, 30*(1), 53-58.

Katz, R., & Tushman, M. (1979). Communication patterns, project performance, and task characteristics: An empirical evaluation and integration in an R & D setting. *Organization Behavior and Group Performance, 23*, 139-162.

Kavanagh, T., Shephard, R.J., Tuck, J.A., & Qureshi, S. (1977). Depression after myocardial infarction: The effects of distance running. *Annals of New York Academy of Sciences, 301*, 1029-1038.

Kazdin, A.E., & Wilcoxon, L.A. (1976). Systematic desensitization and nonspecific effects: A methodological evaluation. *Psychological Bulletin, 83*, 729-758.

Keller, S., & Seraganian, P. (1984). Physical fitness level and autonomic reactivity to psychosocial stress. *Journal of Psychosomatic Research, 28*(4), 279-287.

Kennedy, J.F. (1960, December 26). The soft American. *Sports Illustrated, 13*(2), 15-17.

Kenyon, G.S. (1968a). Conceptual model for characterizing physical activity. *Research Quarterly, 39*, 96-105.

Kenyon, G.S. (1968b). Six scales for assessing attitude toward physical activity. *Research Quarterly, 39*, 566-574.

Kerlinger, F.N. (1973). *Foundations of behavioral research*. New York: Holt Rinehart & Winston.

Key, N. (1986). Abating risk and accidents through communication. *Professional Safety, 31*(11), 25-28.

Kindl, M., & Brown, P. (1976). The team approach—the effective treatment of obesity in the community. *Canadian AHPER Journal, 43*, 39-41.

King, A.C., & Frederiksen, L.W. (1984). Low-cost strategies for increasing exercise behavior. *Behavior Modification, 8*(1), 3-21.

King, A.C., Taylor, C.B., Haskell, W.L., & DeBusk, R.F. (1989). Influence of regular aerobic exercise on psychological health: A randomized, controlled trial of healthy middle-aged adults. *Health Psychology, 8*(3), 305-324.

Kirschenbaum, D.S., & Flanery, R.C. (1983). Behavioral contracting: Outcomes and elements. In M. Hersen, R.M., Eisler, & P.M. Miller (Eds.), *Progress in behavior modification* (Vol. 15, pp. 217-270). New York: Academic Press.

Kirschenbaum, D., & Karoly, P. (1977). When self-regulation fails: Tests of some preliminary hypothesis. *Journal of Consulting and Clinical Psychology, 45*, 1116-1125.

Klein, M.H., Greist, J.H., Gurman, A.S., Neimeyer, R.A., Lesser, D.P., Bushnell, N.J., & Smith, R.E. (1985). A comparative outcome study of group psychotherapy vs. exercise treatment for depression. *International Journal of Mental Health, 13*, 148-177.

Kleinginna, P.R., & Kleinginna, A.M. (1981a). A categorized list of emotion definitions, with suggestions for a consensual definition. *Motivation and Emotion, 5*(4), 345-379.

Kleinginna, P.R., & Kleinginna, A.M. (1981b). A categorized list of motivation definitions, with a suggestion for a consensual definition. *Motivation and Emotion, 5*(3), 263-291.

Knapp, D.N. (1988). Behavioral management techniques and exercise promotion. In R.K.

Dishman (Ed.), *Exercise adherence: Its impact on public health* (pp. 203-235). Champaign, IL: Human Kinetics.

Knapp, D., Gutman, M., Foster, C., & Pollock, M. (1984). Self-motivation among 1984 Olympic speedskating hopefuls and emotional response and adherence to training. *Medicine and Science in Sports and Exercise, 16,* 114-115.

Knapp, D., Gutman, M., Squires, R., & Pollock, M.L. (1983). Exercise adherence among coronary artery bypass surgery (CABS) patients (abstract). *Medicine and Science in Sports and Exercise, 15,* 120.

Knapp, M.L. (1978). *Nonverbal communication in human interaction* (2nd ed.). New York: Holt, Rinehart & Winston.

Knapp, M.R.J. (1977). The activity theory of aging: An examination in the English context. *The Gerontologist, 17*(6), 553-559.

Knight, P.O., Schocken, D.D., Powers, P.S., Feld, S., & Smith, J.T. (1987). Gender comparison in anorexia nervosa and obligate running. *Medicine and Science in Sports and Exercise, 19,* S66.

Kobasa, S.C. (1979). Stressful life events, personality, and health: An inquiry into hardiness. *Journal of Personality and Social Psychology, 37*(1), 1-11.

Kobasa, S.C., Maddi, S.R., & Kahn, S. (1982). Hardiness and health: A prospective study. *Journal of Personality and Social Psychology, 42*(1), 168-177.

Kobasa, S.C., Maddi, S.R., & Puccetti, M.C. (1982). Personality and exercise as buffers in the stress-illness relationship. *Journal of Behavioral Medicine, 5*(4), 391-405.

Kobasa, S.C., Maddi, S.R., Puccetti, M.C., & Zola, M.A. (1985). Effectiveness of hardiness, exercise and social support as resources against illness. *Journal of Psychosomatic Research, 29*(5), 525-533.

Kraus, H., & Hirschland, R.P. (1954). Minimum muscular fitness tests in school children. *Research Quarterly, 25,* 177-188.

Kriesburg, L. (1973). *The sociology of social conflicts.* Englewood Cliffs, NJ: Prentice Hall.

Krotee, M.L., & La Point, J.D. (1979). Sociological perspectives underlying participation in physical activity. In M.L. Krotee (Ed.), *Dimensions of sport sociology* (pp. 205-212). Champaign, IL: Leisure Press.

Kruse, M.S., & Calden, M.E. (1986). Compliance to a clinically prescribed exercise program. *Fitness in Business, 1,* 57-61.

Laffrey, S.C., & Isenberg, M. (1983). The relationship of internal locus of control, value placed on health, perceived importance of exercise, and participation in physical activity. *International Journal of Nursing Studies, 20*(3), 187-196.

Lambert, M.J., Bergin, A.E., & Collins, J.L. (1977). Therapist-induced deterioration in psychotherapy. In A.S. Gurman & A.M. Razin (Eds.), *Effective psychotherapy: A handbook of research* (pp. 452-481). New York: Pergamon Press.

Lassey, W.R., & Sashkin, M. (1983). *Leadership and social change* (3rd ed.). San Diego: University Associates.

Layman, E.M. (1960). Contributions of exercise and sports to mental health and social adjustment. In R. Johnson (Ed.), *Science and medicine of exercise and sport* (pp. 560-599). New York: Harper & Row.

Lazarus, R.S. (1966). *Psychological stress and the coping process.* New York: McGraw-Hill.

Lazarus, R.S. (1976). *Patterns of adjustment.* New York: McGraw-Hill.

Lebow, J. (1982). Consumer satisfaction with mental health treatment. *Psychological Bulletin, 91,* 244-259.

Legwold, G. (1987). Incentives for fitness programs. *Fitness in Business, 2,* 131-133.

Leon, G.R., & Roth, L. (1977). Obesity: Psychological causes, correlations, and speculations. *Psychological Bulletin, 84*(1), 117-139.

Levitz, L., & Stunkard, A.J. (1974). A therapeutic coalition for obesity: Behavior modification and patient self-help. *American Journal of Psychiatry, 131,* 423-427.

Lewin, K. (1948). *Resolving social conflicts: Selected papers on group dynamics.* New York: Harper & Row.

Lewin, K. (1951). *Field theory in social science.* New York: Harper & Row.

Lewin, K., Lippitt, R., & White, R. (1939). Patterns of aggressive behavior in experimentally created "social climates." *Journal of Social Psychology, 10,* 271-299.

Lewis, H.S. (1974). *Leaders and followers: Some anthropological perspectives.* Reading, MA: Addison-Wesley.

Lichtenstein, E. (1982). The smoking problem: A behavioral perspective. *Journal of Consulting and Clinical Psychology, 50,* 804-819.

Lichtenstein, E., & Penner, M.D. (1977). Long-term effects of rapid smoking treatment for dependent cigarette smokers. *Addictive Behaviors, 2,* 109-112.

Lichtman, S., & Poser, E.G. (1983). The effects of exercise on mood and cognitive functioning. *Journal of Psychosomatic Research, 27,* 43-52.

Lindsay-Reid, E., & Osborn, R.W. (1980). Readiness for exercise adoption. *Social Science and Medicine, 14*, 139-146.

Lindskold, S. (1978). Trust development, the GRIT proposal, and the effects of conciliatory acts on conflict and cooperation. *Psychological Bulletin, 85*, 772-793.

Lion, L. (1978). Psychological effects of jogging: A preliminary study. *Perceptual and Motor Skills, 47*, 1215-1218.

Little, J.C. (1969). The athlete's neurosis: A deprivation crisis. *Acta Psychiatrica Scandinavica, 45*, 187-197.

Little, J.C. (1979). Neurotic illness in fitness fanatics. *Psychiatric Annals, 9*(3), 49-57.

Lobstein, D.D., Mosbacher, B.J., & Ismail, A.H. (1983). Depression as a powerful discriminator between physically active and sedentary middle-aged men. *Journal of Psychosomatic Research, 27*(1), 69-76.

Locke, E.A., & Latham, G.P. (1985). The application of goal setting to sports. *Journal of Sport Psychology, 7*(3), 205-222.

Locke, E.A., Shaw, K.N., Saari, L.M., & Latham, G.P. (1981). Goal setting and task performance: 1969-1980. *Psychological Bulletin, 90*(1), 125-152.

Long, B.C. (1984). Aerobic conditioning and stress inoculation: A comparison of stress-management interventions. *Cognitive Therapy and Research, 8*(5), 517-542.

Long, B.C. (1985). Stress management interventions: A 15 month follow-up of aerobic conditioning and stress inoculation training. *Cognitive Therapy and Research, 9*(4), 471-478.

Long, B.C. (1988). Stress management for school personnel: Stress inoculation training and exercise. *Psychology in the Schools, 25*, 314-324.

Long, B.C., & Haney, C.J. (1986). Enhancing physical activity in sedentary women: Information, locus of control, and attitudes. *Journal of Sport Psychology, 8*, 8-24.

Long, B.C., & Haney, C.J. (1988a). Coping strategies for working women: Aerobic exercise and relaxation interventions. *Behavior Therapy, 19*, 75-83.

Long, B.C., & Haney, C.J. (1988b). Long-term follow-up of stressed working women: A comparison of aerobic exercise and progressive relaxation. *Journal of Sport and Exercise Psychology, 10*, 461-470.

Luft, J. (1969). *Of human interaction*. Palo Alto, CA: Mayfield.

Lynn, R.W., Phelan, J.G., & Kiker, V.L. (1969). Beliefs in internal-external control of re-inforcement and participation in group and individual sports. *Perceptual and Motor Skills, 29*, 551-553.

Mager, R.F. (1968). *Developing attitude toward learning*. Palo Alto, CA: Fearon.

Mahoney, M. (1974). *Cognition and behavior modification*. Cambridge, MA: Ballinger.

Mahoney, M., & Arnkoff, D.B. (1978). Cognitive and self-control therapies. In S.L. Garfield & A.E. Bergin (Eds.), *Handbook of psychotherapy and behavior change* (2nd ed., pp. 689-722). New York: Wiley.

Malley, P.B. (1988). Ethical and legal guidelines. In J.C. Boylan, P.B. Malley, & J. Scott (Eds.), *Practicum and internship: Textbook for counseling and psychotherapy* (pp. 213-239). Muncie, IN: Accelerated Development.

Mandell, A.J. (1981). The second second wind. In M.H. Sacks & M.L. Sachs (Eds.), *Psychology of running* (pp. 211-223). Champaign, IL: Human Kinetics.

Marinelli, R.P., & Orto, A.E.D. (1984). *The psychological and social impact of physical disability*. New York: Springer.

Markoff, R.A., Ryan, P., & Young, T. (1982). Endorphins and mood changes in long-distance running. *Medicine and Science in Sports and Exercise, 14*(1), 11-15.

Marlatt, G.A., & Gordon, J.R. (1978). Craving for alcohol, loss of control, and relapse: A cognitive-behavioral analysis. In P.E. Nathan, G.A. Marlatt, & T. Loberg (Eds.), *Alcoholism: New directions in behavioral research and treatment* (pp. 271-314). New York: Plenum Press.

Marlatt, G.A., & Gordon, J.R. (1980). Determinants of relapse: Implications for the maintenance of behavior change. In P.O. Davidson & S.M. Davidson (Eds.), *Behavioral medicine: Changing health lifestyles* (pp. 410-452). Elmsford, NY: Guilford Press.

Marlatt, G.A., & Gordon, J.R. (1985). *Relapse prevention: Maintenance strategies in addictive behavior change*. New York: Guilford Press.

Marsh, H.W., & Jackson, S.A. (1986). Multidimensional self-concepts, masculinity, and femininity as a function of women's involvement in athletics. *Sex Roles, 15*(7/8), 391-415.

Marsh, H.W., & Peart, N.D. (1988). Competitive and cooperative physical fitness training programs for girls: Effects on physical fitness and multidimensional self-concepts. *Journal of Sport and Exercise Psychology, 10*, 390-407.

Marsh, H.W., Richards, G.E., & Barnes, J. (1986). Multidimensional self-concepts: A long term follow up of the effect of participation in an outward bound program. *Personality and Social Psychology Bulletin, 12*(4), 475-492.

Marsh, H.W., & Shavelson, R. (1985). Self-concept: Its multifaceted, hierarchical structure. *Educational Psychologist, 20*(3), 107-123.

Martin, G., & Pear, J. (1978). *Behavior modification: What it is and how to do it*. New York: Prentice Hall.

Martin, J.E., & Dubbert, P.M. (1982). Exercise applications and promotion in behavioral medicine. *Journal of Consulting and Clinical Psychology, 50*(6), 1004-1017.

Martin, J.E., & Dubbert, P.M. (1984). Behavioral management strategies for improving health and fitness. *Journal of Cardiac Rehabilitation, 4*, 200-208.

Martin, J.E., & Dubbert, P.M. (1985). Adherence to exercise. In R.L. Terjung (Ed.), *Exercise and sport sciences reviews* (pp. 137-167). New York: Macmillan.

Martin, J.E., & Dubbert, P.M. (1987). Exercise promotion. In J.A. Blumenthal & D.S. McKee (Eds.), *Applications in behavioral medicine and health psychology: A clinician's source book* (pp. 361-398). Sarasota, FL: Professional Resource Exchange.

Martin, J.E., Dubbert, P.M., Katell, A.D., Thompson, J.K., Raczynski, J.R., Lake, M., Smith, P.O., Webster, J.S., Sikora, T., & Cohen, R.E. (1984). Behavioral control of exercise in sedentary adults: Studies 1 through 6. *Journal of Consulting and Clinical Psychology, 52*(5), 795-811.

Martinsen, E.W. (1990). Benefits of exercise for the treatment of depression. *Sports Medicine, 9*(6), 381-389.

Martinsen, E.W., Hoffart, A., & Solberg, O. (1989). Aerobic and non-aerobic forms of exercise in the treatment of anxiety disorders. *Stress Medicine, 5*, 115-120.

Maslow, A.H. (1968). *Toward the psychology of being* (2nd ed.). New York: D. Van Nostrand.

Massie, J.F., & Shephard, R.J. (1971). Physiological and psychological effects of training. *Medicine and Science in Sports, 3*(3), 110-117.

Matarazzo, J.D. (1980). Behavioral health and behavioral medicine: Frontiers for a new health psychology. *American Psychologist, 35*, 807-817.

Matheny, K.B., Aycock, D.W., Pugh, J.L., Curlette, W.L., & Cannella, K.A. (1986). Stress coping: A qualitative and quantitative synthesis with implications for treatment. *The Counseling Psychologist, 14*(4), 499-549.

Mathes, S.A., & Battista, R. (1985). College men's and women's motives for participation in physical activity. *Perceptual and Motor Skills, 61*, 719-726.

Matson, J.L. (1977). Social reinforcement by the spouse in weight control. *Journal of Behavioral Therapy and Experimental Psychiatry, 8*, 327-328.

May, R. (1977). *Meaning of anxiety*. New York: Norton.

Mayer, J. (1968). *Overweight: Causes, cost, & control*. Englewood Cliffs, NJ: Prentice Hall.

Mayou, R. (1980). Effectiveness of cardiac rehabilitation. *Journal of Psychosomatic Research, 23*, 423-427.

McCann, I.L., & Holmes, D.S. (1984). Influence of aerobic exercise on depression. *Journal of Personality and Social Psychology, 46*(5), 1142-1147.

McCready, M.L., & Long, B.C. (1985). Locus of control, attitudes toward physical activity, and exercise adherence. *Journal of Sport Psychology, 7*, 346-359.

McCullagh, P., North, T.C., & Mood, D. (1988, June). *Exercise as a treatment for depression: A meta-analysis*. Paper presented at the meeting of the North American Society for the Psychology of Sport and Physical Activity, Knoxville, TN.

McGilley, B.M., & Holmes, D.S. (1988). Aerobic fitness and response to psychological stress. *Journal of Research in Personality, 22*, 129-139.

McKenzie, T.L., & Rushall, B.S. (1974). Effects of self-recording on attendance and performance in a competitive swimming training environment. *Journal of Applied Behavioral Analysis, 7*(2), 199-206.

McNair, D.M., Lorr, M., & Droppleman, L.F. (1971). *Manual for the profile of mood states*. San Diego: Educational and Industrial Testing Service.

McPherson, B.D. (1986). Sport, health, well-being and aging: Some conceptual and methodological issues and questions for sport scientists. In B.D. McPherson (Ed.), *Sport and aging* (pp. 3-23). Champaign, IL: Human Kinetics.

McPherson, B.D., Paivio, A., Yuhasz, M.S., Rechnitzer, P.A., Pickard, H.A., & Lefcoe, N.M. (1967). Psychological effects of an exercise program for post-infarction and normal adult men. *Journal of Sports Medicine, 7*, 95-101.

Mehrabian, A. (1971). *Silent messages*. Belmont, CA: Wadsworth.

Meichenbaum, D. (1972). Examination of model characteristics in reducing avoidance behavior. *Journal of Behavior Therapy and Experimental Psychiatry, 31*, 225-227.

Meichenbaum, D. (1974). *Cognitive behavior modification*. Morristown, NJ: General Learning Press.

Meichenbaum, D. (1977). *Cognitive-behavior modification: An integrative approach*. New York: Plenum Press.

Meichenbaum, D. (1986). Cognitive-behavior modification. In F.H. Kanfer & A.P. Goldstein (Eds.), *Helping people change: A textbook of methods* (pp. 346-380). New York: Pergamon Press.

Mendelson, M. (1966). Psychological aspects of obesity. *International Journal of Psychiatry, 2*, 599-612.

Michael, E.D. (1957). Stress adaptation through exercise. *Research Quarterly, 28*(1), 50-54.

Miller, M.J. (1979). Jogotherapy also applies to the elementary child. *Personnel and Guidance Journal, 57*(9), 495.

Miller Brewing Company. (1983). *The Miller Lite report on American attitudes toward sports*. Milwaukee: Author.

Molloy, D.W., Beerschoten, D.A., Borrie, M.J., Crilly, R.J., & Cape, R.D.T. (1988). Acute effects of exercise on neuropsychological function in elderly subjects. *American Geriatrics Society, 36*, 29-33.

Monahan, T. (1986). Family exercise means relative fitness. *The Physician and Sportsmedicine, 14*(10), 202-206.

Moore, M.E., Stunkard, A., & Srole, L. (1962). Obesity, social class, and mental illness. *Journal of the American Medical Association, 181*(11), 138-142.

Moos, R.H., & Finney, J.W. (1983). The expanding scope of alcoholism treatment evaluation. *American Psychologist, 38*, 1036-1044.

Morgan, W.P. (April, 1978). The mind of the marathoner. *Psychology Today, 11*, 38-40.

Morgan, W.P. (1979). Negative addiction in runners. *The Physician and Sportsmedicine, 7*(2), 57-70.

Morgan, W.P. (1980). The trait psychology controversy. *Research Quarterly for Exercise and Sport, 51*(1), 50-76.

Morgan, W.P. (1985a). Affective beneficence of vigorous physical activity. *Medicine and Science in Sports and Exercise, 17*(1), 94-101.

Morgan, W.P. (1985b). Psychogenic factors and exercise metabolism: A review. *Medicine and Science in Sports and Exercise, 17*(3), 309-316.

Morgan, W.P., Costill, D.L., Flynn, M.G., Raglin, J.S., & O'Connor, P.J. (1988). Mood disturbance following increased training in swimmers. *Medicine and Science in Sports and Exercise, 20*, 408-414.

Morgan, W.P., & Goldston, S.E. (1987). Summary. In W.P. Morgan & S.E. Goldston (Eds.), *Exercise and mental health* (pp. 155-159). New York: Hemisphere.

Morgan, W.P., Shephard, R.J., Finucane, R., Schimmelfing, L., & Jazmaji, V. (1984). Health beliefs and exercise habits in an employee fitness program. *Canadian Journal of Applied Sport Sciences, 9*(2), 87-93.

Morris, R.J. (1986). Fear reduction methods. In F.H. Kanfer & A.P. Goldstein (Eds.), *Helping people change: A textbook of methods* (pp. 145-190). New York: Pergamon Press.

Motivation a key to participation. (1981). *Athletic Purchasing and Facilities, 5*, 11-14.

Myers, I.B. (1962). *Manual for the Myers-Briggs type indicator*. Palo Alto, CA: Consulting Psychologists Press.

Napier, R.W., & Gershenfeld, M.K. (1987). *Groups: Theory and experience*. Boston: Houghton Mifflin.

Naughton, J., Bruhn, J.G., & Lategola, M.T. (1968). Effects of physical training on physiologic and behavioral characteristics of cardiac patients. *Archives of Physical Medicine and Rehabilitation, 49*, 131-137.

Neale, D.C., Sonstroem, R.J., & Metz, K.F. (1969). Physical fitness, self-esteem, and attitudes toward physical activity. *Research Quarterly, 40*, 743-749.

Nelson, J.K. (1978). Motivation effects of the use of norms and goals with endurance testing. *Research Quarterly, 49*(3), 317-321.

New ideal of beauty. (1982, August 30). *Time, 120*(9), 72-77.

Newcomb, T.M. (1943). *Personality and social change*. New York: Dryden.

Nieman, D.C., & George, D.M. (1987). Personality traits that correlate with success in distance running. *Journal of Sports Medicine, 27*, 345-356.

Nisbett, R.E. (1968). Determinants of food intake in human obesity. *Science, 159*, 1254-1255.

Noland, M.P., & Feldman, R.H.L. (1984). Factors related to the leisure exercise behavior of returning women college students. *Health Education, 15*(2), 32-36.

Noland, M.P., & Feldman, R.H.L. (1985). An empirical investigation of leisure exercise behavior in adult women. *Health Education, 16*(5), 29-34.

North, T.C., & McCullagh, P. (1988, October). *Aerobic and anaerobic exercise as a treatment for depression: A meta-analysis*. Paper presented at the meeting of the Association for the Advancement of Applied Sport Psychology, Nashua, NH.

Norval, J.D. (1980). Running anorexia [Letter to the editor]. *South African Medical Journal, 58,* 1024.

Nowicki, S., & Strickland, B.R. (1973). A locus of control scale for children. *Journal of Consulting and Clinical Psychology, 40*(1), 148-154.

O'Connell, J.K., & Price, J.H. (1982). Health locus of control of physical fitness program participants. *Perceptual and Motor Skills, 55,* 925-926.

O'Connell, J.K., Price, J.H., Roberts, S.M., Jurs, S.G., & McKinley, R. (1985). Utilizing the health belief model to predict dieting and exercising behavior of obese and nonobese adolescents. *Health Education Quarterly, 12*(4), 343-351.

Oja, P., Teraslinna, P., Partenen, T., & Karava, R. (1974). Feasibility of an 18 month's physical training program for middle-aged men and its effects on physical fitness. *American Journal of Public Health, 64,* 459-465.

Oldridge, N.B. (1977). What to look for in an exercise class leader. *Physician and Sportsmedicine, 5,* 85-88.

Oldridge, N.B. (1979a). Compliance of post myocardial infarction patients to exercise programs. *Medicine and Science in Sports, 11*(4), 373-375.

Oldridge, N.B. (1979b). Compliance with exercise programs. In M.L. Pollock & D.H. Schmidt (Eds.), *Heart disease and rehabilitation* (pp. 619-627). Boston: Houghton Mifflin.

Oldridge, N.B. (1982). Compliance and exercise in primary and secondary prevention of coronary heart disease: A review. *Preventive Medicine, 11,* 56-70.

Oldridge, N.B. (1984a). Adherence to adult exercise fitness programs. In J.D. Matarazzo, C.M. Weiss, J.A. Herd, N.E. Miller, & S.M. Weiss (Eds.), *Behavioral health: A handbook of health enhancement and disease prevention* (pp. 467-487). New York: Wiley.

Oldridge, N.B. (1984b). Compliance and dropout in cardiac exercise rehabilitation. *Journal of Cardiac Rehabilitation, 4,* 166-177.

Oldridge, N.B. (1988a). Cardiac rehabilitation exercise programme: Compliance and compliance-enhancing strategies. *Sports Medicine, 6,* 42-55.

Oldridge, N.B. (1988b). Compliance with exercise in cardiac rehabilitation. In R.K. Dishman (Ed.), *Exercise adherence: Its impact on public health* (pp. 283-303). Champaign, IL: Human Kinetics.

Oldridge, N.B., Donner, A.P., Buck, C.W., Jones, N.L., Andrew, G.M., Parker, J.O., Cunningham, D.A., Kavanagh, T., Rechnitzer, P.A., &

Sutton, J.R. (1983). Predictors of dropout from cardiac exercise rehabilitation: Ontario exercise-heart collaborative study. *American Journal of Cardiology, 51,* 70-74.

Oldridge, N.B., Guyatt, G.H., Fisher, M.E., & Rimm, A.A. (1988). Cardiac rehabilitation after myocardial infarction. *Journal of the American Medical Association, 260*(7), 945-950.

Oldridge, N.B., & Jones, N.L. (1983). Improving patient compliance in cardiac exercise rehabilitation: Effects of written agreement and self-monitoring. *Journal of Cardiac Rehabilitation, 3,* 257-262.

Oldridge, N.B., & Spencer, J. (1985). Exercise habits and perceptions before and after graduation or dropout from supervised cardiac exercise rehabilitation. *Journal of Cardiopulmonary Rehabilitation, 5,* 313-319.

Oldridge, N.B., Wicks, J.R., Hanley, C., Sutton, J.R., & Jones, N.L. (1978). Noncompliance in an exercise rehabilitation program for men who have suffered a myocardial infarction. *Canadian Medical Association Journal, 118,* 361-364.

O'Leary, A. (1985). Self-efficacy and health. *Behavioral Research and Therapy, 23,* 437-451.

Ostrow, A.C. (1984). *Physical activity and the older adult.* Princeton, NJ: Princeton Book Company.

Ostrow, A.C., & Dzewaltowski, D.A. (1986). Older adults perceptions of physical activity participation based on age-role and sex-role appropriateness. *Research Quarterly for Exercise and Sport, 57*(2), 167-169.

Ostrow, A.C., Jones, D.C., & Spiker, D.D. (1981). Age role expectations and sex role expectations for selected sport activities. *Research Quarterly for Exercise and Sport, 52*(2), 216-227.

Pagell, W., Carkhuff, R.R., & Berenson, B.G. (1967). The predicted differential effects of the level of counselor functioning upon the level of functioning of outpatients. *Journal of Clinical Psychology, 23,* 510-512.

Parent, C.J., & Whall, A.L. (1984). Are physical activity, self-esteem and depression related? *Journal of Gerontological Nursing, 10*(9), 8-11.

Pargman, D. (1980). The way of the runner: An examination of motives for running. In R.M. Suinn (Ed.), *Psychology in sports: Methods and applications* (pp. 90-98). Edina, MN: Burgess International.

Passer, M.W. (1982). Children in sport: Participation motives and psychological stress. *Quest, 33*(2), 231-244.

Patrick, G.D. (1986). The effects of wheelchair competition on self-concept and acceptance of disability in novice athletes. *Therapeutic Recreation Journal,* **20**(4), 61-71.

Patterson, L.E., & Eisenberg, S. (1983). *The counseling process* (3rd ed.). Boston: Houghton Mifflin.

Patterson, W.M., Dohn, H.H., Bird, J., & Patterson, G.A. (1983). Evaluation of suicidal patients: The SAD Person's scale. *Psychosomatics,* **24**, 343-348.

Pechacek, T.F., & Danaher, B.G. (1979). How and why people quit smoking: A cognitive-behavioral analysis. In P.C. Kindall & S.D. Hollon (Eds.), *Cognitive-behavioral interventions: Theory, research, and procedures.* New York: Academic Press.

Peele, S. (1981). *How much is too much?* Englewood Cliffs, NJ: Prentice Hall.

Pemberton, C. (1984). Clinical assessment. In J. Storlie & H.A. Jordan (Eds.), *Evaluation and treatment of obesity* (pp. 82-87). Champaign, IL: Life Enhancement.

Pender, N.J., & Pender, A.R. (1986). Attitudes, subjective norms, and intentions to engage in health behaviors. *Nursing Research,* **35**(1), 15-18.

Pennebaker, J.W., & Lightner, J.M. (1980). Competition of internal and external information in an exercise setting. *Journal of Personality and Social Psychology,* **39**(1), 165-174.

Penny, G.D., & Rust, J.O. (1980). Effect of a walking-jogging program on personality characteristics of middle aged females. *Journal of Sports Medicine,* **20**, 221-226.

Perkins, K.A., Rapp, S.R., Carlson, C.R., & Wallace, C.E. (1986). A behavioral intervention to increase exercise among nursing home residents. *The Gerontologist,* **26**(5), 479-481.

Perri, M.G., Lauer, J.B., McAdoo, W.G., McAllister, D.A., & Yancy, D.Z. (1986). Enhancing the efficacy of behavior therapy for obesity: Effects of aerobic exercise and a multicomponent maintenance program. *Journal of Consulting and Clinical Psychology,* **54**(5), 670-675.

Perri, M.G., Richards, C.S., & Schultheis, K.R. (1977). Behavioral self-control and smoking reduction: A study of self-initiated attempts to reduce smoking. *Behavior Therapy,* **8**, 360-365.

Perri, S., II, & Templer, D.I. (1985). The effects of an aerobic exercise program on psychological variables in older adults. *International Journal of Aging and Human Development,* **20**(3), 167-172.

Perry, M.A., & Furukawa, M.J. (1986). Modeling methods. In F.H. Kanfer & A.P. Goldstein (Eds.), *Helping people change: A textbook of methods* (pp. 66-110). New York: Pergamon Press.

Perry, P. (1987). Are we having fun yet? *American Health,* **6**(2), 58-63.

Peterson, L.H. (1983). Introduction, philosophy, and scope. In L.H. Peterson (Ed.), *Cardiovascular rehabilitation: A comprehensive approach* (pp. 1-9). New York: Macmillan.

Petri, H.L. (1986). *Motivation: Theory and research* (2nd ed.). Belmont, CA: Wadsworth.

Piaget, J. (1954). *Constructions of reality in the child.* New York: Basic Books.

Pollock, M.L. (1978). How much exercise is enough? *Physician and Sportsmedicine,* **8**, 50-64.

Pollock, M.L., Foster, C., Salisbury, R., & Smith, R. (1982). Effects of YMCA starter fitness program. *Physician and Sportsmedicine,* **10**(1), 89-100.

Polly, S., Turner, R.D., & Sherman, A. (1976). A self-control program for the treatment of obesity. In J.D. Krumboltz & C.E. Thoresen (Eds.), *Counseling methods* (pp. 106-117). New York: Holt Rinehart & Winston.

Pomerleau, O.F., Adkins, D., & Pertschik, M. (1978). Predictors of outcome and recidivism in smoking cessation treatment. *Addictive Behaviors,* **3**, 65-70.

Powell, K.E. (1988). Habitual exercise and public health: An epidemiological view. In R.K. Dishman (Ed.), *Exercise adherence: Its impact on public health* (pp. 15-39). Champaign, IL: Human Kinetics.

Powell, R.P. (1974). Psychological effects of exercise therapy upon institutionalized geriatric mental patients. *Journal of Gerontology,* **29**(2), 157-161.

Powell, R.R., & Pohndorf, R.H. (1971). Comparison of adult exercisers and nonexercisers on fluid intelligence and selected physiological variables. *Research Quarterly,* **42**(1), 70-77.

Presbie, R.J., & Brown, P.L. (1977). *Physical education: The behavior modification approach.* Washington, DC: National Education Association.

Price, J.H., Galli, N., & Slenker, S. (1985). *Consumer health: Contemporary issues and choices.* Dubuque, IA: Brown.

Prosser, G., Carson, P., & Phillips, R. (1985). Exercise after myocardial infarction: Long term rehabilitation effects. *Journal of Psychosomatic Research,* **29**(5), 535-540.

Prosser, G., Carson, P., Phillips, R., Gelson, A., Buch, N., Tucker, H., Neophytou, M., Lloyd, M., & Simpson, T. (1981). Morale in coronary patients following an exercise program. *Journal of Psychosomatic Research,* **25**, 587-593.

Public Health Service. (1989). *Promoting Health/ Preventing Disease: Year 2000 Objectives for the*

Nation. Washington, DC: U.S. Department of Health and Human Services.

Raglin, J.S., & Morgan, W.P. (1987). Influence of exercise and quiet rest on state anxiety and blood pressure. *Medicine and Science in Sports and Exercise,* **19**(5), 456-463.

Rao, V.V.P., & Overman, S.J. (1986). Psychological well-being and body image: A comparison of black women athletes and nonathletes. *Journal of Sport Behavior,* **9**(2), 79-90.

Ray, R.O., Gissal, M.L., & Smith, E.L. (1982). The effect of exercise on morale of older adults. *Physical and Occupational Therapy in Geriatrics,* **2**(2), 53-62.

Reid, E.L., & Morgan, R.W. (1979). Exercise prescription: A clinical trial. *American Journal of Public Health,* **69**(6), 591-595.

Riddick, C.C., & Daniel, S.N. (1984). The relative contribution of leisure activities and other factors to the mental health of older women. *Journal of Leisure Research,* **16**(2), 136-147.

Riddle, P.K. (1980). Attitudes, beliefs, behavioral intentions, and behaviors of women and men toward regular jogging. *Research Quarterly for Exercise and Sport,* **51**(4), 663-674.

Robbins, J.M., & Joseph, P. (1980). Commitment to running: Implications for the family and work. *Sociological Symposium* **80,** 87-108.

Robbins, J.M., & Joseph, P. (1985). Experiencing exercise withdrawal: Possible consequences of therapeutic and mastery running. *Journal of Sport Psychology,* **7,** 23-39.

Rodin, J., Elman, D., & Schacter, S. (1974). Emotionality and obesity. In S. Schacter & J. Rodin (Eds.), *Obese humans and rats.* Washington, DC: Erlbaum/Wiley.

Rogers, C. (1957). The necessary and sufficient conditions of therapeutic personality change. *Journal of Consulting Psychology,* **321,** 95-103.

Rogers, C. (1967). *The therapeutic relationship and its impact.* Westport, CT: Greenwood Press.

Rogers, R.W. (1983). Cognitive and physiological processes in fear appeals and attitude change: A revised theory of protection motivation. In J.T. Cacioppo & R.E. Petty (Eds.), *Social psychology: A sourcebook* (pp. 153-176). New York: Guilford.

Rosenberg, M. (1979). *Conceiving the self.* New York: Basic Books.

Rosenberg, S.W., & Wolfsfeld, G. (1977). International conflict and the problem of attribution. *Journal of Conflict Resolution,* **21,** 75-103.

Rosenstock, I.M. (1974). The health belief model and preventative health behavior. *Health Education Monographs,* **2**(4), 355-387.

Roskies, E. (1983). Stress management for Type A individuals. In D. Meichenbaum & M.E. Jarenko (Eds.), *Stress reduction and perception* (pp. 261-288). New York: Plenum Press.

Roskies, E., Kearney, H., Spevack, M., & Surkis, A. (1979). Generalizability and durability of treatment effects in an intervention program for coronary-prone Type A managers. *Journal of Behavioral Medicine,* **2**(2), 195-207.

Roskies, E., Seraganian, P., Oseasohn, R., Hanley, J.A., Collu, R., Martin, N., & Smilga, C. (1986). The Montreal Type A intervention project: Major findings. *Health Psychology,* **5**(1), 45-69.

Ross, L. (1977). The intuitive psychologist and his shortcomings: Distortions in the attribution process. In L. Berkowitz (Ed.), *Advances in experimental social psychology* (pp. 173-220). New York: Academic Press.

Roth, D.L., & Holmes, D.S. (1985). Influence of physical fitness in determining the impact of stressful life events on physical and psychologic health. *Psychosomatic Medicine,* **47**(2), 164-173.

Roth, D.L., & Holmes, D.S. (1987). Influence of aerobic exercise training and relaxation training on physical psychologic health following stressful life events. *Psychosomatic Medicine,* **49,** 355-365.

Roth, W.T. (1974). Some motivational aspects of exercise. *Journal of Sports Medicine,* **14,** 40-47.

Rotter, J.B. (1966). Generalized expectancies for internal versus external control of reinforcement. *Psychological Monographs: General and Applied,* **80**(1, Whole No. 609), 1-28.

Rotter, J.B. (1975). Some problems and misconceptions related to the construct of internal versus external control of reinforcement. *Journal of Consulting and Clinical Psychology,* **43**(1), 56-67.

Rubin, J.J. (1980). Experimental research on third-party intervention in conflict: Toward some generalizations. *Psychological Bulletin,* **87,** 379-391.

Rudnicki, J., & Wankel, L.M. (1988). Employee fitness program effects upon long-term fitness involvement. *Fitness in Business,* **3,** 123-129.

Rushall, B.S. (1980). Using applied behavior analysis for altering motivation. In R.M. Suinn (Ed.), *Psychology in sports: Methods and implications* (pp. 63-72). Edina, MN: Burgess International.

Rushall, B.S., & Pettinger, J. (1969). An evaluation of the effect of various reinforcers used as motivators in swimming. *Research Quarterly,* **2**(3), 540-545.

Russell, P.O., Epstein, L.H., & Erickson, K.T. (1983). Effects of acute exercise and cigarette smoking on autonomic and neuromuscular responses to a cognitive stressor. *Psychological Reports, 53*, 199-206.

Russell, R.V. (1987). The importance of recreation satisfaction and activity participation to the life satisfaction of age segregated retirees. *Journal of Leisure Research, 19*(4), 273-283.

Sachs, M.L. (1981). Running addiction. In M. Sacks & M. Sachs (Eds.). *Psychology of running* (pp. 116-127). Champaign, IL: Human Kinetics.

Sachs, M.L. (1984). The runner's high. In M. Sacks & M. Sachs (Eds.) *Running as therapy* (pp. 273-287). Lincoln, NE: University of Nebraska Press.

Sachs, M.L., & Pargman, D. (1984). Running addiction. In M. Sachs & G.W. Buffone (Eds.), *Running as therapy* (pp. 231-253). Lincoln, NE: University of Nebraska Press.

Safrit, M.J., Wood, T.M., & Dishman, R.K. (1985). The factorial validity of the physical estimation and attraction scales for adults. *Journal of Sport Psychology, 7*, 166-190.

Sallis, J.F., Haskell, W.L., Fortmann, S.P., Vranizan, M.S., Taylor, C.B., & Solomon, D.S. (1986). Predictors of adoption and maintenance of physical activity in a community sample. *Preventive Medicine, 15*(4), 331-341.

Saul, S. (1974). *Aging: An album of old people*. New York: Wiley.

Schacter, S. (1971). *Emotion, obesity, and crime*. New York: Academic Press.

Schacter, S., Goldman, R., & Gordon, A. (1968). Effects of fear, food deprivation, and obesity on eating. *Journal of Personality and Social Psychology, 10*, 91-97.

Schacter, S., & Rodin, J. (1974). *Obese humans and rats*. Hillsdale, NJ: Erlbaum.

Schelling, T.C. (1960). *The strategy of conflict*. Cambridge, MA: Harvard University Press.

Scherf, J., & Franklin, B. (1987). Exercise compliance: A data documentation system. *Journal of Physical Education, Recreation and Dance, 58*, 26-28.

Schifter, D.E., & Ajzen, I. (1985). Intention, perceived control, and weight loss: An application of the theory of planned behavior. *Journal of Personality and Social Psychology, 49*(3), 843-851.

Schreshum, J. (1980). The social context of leader-subordinate relations: An investigation of the effects of group cohesiveness. *Journal of Applied Psychology, 65*, 183-194.

Schwartz, G.E., Davidson, R.J., & Goleman, D.J. (1978). Patterning of cognitive and somatic processes in the self-regulation of anxiety: Effects of meditation versus exercise. *Psychosomatic Medicine, 40*(4), 321-327.

Schwartz, G.E., & Weiss, S. (1977). What is behavioral medicine? *Psychosomatic Medicine, 36*, 377-381.

Secord, P.F., & Jourard, S.M. (1953). The appraisal of body-cathexis: Body-cathexis and the self. *Journal of Consulting Psychology, 17*(5), 343-354.

Sexton, H., Maere, A., & Dahl, N.H. (1989). Exercise intensity and reduction in neurotic symptoms. *Acta Psychiatrica Scandinavica, 80*, 231-235.

Shamoian, C.A. (1983). Psychogeriatrics. *Medical Clinics of North America, 67*(2), 361-378.

Sharp, M.W., & Reilley, R.R. (1975). The relationship of aerobic physical fitness to selected personality traits. *Journal of Clinical Psychology, 31*, 428-430.

Shaver, P., & Freedman, J. (1976). Your pursuit of happiness. *Psychology Today*, 27-32.

Shaw, L.W. (1981). Effects of a prescribed supervised exercise program on mortality and cardiovascular morbidity in patients after a myocardial infarction. *American Journal of Cardiology, 48*, 39-46.

Shaw, M. (1964). Communication networks. In L. Berkowitz (Ed.), *Advances in experimental social psychology, Volume 1* (pp. 111-147). New York: Academic Press.

Shaw, M. (1981). *Group dynamics: The psychology of small group behavior*. (3rd ed.). New York: McGraw-Hill.

Shephard, R.J. (1988a). Exercise adherence in corporate settings: Personal traits and program barriers. In R.K. Dishman (Ed.), *Exercise adherence: Its impact on public health* (pp. 305-319). Champaign, IL: Human Kinetics.

Shephard, R.J. (1988b). Fitness boom or bust—A Canadian perspective. *Research Quarterly for Exercise and Sport, 59*(3), 265-269.

Shephard, R.J. (1990). *Fitness in special populations*. Champaign, IL: Human Kinetics.

Shephard, R.J., Corey, P., & Kavanagh, T. (1981). Exercise compliance and the prevention of a recurrence of myocardial infarction. *Medicine and Science in Sports and Exercise, 13*(1), 1-5.

Shephard, R.J., & Cox, M. (1980). Some characteristics of participants in an industrial fitness programme. *Canadian Journal of Applied Sport Science, 5*(2), 69-76.

Shephard, R.J., Kavanagh, T., & Klavora, P. (1985). Mood state during postcoronary cardiac rehabilitation. *Journal of Cardiopulmonary Rehabilitation, 5*, 480-484.

Shipman, W.M. (1984). Emotional and behavioral effects of long distance running on children. In M. Sachs & G.W. Buffone (Eds.), *Running as therapy* (pp. 125-138). Lincoln, NE: University of Nebraska Press.

Sidney, K.H., & Shephard, R.J. (1976). Attitudes towards health and physical activity in the elderly: Effects of a physical training program. *Medicine and Science in Sports*, **8**(4), 246-252.

Siegel, M. (1979). Privacy, ethics and confidentiality. *Professional Psychology*, **10**, 249-258.

Silverstein, B., Peterson, B., & Perdue, L. (1986). Some correlates of the thin standard of bodily attractiveness for women. *International Journal of Eating Disorders*, **5**(5), 895-905.

Silverstone, J.T. (1968). Obesity. *Proceedings of the Royal Society of Medicine*, **61**, 371-375.

Sime, W.E. (1984). Psychological benefits of exercise training in the healthy individual. In J.D. Matarazzo, S.M. Weiss, J.A. Herd, W.E. Miller, & S.M. Weiss (Eds.), *Behavioral health: A handbook of health enhancement and disease prevention* (pp. 488-507). New York: Wiley.

Simons, A.D., Epstein, L.H., McGowen, C.R., Kupfer, D.J., & Robertson, R.J. (1985). Exercise as a treatment for depression: An update. *Clinical Psychology Review*, **5**, 553-568.

Sinyor, D., Schwartz, S.G., Peronnet, F., Brisson, G., & Seraganian, P. (1983). Aerobic fitness level and reactivity to psychosocial stress: Physiological, biochemical, and subjective measures. *Psychosomatic Medicine*, **45**(3), 205-217.

Slenker, S.E., Price, H.J., & O'Connell, J.K. (1985). Health locus of control of joggers and nonexercisers. *Perceptual and Motor Skills*, **61**, 323-328.

Slenker, S.E., Price, H.J., Roberts, S.M., & Jurs, S.G. (1984). Joggers versus nonexercisers: An analysis of knowledge, attitudes and beliefs about jogging. *Research Quarterly for Exercise and Sport*, **55**(4), 371-378.

Smith, E.L. (1984). Special considerations in developing exercise programs for the older adult. In J.P. Matarazzo, S.M. Weiss, J.A. Herd, & N.E. Miller (Eds.), *Behavioral health: A handbook of health enhancement and disease prevention* (pp. 525-546). New York: Wiley.

Smith, N.J. (1980). Excessive weight loss and food aversion in athletes simulating anorexia nervosa. *Pediatrics*, **66**(1), 139-142.

Snodgrass, S.E., Higgins, J.G., & Todisco, L. (1986, August). Paper presented at the meeting of the American Psychological Association, Washington, DC.

Snyder, E.E., & Kivlin, J.E. (1975). Women athletes and aspects of psychological well being and body image. *Research Quarterly*, **46**(2), 191-199.

Snyder, E.E., & Spreitzer, E.A. (1974). Involvement in sports and psychological well-being. *International Journal of Sport Psychology*, **5**, 28-39.

Snyder, E.E., & Spreitzer, E. (1979). Lifelong involvement in sport as a leisure pursuit: Aspects of role construction. *Quest*, **31**(1), 57-70.

Snyder, E.E., & Spreitzer, E. (1984). Patterns of adherence to a physical conditioning program. *Sociology of Sport Journal*, **1**, 103-116.

Snyder, G., Franklin, B., Foss, M., & Rubenfire, M. (1982). Characteristics of compliers and noncompliers to cardiac exercise therapy program. *Medicine and Science in Sports and Exercise*, **14**, 179.

Snyder, J.T. (1989). *Health psychology and behavioral medicine*. Englewood Cliffs, NJ: Prentice Hall.

Soloff, P.H., & Bartel, A.G. (1979). Effects of denial on mood and performance in cardiovascular rehabilitation. *Journal of Chronic Disease*, **32**, 307-313.

Song, T.K., Shephard, R.J., & Cox, M. (1983). Absenteeism, employee turnover and sustained exercise participation. *Journal of Sportsmedicine and Physical Fitness*, **22**, 392-399.

Sonstroem, R.J. (1974). Attitude testing examining certain psychological correlates of physical activity. *Research Quarterly*, **45**(2), 93-103.

Sonstroem, R.J. (1976). The validity of self-perceptions regarding physical and athletic ability. *Medicine and Science in Sports*, **8**(2), 126-132.

Sonstroem, R.J. (1978). Physical estimation and attraction scales: Rationale and research. *Medicine and Science in Sports*, **10**(2), 97-102.

Sonstroem, R.J. (1982). Attitudes and beliefs in the prediction of exercise participation. In R.C. Cantu & W.J. Gillespie (Eds.), *Sports medicine, sport science* (pp. 3-16). Lexington, MA: Heath.

Sonstroem, R.J. (1984). Exercise and self-esteem. In R.L. Terjung (Ed.), *Exercise and sport science reviews* (pp. 123-155). Toronto: Collare.

Sonstroem, R.J. (1988). Psychological models. In R.K. Dishman (Ed.), *Exercise adherence: Its impact on public health* (pp. 125-153). Champaign, IL: Human Kinetics.

Sonstroem, R.J., & Kampper, K.P. (1980). Prediction of athletic participation in middle school males. *Research Quarterly for Exercise and Sport*, **51**(4), 685-694.

Sonstroem, R.J., & Morgan, W.P. (1989). Exercise and self-esteem: Rationale and model. *Medicine and Science in Sports and Exercise*, **21**(3), 329-337.

Sonstroem, R.J., & Walker, M.I. (1973). Relationships of attitudes and locus of control to exercise and physical fitness. *Perceptual and Motor Skills*, **36**, 1031-1034.

Speaker, J.G., Schultz, C., Grinker, J.A., & Stern, J.S. (1983). Body size estimation and locus of control in obese adolescent boys. *International Journal of Obesity*, **7**, 73-83.

Spielberger, C.D. (1972). Anxiety as an emotional state. In C.D. Spielberger (Ed.), *Anxiety: Current trends in theory and research* (pp. 23-49). New York: Academic Press.

Spielberger, C.D., Gorsuch, R.L., & Lushene, R.E. (1970). *Manual for the state-trait anxiety inventory*. Palo Alto, CA: Consulting Psychologists Press.

Spino, M. (1971). Running as a spiritual experience. In J. Scott (Ed.), *The athletic revolution* (pp. 222-225). New York: Free Press.

Spirduso, W.W. (1986). Physical activity and the prevention of premature aging. In V. Seefeld (Ed.), *Physical activity and well-being* (pp. 142-160). Reston, VA: American Alliance for Health, Physical Education, Recreation and Dance.

Stamford, B., Hambacher, W., & Fallica, A. (1974). Effects of daily physical exercise on the psychiatric state of institutionalized geriatric mental patients. *Research Quarterly*, **45**, 34-41.

Stephens, T. (1987). Secular trends in adult physical activity: Exercise boom or bust? *Research Quarterly for Exercise and Sport*, **58**(2), 94-105.

Stephens, T., Jacobs, D.R., & White, C.C. (1985). A descriptive epidemiology of leisure-time activity. *Public Health Reports*, **100**(2), 147-158.

Steptoe, A., & Bolton, J. (1988). The short term influence of high and low intensity physical exercise on mood. *Psychology and Health*, **2**, 91-106.

Steptoe, A., & Cox, S. (1988). Acute effects of aerobic exercise on mood. *Health Psychology*, **7**(4), 329-340.

Steptoe, A., Edwards, S., Moses, J., & Mathews, A. (1989). The effects of exercise training on mood and perceived coping ability in anxious adults from the general population. *Journal of Psychosomatic Research*, **33**(5), 537-547.

Steptoe, A., Kearsley, N. (1990). Cognitive and somatic anxiety. *Behavioral Research Therapy*, **28**(1), 75-81.

Stern, J.S. (1983). Diet and exercise. In M.R.C. Greenwood (Ed.), *Obesity* (pp. 65-84). New York: Churchill Livingstone.

Stern, M.J., & Cleary, P. (1981). National exercise and heart disease project: Psychosocial changes observed during a low-level exercise

program. *Archives of Internal Medicine*, **141**, 1463-1467.

Stern, M.J., & Cleary, P. (1982). The national exercise and heart disease project: Long-term psychosocial outcome. *Archives of Internal Medicine*, 1093-1097.

Stern, M.J., Gorman, P.A., & Kaslow, L. (1983). The group counseling vs. exercise therapy study. *Archives of Internal Medicine*, **143**, 1719-1725.

Stiles, M.H. (1967). Motivation for sports participation in the community. *Canadian Medical Association Journal*, **96**, 889-892.

Stogdill, R.M. (1948). Personal factors associated with leadership. *Journal of Psychology*, **23**, 35-71.

Stogdill, R.M. (1974). *Handbook of leadership*. New York: Free Press.

Stones, M.J., Kozma, A., & Stones, L. (1987). Fitness and health evaluations by older exercisers. *Canadian Journal of Public Health*, **78**, 18-20.

Storlie, J. (1984). Techniques of behavioral intervention. In J. Storlie & H.A. Jordan (Eds.), *Behavioral management of obesity* (pp. 19-48). New York: Spectrum Books.

Strecher, V.J., DeVellis, B.M., Becker, M.H., & Rosenstock, I.M. (1986). The role of self-efficacy in achieving health behavior change. *Health Education Quarterly*, **13**(1), 73-92.

Strickland, B.R. (1978). Internal-external expectancies and health related behaviors. *Journal of Consulting and Clinical Psychology*, **46**, 1192-1211.

Strong, S.R. (1968). Counseling: An interpersonal influence process. *Journal of Counseling Psychology*, **15**, 215-224.

Strongman, K.T. (1987). *The psychology of emotion*. New York: Wiley.

Strupp, H.H., Hadley, S.W., & Gomes-Schwartz, B. (1977). *Psychotherapy for better or worse: The problem of negative effects*. New York: Jason Aronson.

Stunkard, A.J. (1979). Behavioral medicine and beyond: The example of obesity. In O.F. Pomerleau & J.P. Brady (Eds.), *Behavioral medicine: Theory and practice* (pp. 279-298). Baltimore: Williams & Wilkins.

Stunkard, A., & Mendelson, M. (1961). Disturbances in body image of some obese persons. *American Journal of Psychiatry*, **123**, 328-331.

Subhan, S., White, J.A., & Kane, J. (1987). The influence of exercise on stress states using psychophysiological indices. *Journal of Sports Medicine*, **27**, 223-229.

Summers, J.J., Machin, V.J., & Sargent, G.I. (1983). Psychosocial factors related to marathon running. *Journal of Sport Psychology*, **5**, 314-331.

Summers, J.J., Sargent, G.I., Levey, A.J., & Murray, K.D. (1982). Middle aged, non elite marathon runners: A profile. *Perceptual and Motor Skills,* **54**, 963-969.

Super, D.E., Starishevisky, R., Matlin, N., & Jordaan, J.P. (1963). *Career development: Self-concept theory.* New York: College Entrance Examination Board.

Taylor, C.B., Bandura, A., Ewart, C.K., Miller, N.H., & DeBusk, R.F. (1985). Exercise testing to enhance wives' confidence in their husbands' cardiac capability soon after clinically uncomplicated acute myocardial infarction. *American Journal of Cardiology,* **55**, 635-638.

Taylor, C.B., Sallis, J.F., & Needle, R. (1985). The relation of physical activity and exercise to mental health. *Public Health Reports,* **100**(2), 195-202.

Teraslinna, P., Partanen, T., Koskela, A., & Oja, P. (1969). Characteristics affecting willingness of executives to participate in an activity program aimed at coronary heart disease prevention. *Journal of Sports Medicine and Physical Fitness,* **17**, 224-229.

Thackeray, M.G., Skidmore, R.A., & Farley, O.W. (1979). *Introduction to mental health: Field and practice.* Englewood Cliffs, NJ: Prentice Hall.

Tharion, W.J., Strowman, S.R., & Rauch, T.M. (1988). Profile changes in moods of ultramarathoners. *Journal of Sport and Exercise Physiology,* **10**, 229-235.

Thaxton, L. (1982). Physiological and psychological effects of short term exercise addiction on habitual runners. *Journal of Sport Psychology,* **4**(1), 73-80.

Thompson, C.E., & Wankel, L.M. (1980). The effects of perceived activity choice upon frequency of exercise behavior. *Journal of Applied Social Psychology,* **10**(5), 436-443.

Thompson, J.K., & Blanton, P. (1987). Energy conservation and exercise dependence: A sympathetic arousal hypothesis. *Medicine and Science in Sports and Exercise,* **19**(2), 91-99.

Thompson, J.K., Jarvie, G.J., Lahey, B.B., & Cureton, K.J. (1982). Exercise and obesity: Etiology, physiology, and interventions. *Psychological Bulletin,* **91**, 55-79.

Thoresen, C.E., & Eagleston, J.R. (1985). Counseling for health. *Counseling Psychologist,* **13**(1), 15-87.

Thoresen, C.E., & Mahoney, M.J. (1974). *Behavioral self-control.* New York: Holt Rinehart & Winston.

Tirrell, B.E., & Hart, L.K. (1980). The relationship of health beliefs and knowledge to exercise compliance in patients after coronary bypass. *Heart and Lung,* **9**, 487-493.

Tomarken, A.J., & Kirschenbaum, D.S. (1982). Self-regulatory failure: Accentuate the positive? *Journal of Personality and Social Psychology,* **43**(3), 584-597.

Truax, C.B., & Carkhuff, R.R. (1967). *Toward effective counseling and psychotherapy: Training and practice.* Chicago: Aldine.

Tu, J., & Rothstein, A.L. (1979). Improvement of jogging performance through application of personality specific motivational techniques. *Research Quarterly,* **50**(1), 97-103.

Tucker, L.A. (1983). Muscular strength and mental health. *Journal of Personality and Social Psychology,* **45**(6), 1355-1360.

Tucker, L.A. (1984). Trait psychology and performance: A credulous viewpoint. *Journal of Human Movement Studies,* **10**, 53-62.

Tucker, L.A., Cole, G.E., & Friedman, G.M. (1986). Physical fitness: A buffer against stress. *Perceptual and Motor Skills,* **63**, 955-961.

Tuckman, B.W., & Jensen, M.A.C. (1977). Stages of small group development revisited. *Group and Organizational Studies,* **2**, 419-427.

Turk, D.C., Meichenbaum, D., & Genest, M. (1983). *Pain and behavioral medicine: A cognitive-behavioral perspective.* New York: Guilford Press.

Valliant, P.M., & Asu, M.E. (1985). Exercise and its effects on cognition and physiology in older adults. *Perceptual and Motor Skills,* **61**, 1031-1038.

Valliant, P.M., Bezzubyk, I., Daley, L., & Asu, M.E. (1985). Psychological impact of sport on disabled athletes. *Psychological Reports,* **56**, 923-927.

Valois, P., Shephard, R.J., & Godin, G. (1986). Relationship of habit and perceived physical ability to exercise behavior. *Perceptual and Motor Skills,* **62**, 811-817.

Van Hoose, W.H., & Kottler, J. (1985). *Ethical and legal issues in counseling and psychotherapy* (2nd ed.). San Francisco: Jossey-Bass.

Vitulli, W.F. (1987). Manifest reasons for jogging. *Perceptual and Motor Skills,* **64**, 650.

Vroom, V.H. (1973). A new look at managerial decision-making. *Organizational Dynamics,* **1**, 66-80.

Waldstreicher, J. (1985). Anorexia nervosa presenting as morbid exercising. *Lancet,* **1**(8435), 987.

Wallston, B.S., & Wallston, K.A. (1978). Locus of control and health: A review of the literature. *Health Education Monographs,* **6**(2), 107-117.

Wallston, B.S., Wallston, K.A., Kaplan, G.D., & Maides, S.A. (1976). Development and validation of the health locus of control (HLC) scale.

Journal of Consulting and Clinical Psychology, **44**(4), 580-585.

Wallston, K.A., Wallston, B.S., & DeVellis, R. (Eds.) (1978). Development of the multidimensional health locus of control scales (MHLC). *Health Education Monographs,* **6**(2), 160-170.

Wankel, L.M. (1984). Decision-making and social-support strategies for increasing exercise involvement. *Journal of Cardiac Rehabilitation,* **4**(4), 124-135.

Wankel, L.M. (1985). Personal and situational factors affecting exercise involvement: The importance of enjoyment. *Research Quarterly for Exercise and Sport,* **56**(3), 275-282.

Wankel, L.M. (1987). Enhancing motivation for involvement in voluntary exercise programs. In M.L. Maehr (Ed.), *Advances in motivation and achievement: Enhancing motivation* (Vol. 5, pp. 239-286). Greenwich, CT: JAI Press.

Wankel, L.M., & Kreisel, P.S.J. (1985). Factors underlying enjoyment of youth sports: Sport and age group comparisons. *Journal of Sport Psychology,* **7**(1), 51-64.

Wankel, L.M., & Sefton, J.M. (1989). A season-long investigation of fun in youth sports. *Journal of Sport and Exercise Psychology,* **11**, 355-366.

Wankel, L.M., & Thompson, C. (1977). Motivating people to be physically active: Self-persuasion vs. balanced decision making. *Journal of Applied Social Psychology,* **7**(4), 332-340.

Wankel, L.M., Yardley, J.K., & Graham, J. (1985). The effects of motivational interventions upon the exercise adherence of high and low self-motivated adults. *Canadian Journal of Applied Sport Sciences,* **10**(3), 147-156.

Ward, A. (1984, November). Aging athletes: Older but fitter. *New York Times Magazine,* pp. 93-96.

Ward, A., & Morgan, W. (1984). Adherence patterns of healthy men and women enrolled in an adult exercise program. *Journal of Cardiac Rehabilitation,* **4**, 143-152.

Wax, R.H., & Wax, M.L. (1978). How people stop smoking: An exploratory study. *Mid-American Review of Sociology,* **3**, 1-15.

Weber, R.J. (1953). Relationship of physical fitness to success in college and personality. *Research Quarterly,* **24**, 471-474.

Weight, L.M., & Noakes, T.D. (1987). Is running an analog of anorexia?: A survey of the incidence of eating disorders in female distance runners. *Medicine and Science in Sports and Exercise,* **19**(3), 213-217.

Weinberg, R., Gould, D., & Jackson, A. (1979). Expectations and performance: An empirical test of Bandura's self-efficacy theory. *Journal of Sport Psychology,* **11**(4), 320-340.

Weinberg, R.S., Gould, D., Yukelson, D., & Jackson, A. (1981). The effect of preexisting and manipulated self efficacy on a competitive muscular endurance task. *Journal of Sport Psychology,* **1**(4), 345-354.

Weinberg, R.S., Jackson, A., & Kolodny, K. (1988). The relationship of massage and exercise to mood enhancement. *The Sport Psychologist,* **2**, 202-211.

Weiner, B. (1979). A theory of motivation for some classroom experiences. *Journal of Educational Psychology,* **71**, 3-25.

Weiner, B. (1986). *An attributional theory of motivation and emotion.* New York: Springer-Verlag.

Weinstein, W.S., & Meyers, A.W. (1983). Running as treatment for depression: Is it worth it? *Journal of Sport Psychology,* **5**, 288-301.

Wessman, A.E., & Ricks, D.F. (1966). *Mood and personality.* New York: Holt Rinehart & Winston.

Wheeler, G.C., Wall, S.R., Belcastro, A.N., Conger, P., & Cumming, D.C. (1986). Are anorexic tendencies prevalent in the habitual runner? *British Journal of Sports Medicine,* **20**(2), 77-81.

White, R.W. (1959). Motivation reconsidered: The concept of competence. *Psychological Review,* **66**(5), 297-333.

Whitehead, J., & Corbin, C.B. (1988). Multidimensional scales for the measurement of locus of control of reinforcements for physical fitness behaviors. *Research Quarterly for Exercise and Sport,* **59**(2), 108-117.

Whitehouse, F.A. (1977). Motivation for fitness. In R. Harris & L.J. Frankel (Eds.), *Guide to fitness after fifty* (pp. 171-189). New York: Plenum Press.

Whiting, H.T.A., & Stembridge, D.E. (1965). Personality and the persistent non-swimmer. *Research Quarterly,* **36**(3). 348-356.

Wiggins, J., & Weslander, D. (1979). Personality characteristics of counselors rated as effective or ineffective. *Journal of Vocational Behavior,* **15**, 175-185.

Wilfley, D., & Kunce, J. (1986). Differential physical and psychological effects of exercise. *Journal of Counseling Psychology,* **33**(3), 337-342.

Williams, R.L., & Long, J.D. (1975). *Toward a self-managed lifestyle.* Boston: Houghton-Mifflin.

Wilson, G.T., & Brownell, K.D. (1980). Behavior therapy for obesity: An evaluation of treatment outcome. *Advances in Behavior Research and Therapy,* **3**, 49-86.

Wilson, P.K. (1988). Cardiac rehabilitation: Then and now. *Physician and Sports Medicine,* **16**(9), 75-81.

Wilson, V.E., Morley, N.C., & Bird, E.I. (1980). Mood profiles of marathon runners, joggers, and non-exercisers. *Perceptual and Motor Skills,* **50**, 117-118.

Winston, R.B., Jr., Bonney, W.C., Miller, T.K., & Dagley, J.C. (1988). *Promoting student development through intentionally structured groups.* San Francisco: Jossey-Bass.

Wishnie, H.A., Hackett, T.P., & Cassem, N.H. (1971). Psychological hazards of convalescence following myocardial infarction. *Journal of the American Medical Association,* **215**(8), 1292-1296.

Wood, D.T. (1977). The relationship between anxiety and acute physical activity. *American Corrective Therapy Journal,* **31**(3), 67-69.

Wooley, O.W., & Wooley, S. (1982). The Beverly Hills eating disorder: The mass marketing of anorexia nervosa [Editorial]. *International Journal of Eating Disorders,* **1**(3), 57-69.

Wright, B.A. (1983). *Physical disability: A psychosocial approach.* Philadelphia: Harper & Row.

Wrightsman, L.S. (1972). *Social psychology in the seventies.* Belmont, CA: Brooks/Cole.

Wurtele, S.K., & Maddux, J.E. (1987). Relative contributions of protection motivation theory components in predicting exercise intentions and behavior. *Health Psychology,* **6**(5), 453-466.

Yates, A. (1987). Eating disorders and long-distance running: The ascetic condition. *Integrated Psychiatry,* **5**, 201-211.

Yates, A., Leehey, K., & Shisslak, C.M. (1983). Running—An analogue of anorexia. *New England Journal of Medicine,* **308**, 251-255.

Yoesting, D.R., & Burkhead, D.L. (1973). Significance of childhood recreation experiences on adult leisure behavior: An exploratory analysis. *Journal of Leisure Research,* **17**(5), 25-36.

Young, P.T. (1973). Feeling and emotion. In B.B. Wolman (Ed.), *Handbook of general psychology* (pp. 749-771). Englewood Cliffs, NJ: Prentice Hall.

Young, R.J., & Ismail, A.H. (1977). Comparison of selected personality variables in regular and nonregular adult male exercisers. *Research Quarterly,* **48**, 617-622.

Name Index

Subject Index

Page numbers in italics indicate figures or tables.